19TH EDITION

W9-AXS-336

The Comprehensive NCLEX-PN® Review

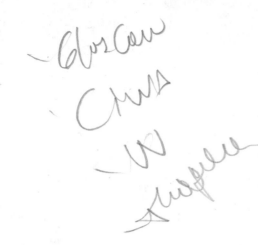

Contributors

Lawrette Axley, PhD, RN, CNE

Adrienne Blanks, DNP, MSN, RN

Bridgette Bryan, DNP, MS, RN

Nicole Hancock, EdD, MSN, RN

Deborah Cardi, MSN, RN

Alison DeLong, MS, RN

Jo Ellen Greischar-Billiard, MS, RN

Dianne Harris, Ed.D., MSN, RN, CNE

Teresa LaFave, NP, MS, RN

Japonica Morris, EdD, MSN, RN

Rhonda Payne, PhD, RN, CNE

Shari Payne, MSN, RN

Sheri Shields, RN, MSN

Faye Sigman, PhD, MSN, RN

Joy Weller, MS, RN

Intellectual Property Notice

REPRINTED MAY 2021

Director of development: Derek Prater

Project management: Nicole Burke

Coordination of content review: Lawrette Axley

Copy editing: Kya Rodgers, Kelly Von Lunen

Layout: Bethany Phillips, Spring Lenox

Cover design: Jason Buck

Important Notice to the Reader

User's Guide and Organization

Congratulations, graduate! You have successfully completed your program of nursing studies and are now eligible to take the licensing exam created by the National Council of State Boards of Nursing (NCSBN®).

Understanding the organizational format of this review book will help guide you through a focused review in preparation for the NCLEX®. The book is intended to accompany a live review presentation and then be used as an outline for continued review prior to taking the NCLEX. Each unit focuses on a specific area of nursing care. Unit 1 offers practical information about the exam, including how to prepare and test-taking strategies. The next eight units review essential content for the exam:

- Coordinated Care
- Community Health Nursing
- Pharmacology in Nursing
- Fundamentals for Nursing
- Adult Medical Surgical Nursing
- Mental Health Nursing
- Maternal and Newborn Nursing
- Nursing Care of Children

Tables and graphics are provided throughout to simplify more challenging content.

The content provided in this book is organized by specific areas of nursing and focuses on descriptions, contributing factors, manifestations, and collaborative care, which includes nursing interventions, diagnostics, medications, therapeutic measures, client education, and referral. The information is presented in a manner that promotes analysis and application of knowledge and reinforces priority of care when managing client care.

In the Practice Questions section, additional NCLEX-style questions are provided. Remember to apply clinical reasoning and use your test-taking strategies to select the correct answers.

It is important for new graduates to stay connected to content and practice questions until the NCLEX is taken. Implementing a focused review will create success on the NCLEX.

Feedback is always welcome. Therefore, please send suggestions for improvement, any noted errors, and personal testimonials of effectiveness to: LRAdmin@atitesting.com.

Table of Contents

UNIT 6   ADULT MEDICAL SURGICAL NURSING   79

UNIT 7   MENTAL HEALTH NURSING   171

Review of Test-Taking Strategies for the NCLEX® Exam

SECTION 1

Information About NCLEX

A. **General Information**

1. The purpose of the NCLEX-PN is to determine whether a candidate is prepared to safely and effectively practice entry-level nursing.

2. The exam is designed to test essential nursing knowledge and a candidate's ability to apply that knowledge to clinical situations.

3. The exam is pass/fail. No other score is given.

B. **Computerized Adaptive Testing (CAT)**

1. CAT is a system that selects test items for you based on answers selected up to that point in the exam.

2. When a question is answered, CAT selects items to administer that match the candidates ability.

3. Passing or failing is determined when you reach a point in the test when minimal competency has been demonstrated.

C. **Exam Schedule**

1. The exam is given all year.

D. **Number of Questions and Time Allowed**

1. There is no minimum amount of time for the exam. The maximum time allowed is 5 hr. The average time for a candidate is 2.5 hr.

2. Candidates who have applied for licensure/registration with a participating board of nursing (BON)/Review Board (RB) will be permitted to take the NCLEX eight times a year, but no more than once in any 45-day period.

3. The computer will automatically stop as soon as one of the following occurs.

   a. The candidate's measure of competency is determined to be above or below the passing standard.

   b. The candidate has answered all 205 test questions.

   c. The maximum amount of time has expired.

4. It is not possible to skip questions or return to previous questions.

5. The NCLEX-PN has a range of 85 to 205 questions. The exam includes 25 questions that are not scored.

6. Breaks are optional and count as part of the total 5 hr. Remember, a fresh mind is more alert!

7. About 2% of NCLEX candidates run out of time on their exams. So be aware of the time, but be sure to give every question your best effort. Do not randomly answer questions to finish quickly, as this can hinder your chance of passing.

SECTION 2

The NCLEX-PN Test Plan

A. **The NCLEX-PN test plan is revised every 3 years.** The current test plan (available at www.ncsbn.org) identifies the major categories and nursing activities that guide the exam's content and questions.

B. **NCLEX questions are distributed and weighted according to client need categories in the current test plan.**

C. **The NCLEX-PN Registration Process**

1. Apply for licensure with one BON.

2. Register and pay fees with Pearson VUE via the Internet (www.pearsonvue.com) or telephone.

3. Receive acknowledgment of receipt of registration from Pearson VUE.

4. The BON determines eligibility in the Pearson VUE system.

5. Receive Authorization to Test (ATT) email from Pearson VUE. (NOTE: Must test during the validity dates on the ATT.)

6. Schedule your exam appointment via the Internet (by accessing your online account) or by telephone.

   a. Arrive 30 minutes before the exam appointment and present acceptable identification. Your signature, photograph, and palm vein scan will be obtained.

   b. Examples of acceptable forms of identification for domestic test centers

      1) Passport books and cards

      2) Driver's license

      3) Provincial/territorial or state identification card

      4) Permanent residence card

      5) Military identification card

   c. The only identifications acceptable for international test centers are passport books and cards.

7. If you are not successful on NCLEX, contact ATI for continued assistance and support.

Visit the Pearson VUE website to take the online NCLEX tutorial at www.pearsonvue.com.

You can learn more about the NCLEX at www.ncsbn.org.

NCLEX-PN Item Types

A. **Items include multiple-choice, multiple response, fill-in-the-blank calculation, ordered response, and hot spots.** All item types can include multimedia (charts, tables, graphics, sound, video).

B. **Multiple Choice**

1. Has four options, only one of which is correct.

2. The correct answer is the **best** answer.

3. The other three options are distractors.

4. Distractors are options made to look like correct answers. They are intended to distract you from selecting the correct answer.

C. **Fill-in-the-Blank**

1. Fill-in-the-blank items are calculation problems. The question might ask for an answer in a specific unit amount or a rounded decimal. If required, perform rounding at the end of the calculation.

2. To answer these questions, a number should be typed into the answer box on the screen. You will not type the unit of measurement.

3. When answering the question, solve for the correct unit value.

4. Write out the calculations on material provided.

5. Click on the calculator button and verify your calculation.

D. **Drag-and-Drop/Ordered Response**

1. Drag-and-drop/ordered response items list steps that must be placed in a correct order (numerical, alphabetical, chronological).

2. Drag options in the left-hand column into the order of performance in the right-hand column.

3. There is only one correct sequence.

E. **Multiple Response (Select All That Apply)**

1. Multiple response questions may have a single correct response, have more than one correct response or require all responses to be correct.

2. To answer these questions, click on all answers that apply.

3. Credit will only be given for completely correct answers. No partial credit is given.

4. Consider each response as a true-false question.

F. **Hot Spot**

1. Hot spot items use a point-and-click method that presents the candidate with a problem and a figure. The test taker selects the correct location on the figure.

2. An X will appear on the area selected. Click on the area that constitutes the landmark to correctly answer the item.

3. Read the question carefully, then analyze the image.

4. The exam will allow you to reclick on the image as many times as necessary.

5. It is very important to remember that the screen is not a mirror image. If the question asks for an answer on the right or left side of the body, make sure to click on the appropriate side.

G. **Multimedia.** Any item formats may include multimedia.

1. Charts or Tables

a. First, read the question carefully. Use the mouse to click on each tab to open the document. When the tab is clicked, a separate window will open to display the data. Analyze the data provided in the charts or tables to correctly answer the question.

2. Graphic Option

a. The item and/or answer options are presented as graphics instead of text.

b. The answers to these items are preceded by circles. Be sure to click on the circle to select the answer.

3. Sound and Video

a. When an audio item is presented on NCLEX, the candidate is prompted to put on headphones. The volume of the audio can be adjusted, and the clip can be replayed as often as needed.

Assess and Remediate

A. **New nursing graduates should review content and questions daily until they take the exam.** Adequate review depends on scores obtained on practice assessments. NCLEX preparation after a Live Review can take from 2 to 8 weeks.

B. **For content review, use this NCLEX-PN review book that outlines content.** Use other nursing reference materials for more detailed information.

C. **Your practice assessment score reports will identify and help direct review of content.**

D. **Begin with areas that are most difficult or least familiar.**

E. **When studying body systems and the associated diseases:**

1. Define the disease in terms of the pathophysiological process that is occurring.

2. Identify a client's early and late manifestations.

3. Identify the most important or life-threatening complications.

4. Review the prescribed medical plan including diagnostic and laboratory tests, expected lab value alterations, medications, and treatments.

5. Identify and prioritize the nursing interventions associated with early and late manifestations.

6. Identify client teaching that the nurse should reinforce to the client/family to prevent or adapt to the disease process or condition.

Test-Taking Strategies

NOTE: Although the majority of NCLEX-PN items are written at the application and analysis level, there are some knowledge and comprehension items on the test. Make certain that you have a broad knowledge in all Client Need categories so that you can demonstrate a minimal level of competency when asked to apply your knowledge to the care of the clients in the scenario presented on the exam.

Example: A nurse prepares to administer medications to a client who has asthma. Which effects should the nurse recognize as an adverse response to bronchodilator therapy?

1. Limited routes of administration
2. Hyperkalemia
3. Increased myocardial oxygen use
4. Hypoglycemia

NOTE: Knowledge-based questions test recall and recognition.

Example: An older adult client reports recurring calf pain after walking one to two blocks that disappears with rest. The client has weak pedal pulses, and the skin on the lower legs is shiny and cool to touch. Which nursing interventions is appropriate at this time?

1. Position the legs dependently.
2. Elevate the left leg above the heart.
3. Immobilize the left leg to prevent further injury.
4. Assess dorsiflexion and extension of the left foot.

NOTE: Application and analysis questions require use of nursing knowledge to solve client problems.

A. **The amount of information in the stem and distractors can be overwhelming.** A useful approach is to break the analysis of the question into a series of steps. Remember to focus on the fact that there is always something you know in the question and answer options. This helps you stay in control of the exam.

B. **Use the STOP (Story, Think, Options, Pick) approach.**

1. **Story:** Identify the issue and client in the question.

   a. The issue in a question is the problem that is presented. Examples of the issue:

      1) Medication: digoxin
      2) Nursing problem: A client who is at risk for infection or in pain
      3) Behavior: Restlessness, agitation
      4) Disorder: Diabetes mellitus, ulcerative colitis
      5) Procedure: Glucose tolerance test, cardiac catheterization
      6) The client in the question usually has a health problem.
      7) The client can also be a relative, significant other, or another member of the health care team with whom the nurse is interacting.
      8) The correct answer to the question must relate to the client in the question.

2. **Think:** About the type of stem and key words.

   a. Identify the type of stem in the question.

      1) True-response stem requires an answer that is a true statement.

         a) Example: A nurse is preparing to administer a bolus feeding to a client through a nasogastric (NG) tube and observes that the exit mark on the tube has moved since the last feeding. Which action should the nurse take?

      2) False-response stem requires an answer that is a false statement.

         a) Example: A newly licensed nurse is preparing to remove a client's abdominal wound sutures. The manager recognizes a need for further education when the nurse does which of the following?

      3) Answering questions that focus on priorities.

         a) The majority of NCLEX questions will be priority-setting questions, which ask the test taker to identify what comes first, is most important, or gets the highest priority.

         b) The NCLEX will use stems that ask, "What will the nurse do **first**?"

            (1) For example:

               (a) What is the nurse's initial response?
               (b) A nurse should give immediate consideration to which of the following?
               (c) Which nursing action should receive the highest priority?
               (d) Which action should the nurse take first?

            (2) Example: A nurse is preparing an automated external defibrillator (AED) for a client receiving CPR after a cardiac arrest. Which action should the nurse perform first?

   b. Key words focus attention on important details.

      1) During the **early** period, which nursing **procedure** is **best**?
      2) The nurse should **expect** to find which characteristics in an **adult** who has **diabetes mellitus**?
      3) Which nursing **action** is **essential**?
      4) Which nursing **action** should the nurse take **first**?

3. **Options:** Consider potential responses/answers.

   a. Develop answers in your mind before looking at the options provided.

   b. Review each answer option one at a time.

4. **Pick:** The correct answer.
   a. Identify the option that best matches your answer or that best answers the question.
   b. Make your selection and do not change it.
5. Apply the STOP strategy to the following question.
   a. A client who has recently undergone surgery for a tracheostomy is now at home. The nurse recognizes a need for immediate intervention when the caregiver does which of the following?
      1) Places an air humidifier at the bedside
      2) Suctions intermittently for 15 seconds
      3) Cuts a 4x4 gauze pad to put around the tracheostomy tube
      4) Removes the ties before cleaning the tracheostomy

C. **Use priority-setting guidelines to answer questions.**
   1. **Maslow's Hierarchy of Needs** indicates that physiological needs come first. Following are safety and security; love and belonging; self-esteem; and self-actualization.
   2. **"ABCs"** (airway, breathing, circulation) needs will frequently take priority. Never perform ABC checks blindly without considering whether ABC issues are acute vs. chronic or stable vs. unstable. For example, a client who has quadriplegia and receiving ventilation has chronic airway/breathing problems. However, if there is not an acute consideration, such as pneumonia, the client should be considered chronic and stable. This client would not be the nurse's first priority.
   3. **Sources of safety and risk reduction** issues need to be identified.
   4. **The nursing process** indicates that assessment is a priority.
   5. Consider options that are **least restrictive or least invasive**.
   6. Determine the survival potential of the client. Is the issue emergent, urgent, nonurgent, or expectant? It is not unusual to want to care for the client who, in your mind, is the sickest. However, this might be an inappropriate choice in a triage situation. Clients who are so sick that they cannot be saved should not be treated first.
   7. **Acute** client problems take priority over **chronic** problems.
   8. Determine if the client is **stable** or **unstable**.

D. **Default test-taking strategies help you make decisions.**
   1. Use time to your advantage.
      a. **Early vs. late signs and symptoms**: Early manifestations are generalized and nonspecific, whereas late signs are specific and serious. Eliminate incorrect answer choices using this strategy.
         1) Example: An adolescent was admitted 12 hr ago following a motor vehicle crash. Multiple skeletal fractures were sustained. The client is in balanced-suspension traction. Which assessment findings require immediate intervention by the nurse?
            1. Disorientation
            2. Shallow respirations
            3. Chest pain with positioning
            4. Bloody drainage at the pin site
      b. **Pre, post, intra**: You might be asked about complications associated with certain procedures. What should you do if you know little or nothing about the procedure? Pay attention to whether the question is asking about preprocedural or postprocedural concerns. Eliminate the options that do not correspond to what is being asked.
         1) Example: A nurse is caring for a client who is scheduled for electroconvulsive therapy (ECT). Which medications should the nurse expect to withhold prior to therapy?
            1. Atropine sulfate
            2. Phenytoin
            3. Methohexital
            4. Succinylcholine
      c. **Time elapsed**: The priority nursing action will change based on the time interval stipulated. The closer the client is to the origination of risk, the higher the risk for complications. The time issue can be stated in terms of hours or days. In other instances, the physical location of the client will tell you how long it has been since the origination of risk. Pay attention. Is the client in the PACU, postsurgical unit, or somewhere else? The time issue buried in those words should help you eliminate incorrect answers that don't match what is being asked.
         1) Example: A home health nurse is performing an admission assessment on a client who had a knee arthroplasty 1 week ago. Which client statement should concern the nurse most?
            1. "I am so glad to be off those blood thinners."
            2. "I will keep a pillow under my knee when I am in bed."
            3. "I am planning to use a wheelchair to help me get around."
            4. "I plan to take ibuprofen instead of the prescribed hydrocodone for pain control."

d. Remember: The **most complete answer** = least room for error.

   1) You'll encounter questions on NCLEX that will ask you to choose the instruction or documentation that is most accurate. What should you do if you don't remember much about the subject matter? Choosing an answer that is most complete will typically result in the least room for error and subsequent delivery of safe and effective care.

   2) To help determine which answer is the most complete, evaluate answer options based on how much objectivity (fact) vs. subjectivity (opinion) there is in the answer choices. A specific value (like a blood pressure) is factual, whereas a client's report of past incidences of "high" blood pressure is subjective. Responses that are subjective are generally not correct.

      a) Example: A client has not voided 8 hr following the removal of an indwelling bladder catheter. Which should be the nurse's initial action?

         1. Increase fluids.

         2. Perform bladder scan.

         3. Place indwelling catheter.

         4. Provide assistance to bathroom.

e. Read the question and options closely for words asking about **direction** or **magnitude**. For instance, stop and concentrate on the terms intra vs. inter; hyper vs. hypo; increase vs. decrease; lesser vs. greater; and gain vs. lose. It is common to misread these terms by simply skimming over them too quickly.

   1) Example: A nurse irrigates a postoperative client's NG tube twice with 30 mL normal saline solution. At the end of the shift, the NG collection device contains 475 mL. Record the amount of NG drainage.

f. When in doubt, choose a nursing action that could **prevent harm to the client**. Even if you don't know whether it is related to the stem, it is still a life-saving maneuver that, in all likelihood, is correct.

   1) Example: A nurse is caring for a client who has a chest tube. The nurse notes that the chest tube has become disconnected from the chest drainage system. Which action should the nurse take?

        1. Reposition the client to a high-Fowler's position.

        2. Increase the suction to the chest drainage system.

        3. Place the client on low flow oxygen via nasal cannula.

        4. Immerse the end of the chest tube in a bottle of sterile water.

g. Seldom will a correct answer have the nurse physically leave the client. Choose an answer that **keeps the nurse with the client**.

   1) Example: When an older adult client dies from complications of a cerebral vascular accident (CVA), the client's partner is present at the bedside. Which action should the nurse take?

        1. Escort the partner to the hallway outside the room.

        2. Ask the chaplain to come be with the partner.

        3. Stay with the partner at the bedside.

        4. Give the partner time alone.

h. In some instances, rule out an option if you know it is associated with something else. For example, you may not know about the laboratory values for warfarin therapy, but you do know the laboratory values for heparin and aspirin. Those values can be eliminated because you are **using what you know.**

   1) Example: A client who has a new diagnosis of rheumatoid arthritis is required to receive 3 months of methotrexate therapy. Which of the following are associated with the therapy? (Select all that apply.)

        1. WBC count 1,200/mm^3

        2. Weight gain 2.27 kg (5 lb)

        3. Oral temperature 37.2° C (99° F)

        4. Urine specific gravity 1.003

        5. Platelets 5,000/mm^3

i. **Safe and effective delegation** of tasks and client care assignments are extremely important when setting priorities for client care.

   1) RNs perform all initial client teaching. The licensed practical nurse (LPN) may reinforce teaching performed by the RN.

   2) RNs should perform all admission assessments and vital signs so that an accurate baseline is established.

   3) Client care assignments are made by the RN, not by support staff.

      a) Example: A nurse is organizing care for a group of clients. Which client should the nurse assign to the assistive personnel (AP)?

         1. Record a client's vital signs during the transfusion of blood.

         2. Assist a client who is requesting a bedpan 1 day following hysterectomy.

         3. Offer a pamphlet regarding advanced directives to a newly admitted client.

         4. Ask a client if pain was relieved after administration of acetaminophen.

j. You might want to answer questions based on the way you saw procedures done while you were in a clinical setting at school, during summer employment, or working as an intern. NCLEX items must be answered to be consistent with nationwide practice standards, not necessarily with what might have been done within a particular institution or geographic area.

The Day of the Exam

A. **Plan for everything.**

B. **Assemble everything needed for the exam the night before.**

C. **Identification:** When candidates arrive at the test center, they are required to present one form of acceptable identification. The first and last names on the ID must exactly match the first and last names on the application sent to the board of nursing. Visit the NCSBN website (www.ncsbn.org) for acceptable forms of ID.

D. **Candidates are required to arrive at least 30 min before the scheduled testing time.**

E. **Verify the route to the exam site, and take a test drive several days prior.**

F. **Pay close attention to your physiological needs.**

　　1. Dress in layers to accommodate your comfort in the testing center. No hats, scarves, gloves, or coats are allowed in the testing room.

　　2. Get a good night's sleep the night before the exam.

　　3. Eat a nourishing meal that includes protein and long-acting carbohydrates.

　　4. Avoid stimulants and depressants.

　　5. Use the restroom as needed prior to the exam.

G. **During the exam**

　　1. Listen to and carefully read the instructions.

　　2. Avoid distraction. Focus on answering one question at a time.

　　3. Think positively.

H. **Manage anxiety.**

　　1. Mild levels of anxiety increase effectiveness.

　　2. Avoid cramming the night before the exam.

　　3. Do something enjoyable and relaxing the night before the exam.

　　4. Learn and practice measures to manage your anxiety level during the exam, as needed.

　　　a. Take a few deep breaths.

　　　b. Tense and relax muscles.

　　　c. Visualize a peaceful scene.

　　　d. Visualize your success.

UNIT TWO

Coordinated Care

Leadership and Management

A. **Leadership:** A way of behaving that influences others to respond—not because they have to, but because they want to. Leaders help others to identify and focus on the achievement of goals. Leadership is an interaction that focuses on the personal development of the members of the group.

1. Essential Components of Leadership
   a. Effective communication
   b. Conflict manager
   c. Knowledge/competence
   d. Role model
   e. Delegation
   f. Identifies goals/objectives
   g. Motivation
   h. Proactive
   i. Flexible

2. **Leadership Styles**
   a. **Authoritative**
   b. **Democratic**
   c. **Laissez-faire**

3. All nurses need leadership skills to initiate and maintain effective working relationships, coordinate care, delegate, and resolve conflict. Transactional leaders focus on immediate problems using rewards as motivation. Transactional leaders empower and motivate followers toward a common vision.

B. **Management:** A problem-oriented process with a focus on the activities needed to achieve a goal; supplying the structure, resources, and direction for the activities of the group. Management involves personal interaction, but the focus is on the group's process. The most effective managers are also effective leaders. The organization grants power and authority to the manager.

1. Functions of Management
   a. Planning
   b. Organizing
   c. Staffing
   d. Directing
   e. Controlling

2. Characteristics of Managers
   a. Hold formal position of authority and power
   b. Coach subordinates
   c. Work toward shared goals of quality, efficiency, and excellence
   d. Promote innovation

3. **Nursing Interventions:** Nurses should learn management skills and identify their own personal leadership styles. Nurses should know the differences between being an authoritative and democratic leader. The most effective management style in a health care environment is the democratic leader who uses an interprofessional approach to encourage open communication and collaboration, which will promote individual autonomy and accountability.

DETERMINE THE LEADERSHIP STYLE
(AUTHORITATIVE, DEMOCRATIC, OR LAISSEZ-FAIRE) USED IN EACH SCENARIO

Scenario 1: A nurse manager does not participate, but delegates the staff scheduling to the nurses on the unit.	☐ AUTHORITATIVE ☐ LAISSEZ-FAIRE ☐ DEMOCRATIC
Scenario 2: A nurse manager allows the staff nurses to participate in trial use of new IV pumps and contribute input when choosing a new product.	☐ AUTHORITATIVE ☐ LAISSEZ-FAIRE ☐ DEMOCRATIC
Scenario 3: A nurse manager makes a decision for the staff to wear blue scrubs without consulting the staff nurses.	☐ AUTHORITATIVE ☐ LAISSEZ-FAIRE ☐ DEMOCRATIC
Scenario 4: A nurse manager allows the staff to choose which holiday they would prefer to take off before completing the work schedule.	☐ AUTHORITATIVE ☐ LAISSEZ-FAIRE ☐ DEMOCRATIC
Scenario 5: A nurse manager instructs the staff nurses to "work out the problem between yourselves" when a conflict arises between two nurses.	☐ AUTHORITATIVE ☐ LAISSEZ-FAIRE ☐ DEMOCRATIC
Scenario 6: A nurse manager changes the policy regarding sterile dressing changes and directs the staff to follow the new procedure.	☐ AUTHORITATIVE ☐ LAISSEZ-FAIRE ☐ DEMOCRATIC

Answer key: 1. Laissez-faire; 2. Democratic; 3. Authoritative; 4. Democratic; 5. Laissez-faire; 6. Authoritative

C. **Professional Communication:** Involves sending, receiving, and interpreting written, face-to-face, and nonverbal information between at least two people.

1. Influence outcomes with good communication.
   a. Reduce errors.
   b. Improve continuity of care.
   c. Build teamwork/collaboration.

2. Coordination of Care
   a. Leadership and Management
   b. Setting priorities
   c. Delegation
   d. Conflict resolution
   e. Problem solving
   f. Documentation
   g. Consultation
   h. Transfers
   i. Discharge

3. **Therapeutic communication:** The purposeful use of communication to build and maintain helping relationships with clients, families, and significant others. Therapeutic communication is client-centered, purposeful, planned, and goal-directed.

4. **Nursing Interventions:** Effective communication requires commitment, effort, focus, and cooperation, especially when dealing with complex clinical issues and people who have diverse backgrounds and perspectives. It is essential to understand and use effective communication skills to successfully manage others.

D. **Conflict:** Arises when there are two or more opposing views, feelings, expectations, or other divergent issues.

1. Types of conflict
   a. Intrapersonal: Individual
   b. Interpersonal: Between two or more people
   c. Intergroup: Between two or more departments or organization

2. Causes of conflict
   a. Ineffective communication
   b. Unmet/unclear expectations
   c. Change
   d. Differences in values/beliefs

3. Conflict management strategies
   a. Avoiding/withdrawing
   b. Cooperating/accommodating
   c. Compromising/negotiating
   d. Competing/coercing
   e. Collaborating
   f. Smoothing

4. **Nursing Interventions:** Nurses should use problem-solving and negotiation strategies to resolve conflict.

Teamwork and Collaboration

A. Foster a culture that values collaboration and cooperation.

B. Communicate that teamwork is expected.

C. Publicly celebrate team success.

D. Offer assistance during crises.

E. Assist team members with client care.

F. Participate in team conferences.

Quality

A. **Quality Improvement:** A philosophy that promotes implementation of a plan to continually improve health care services client outcomes

B. **Performance Improvement (Quality Improvement, Quality Control):** The process used to identify and resolve performance deficiencies focusing on assessment of outcomes to improve delivery of quality care

1. Steps in the performance improvement process
   a. A standard is developed and approved by facility committee.
   b. Standards are made available to employees via policies and procedures.
   c. Quality issues are identified by staff, management, or risk management department.
   d. An interprofessional team is developed to review the issue.
   e. The current state of structure and process related to the issue is analyzed.
   f. Data collection methods are determined.
   g. Data are collected, analyzed, and compared with the established benchmark.
   h. If the benchmark is not met, possible influencing factors are determined. A root cause analysis can be done.
      1) Investigates the consequence and possible causes
      2) Analyzes the possible causes and relationships that might exist
      3) Determines additional influences at each level of relationship
      4) Determines the root cause or causes
   i. Potential solutions or corrective actions are analyzed, and one is selected for implementation.
   j. Educational or corrective action is implemented.
   k. The issue is re-evaluated at a pre-established time to determine the efficacy of the solution or corrective action.

III Variance/Incident/Irregular Occurrence

A variance, or incident, is an event that occurs outside the expected events or activities of the client's stay, unit functioning, or organizational processes.

A. **Nursing Interventions:** Incident or variance reports are not intended to point blame, just to document the facts. Their purpose is to identify situations or system issues that contributed to the occurrence and to engage strategies to prevent reoccurrence or to correct the situation. Generally, the report is confidential communication and cannot be subpoenaed. However, if it is inadvertently disclosed, it can be subpoenaed. The report should not be placed in the chart.

B. **Reportable Incidents**

1. Medication errors

2. Procedure/treatment errors

3. Equipment-related injuries/errors

4. Needlestick injuries

5. Client falls/injuries

6. Visitor/volunteer injuries

7. Threat made to client or staff

8. Loss of property (dentures, jewelry, personal wheelchair)

IV Resource Management

Budgeting and resource allocation are determined based on human, financial, and material resources.

A. **Considerations**

1. Budgeting: Personnel, operational, capital

2. Resource allocation: Distribution of goods and services

3. Cost-effective care: Efficiency without comprise to standards and/or quality

B. **Budget process**

1. **Planning:** Determine what the needs are.

2. **Setting Goals:** Determine what should be accomplished.

3. **Preparation:** Develop a plan (time frame).

4. **Monitoring and approval:** Implement the plan (ongoing monitoring and analysis).

5. **Modification:** Evaluate the outcome (revise and modify as needed).

C. **Nursing Interventions:** A nurse manager must be aware of economic issues in health care. Budgetary terms are fundamental to understanding the financial management of facilities. The more information available to the nurse, the better the decisions and input into long-range planning for the facility.

V Case Management

Case management provides client care coordination with the interprofessional team.

A. The principles of case management include a collaborative process to provide quality and continuity of care by minimizing fragmentation and high cost. Furthermore, the case manager is an advocate for the client and family.

VI Continuity of Care

Focuses on the experience of the client as the client moves through the health care system. Guiding the client through this experience requires coordination, integration, collaboration, and facilitation of all the events along the continuum.

A. **Nursing's Role in Continuity of Care**

1. Coordinate care with the interprofessional team.

2. Act as a liaison and be a client advocate.

3. Complete admission, transfer, discharge, and postdischarge prescriptions.

4. Initiate, revise, and evaluate the plan of care.

5. Report the client's status.

6. Coordinate discharge planning.

7. Facilitate referrals and use of community resources.

VII Consultation and Referral

A. **Consultation:** A professional provides expert advice in a particular area and determines what treatment or services the client requires.

1. Examples of consultation: An orthopedic surgeon for a client who has a hip fracture; a psychiatrist for a client whose risk for suicide must be determined.

2. **Nursing Interventions:** Notify the primary care provider of the client's needs, provide the consultant with pertinent information, include the consultant's information in the plan of care, and facilitate coordination with other providers to protect the client from conflicting and potentially dangerous prescriptions.

B. **Referral:** A formal request for a specific service by another provider so that the client can access the care identified by the primary care provider or consultant. The intervention becomes that specialist's responsibility, but the nurse continues to be responsible for monitoring the client's response and progress.

1. Examples of referrals: Inpatient—physical therapy, wound care nurse; outside of the facility—hospice

C. **Nursing Interventions:** The processes of consultation and referral are integral for effective use of services along the continuum, and they establish collaboration with the interprofessional team. The nurse should support the client/family with appropriate consultation and referral to contacts in the community.

Delegation and Prioritization

I Delegation/Assignment/ Supervision/Accountability

A. **Delegating:** Transferring the authority to perform a selected nursing task in a selected situation to another team member while maintaining accountability.

B. **Assigning:** Transferring the authority, accountability, and responsibility to another member of the health care team (such as when an RN directs another RN to assess a client, the second RN is already authorized to assess clients in the RN scope of practice).

C. **Supervising:** Monitoring the progress toward completion of delegated tasks. The amount of supervision required depends on the direction of the delegation, the abilities of the person being delegated to, and the location of the ultimate responsibility for outcomes.

D. **Accountability:** Moral responsibility for consequences of actions.

E. **Five Rights of Delegation**

1. Right person
2. Right task
3. Right circumstances
4. Right direction and communication
5. Right supervision and evaluation

F. **Nursing Interventions:** It is essential for a nurse to understand legal responsibilities when managing and delegating nursing care to a wide variety of health care workers. The nurse must delegate activities thoughtfully, taking into account individual job descriptions, knowledge base, and skills demonstrated. Remember, the professional nurse is accountable for determining the extent and complexity of client needs and for assigning work that is consistent with the individual's position, description, and duties.

G. **The RN Cannot Delegate**

1. Nursing process
2. Client education
3. Tasks that require nursing judgment (including care of unstable clients)

DELEGATION WORKSHEET

Which tasks are most appropriately delegated to a licensed practical nurse (LPN) or assistive personnel (AP)?

1. Activities of daily living	☐ LPN	☐ AP
2. Ambulating	☐ LPN	☐ AP
3. Tracheostomy care	☐ LPN	☐ AP
4. Suctioning	☐ LPN	☐ AP
5. Feeding	☐ LPN	☐ AP
6. Positioning	☐ LPN	☐ AP
7. Inserting urinary catheter	☐ LPN	☐ AP
8. Checking nasogastric tube patency	☐ LPN	☐ AP
9. Medication administration	☐ LPN	☐ AP
10. Sterile specimen collection	☐ LPN	☐ AP
11. Vital signs (on stable clients)	☐ LPN	☐ AP
12. Intake and output	☐ LPN	☐ AP
13. Reinforcing client teaching	☐ LPN	☐ AP

Answer Key: 1. AP; 2. AP; 3. LPN; 4. LPN; 5. AP; 6. AP; 7. LPN; 8. LPN; 9. LPN; 10. LPN; 11. AP; 12. AP; 13. LPN

II Roles and Responsibilities for Levels of Staff

A. **Assistive Personnel (AP)/ Unlicensed Assistive Personnel (UAP)**

1. Training is often on the job.
2. An AP can complete a certification program (certified nursing assistant).
3. An AP functions under the direction of the licensed practical nurse (LPN) or RN.
4. Skills
   a. Performs basic hygiene care and grooming
   b. Reports to the LPN or RN
   c. Provides assistance with ADLs (nutrition, elimination, mobility)
   d. Performs basic skills, such as taking vital signs (including pulse oximetry) and calculating I&O
   e. Emphasis is on maintaining a safe environment and recognizing situations to report to immediate superior
   f. Performs skills that are noninvasive and do not require sterile technique

B. **Licensed Practical Nurse (LPN)/**
   Licensed Vocational Nurse (LVN)

   1. Education is approximately 12 to 18 months in an accredited program.

   2. LPNs must complete and pass the NCLEX-PN® exam for licensure.

   3. Supervised by the RN or provider.

   4. Scope of practice is determined by nurse practice acts, which vary by state. (Requirements to maintain an active license are determined by each state.)

      a. Meets the health needs of clients

      b. Cares for clients whose condition is considered to be stable or chronic with an expected outcome

      c. Performs reinforcement teaching

      d. Contributes to care plan through discussing client problems/findings with the RN

      e. Calculates and monitors IV flow rate

      f. Administers IVPB medications

      g. Monitors IV fluids

C. **Registered Nurse (RN)**

   1. Can have a diploma, associate degree, baccalaureate degree, or higher.

   2. Education is 2 or more years.

   3. RNs must pass the NCLEX-RN® exam for licensure.

   4. Functions under the direction of the provider.

   5. Advanced clinical skills in caring for the acute client who has complex care needs; outcome uncertain.

   6. Scope of practice is determined by nurse practice acts, which vary by state. (Requirements to maintain an active license are determined by each state.)

D. **Advanced Practice Nurse**

   1. Can be non-degree, master's degree, or higher.

   2. Education ranges from 18 months to more than 4 years (in addition to basic RN program).

   3. Must complete and pass a certification exam (in addition to the NCLEX-RN exam) applicable to the specialty and practice (adult nurse practitioner, diabetic educator).

   4. Functions vary according to the state practice act, which can be either autonomous or under the direct or indirect supervision of a provider.

   5. Skills vary according to the state practice act and can include the ability to prescribe, diagnose, and treat.

E. **Health Care Provider**

   1. Can be a provider, provider's assistant, or nurse practitioner.

   2. In general, only an attending provider has admitting privileges to a facility, although another care provider in the practice can direct the care given to the client.

III Prioritization Principles

A. **Nurses must continually set and reset priorities in order to safely care for multiple clients.**

   1. Assessments are completed.

   2. Interventions are provided.

   3. Steps in a client procedure are completed.

   4. Components of client care are completed.

B. **Establishing priorities in nursing practice requires that these decisions be made based on evidence obtained**

   1. During shift reports and other communications with members of the health care team

   2. Through careful review of documents

   3. By continually and accurately collecting client data

PRIORITIZATION PRINCIPLES IN CLIENT CARE

PRINCIPLE	EXAMPLES
Prioritize systemic before local ("life before limb").	Prioritizing interventions for a client in shock over interventions for a client who has a localized limb injury
Prioritize acute (less opportunity for physical adaptation) before chronic (greater opportunity for physical adaptation).	Prioritizing the care of a client who has a new injury/illness (confusion, chest pain) or an acute exacerbation of a previous illness over the care of client who has a long-term chronic illness
Prioritize actual problems before potential future problems.	Prioritizing administration of medication to a client experiencing acute pain over ambulation of a client at risk for thrombophlebitis
Prioritize according to Maslow's Hierarchy of Needs.	Prioritizing the care of the client needs according to Maslow's Hierarchy (physiological needs, such as nutrition, are a higher priority than self-esteem)
Recognize and respond to trends vs. transient findings.	Recognizing a gradual deterioration in a client's level of consciousness or Glasgow Coma Scale score
Recognize signs of emergencies and complications vs. expected findings.	Recognizing signs of increasing intracranial pressure in a client who has a new diagnosis of a stroke vs. the findings expected following a stroke
Apply clinical knowledge to procedural standards to determine the priority action.	Recognizing that the timing of administration of antidiabetic and antimicrobial medications is more important than administration of some other medications

PRIORITIZATION WORKSHEET

Select the client from each group that the nurse should tend to first after morning report and select a principle of prioritization that applies to that client.

Group A

- ☐ 1. A client receiving morphine sulfate via a PCA pump with respirations of 8/min
- ☐ 2. A client 2 days postoperative following right knee replacement who has not had a bowel movement
- ☐ 3. A client who has a left below-the-knee amputation who is having difficulty with body image
- ☐ 4. A client who has a heart rate of 110/min after an albuterol respiratory treatment

Group B

- ☐ 1. A client who has diabetes mellitus and whose capillary blood glucose is 150 mg/dL before breakfast
- ☐ 2. A client 2 days postoperative following colon resection with an oral temperature of 39.8° C (103.6° F)
- ☐ 3. A client in Buck's traction who refuses to take the daily prescribed stool softener
- ☐ 4. A client who has a cervical fusion and needs to ambulate the length of the hallway

Group C

- ☐ 1. A client who has chronic kidney disease and a creatinine level of 2.3
- ☐ 2. A client who is 2 hr postoperative following cardiac catheterization who has capillary refill less than 3 seconds
- ☐ 3. A client who has a swollen, reddened, and painful intravenous site after receiving antibiotics
- ☐ 4. A client who has expiratory wheezes after receiving intravenous contrast for a CT scan

Answer Key

Group A: The client receiving morphine should be seen first. Respiratory depression is an adverse effect of morphine. Several principles can be used in the scenario: ABCs, which includes airway and breathing; unexpected problem before an expected problem; actual problem before potential problem; and physiological needs from Maslow's Hierarchy of Needs. Place this client as the highest priority. The postoperative client who has not had a bowel movement has a potential problem but not an actual problem at this point. A client who has impaired body image falls under self-esteem or socialization in Maslow's Hierarchy of Needs,. The client who has a heart rate of 110/min after an albuterol treatment is experiencing an expected reaction to this medication.

Group B: The client 2 days postoperative following colon resection who has a temperature of 39.8° C (103.6° F) should be seen first. An elevated temperature in the first few days postoperative can indicate an infection and should be addressed immediately. This is a safety issue according to Maslow's Hierarchy of Needs, and it is an unexpected event. It also could be systemic and cause sepsis. Capillary blood sugar glucose 150 mg/dL is elevated but expected for most clients who have diabetes mellitus. The client in Buck's traction who refuses to take his stool softener might have a potential problem, but does not have an actual problem at this time. A client who has cervical fusion and needs to ambulate also has a potential problem of thrombosis, but does not have an actual problem. Actual problems are higher priority than potential problems.

Group C: The client who has expiratory wheezes should be seen first, as the finding can indicate allergic reaction to the contrast. The client has an actual airway problem (ABCs and Maslow's physiological needs), which is an unexpected finding indicating a systemic complication and places this client at highest priority. The client who has chronic kidney disease and a creatinine level of 2.3 mg/dL has an expected elevation for the condition. The client who has a capillary refill of less than 3 seconds has an expected outcome. A client who has a swollen, reddened, and painful IV site has an actual safety problem (Maslow's Hierarchy of Needs), but the condition is local, not systemic.

Ethical Issues

I Ethical Practice

A. **Ethical Principles**

1. **Autonomy:** The right to make one's own decisions

2. **Beneficence:** The obligation to do good for others

3. **Confidentiality:** The obligation to observe the privacy of another and maintain strict confidence

4. **Fidelity:** The obligation to be faithful to agreements and responsibilities, to keep promises

5. **Justice:** The obligation to be fair to all people (when allocating limited resources)

6. **Nonmaleficence:** The obligation not to harm others (Hippocrates states, "First, do no harm.")

7. **Paternalism:** Assuming the right to make decisions for another

8. **Veracity:** The obligation to tell the truth

B. **Ethical Dilemmas:** Ethical dilemmas are problems for which more than one choice can be made, and the choice is influenced by the values and beliefs of the decision makers. Ethical dilemmas are very common in health care, and nurses must be prepared to apply ethical theory and decision-making.

C. **The American Nurses Association's (ANA) *Code of Ethics for Nurses*:** Sets guidelines to use when providing client care, outlines the nurse's responsibility to the client and the profession of nursing, and assists the nurse in making ethical decisions.

D. **Ethical Decision-Making:** A process in which the nurse, client, client's family, and health care team make decisions, taking into consideration personal and philosophical viewpoints, the ANA *Code of Ethics for Nurses*, and ethical principles. Frequently, this requires that a balance be struck between science and morality.

E. **Advocacy:** A process by which the nurse assists the client to grow and develop toward self-actualization. Advocacy is a critical leadership role and emphasizes the values of caring, autonomy, respect, and empowerment.

II Organ Donation

A. **Organ and tissue donation is regulated by state and federal laws.** Facilities will have specific policies and procedures to follow during the process.

B. Federal law requires health care facilities to provide access to trained specialists who make the request to clients and/or family members and provide information regarding consent, organ and tissues that can be donated, and how burial or cremation will be affected by donation.

C. Provide emotional support and answer questions.

III Advance Directives

A document in which a client who is competent can express wishes regarding future acceptable health care (including the desire for extraordinary lifesaving measures: resuscitation, intubation, and artificial hydration and nutrition) and/or designate another person to make decisions when the client becomes physically or mentally unable to do so. The Patient Self-Determination Act requires all clients admitted to a health care facility be asked if they have advance directives.

A. **Planning guides for seriously ill clients**

1. **Living will:** Legal document that instructs providers and family members about what, if any, life-sustaining treatment an individual wants if at some time the individual is unable to make decisions.

2. **Durable power of attorney for health care:** Legal document that designates another person to make health care decisions for the client when the client becomes unable to make decisions independently.

3. **Nursing Interventions:** Ensure communication to the health care team when clients have provided advance directives (available in the medical record). Clients who do not have advance directives must be given written information outlining rights related to health care decisions.

Legal Issues

I Informed Consent

Obtained after a client receives complete disclosure of all pertinent information provided by the provider regarding the surgery or procedure to be performed. Obtained only if the client understands the potential benefits and risks associated with the surgery or procedure.

A. **Elements of Informed Consent**

1. Individual giving consent must fully understand the procedure that will be performed, the risks involved, expected/desired outcomes, expected complications/side effects, and alternate treatments or therapies available.

2. Consent is given by a competent adult, legal guardian, designated power of attorney (DPOA), emancipated or married minor, parent of a minor, or a court order.

3. A trained medical interpreter must be provided when the person giving consent is unable to communicate due to a language barrier.

B. **Nurse's Role:** Witness the client's signature and ensure the provider gave the necessary information and that the client understood and is competent to sign. Notify the provider if clarification is needed.

C. **Documentation:** Thorough documentation includes reinforcement of information given by the provider, any irregular occurrences, and use of an interpreter.

II Client Rights

A. **Patient Bill of Rights:** Right to humane care and treatment

B. **Americans with Disabilities Act (ADA):** Eliminates discrimination against Americans who have physical or mental disabilities

C. **Confidentiality:** The right to privacy with respect to one's personal medical information

  1. **Legislation:** Health Insurance Portability and Accountability Act (HIPAA) of 1996

     a. A uniform, federal act providing privacy protection for health consumers

     b. State laws that can provide additional protections to consumers are not affected by HIPAA

     c. Guarantees that clients are able to access their medical records

     d. Provides clients with control over how their personal health information is used and disclosed

     e. Outlines limited circumstances in which personal health information can be disclosed without first obtaining consent of the client or the client's family

        1) Suspicion of child or elder abuse

        2) When otherwise required by law (such as suspicion of criminal activity)

        3) Incidences of state agency or health department requirements; reportable communicable disease

III Legal Responsibilities

A. **Sources of Law:** The Constitution, statutes, administrative agencies, and court decisions

B. **Types of Laws and Courts**

  1. Criminal law

     a. Felony: Serious crime

     b. Misdemeanor: Less serious crime

  2. Civil laws

     a. Tort law

        1) **Unintentional torts:** Negligence, malpractice

        2) **Quasi-intentional torts:** Breach of confidentiality, defamation of character

        3) **Intentional torts:** Assault, battery, false imprisonment

  3. State laws: Nursing practice is regulated by state law. Each state's board of nursing has rules, regulations, and standards that vary based on statutes defining practice.

C. **Nurse Practice Acts**

  1. Vary from state to state

D. **Good Samaritan Law**

  1. Health care providers are protected from potential liability if volunteering away from their place of employment, as long as the nurse's actions are not grossly negligent.

E. **Mandatory Reporting**

  1. Abuse

     a. Nurses are mandated to report abuse of vulnerable populations (children, older adults). Any suspicion of abuse must be reported based on facility policy.

  2. Communicable Disease

     a. A complete list is available from the CDC. Report to the public health department to ensure appropriate medical treatment. Plan for prevention and control, including public education.

F. **Impaired Coworker**

  1. A nurse who suspects a coworker of using drugs or alcohol while working has the duty to report to the appropriate supervisory personnel according to institutional policy

G. **Malpractice (Professional Negligence)**

  1. The failure of a person who has professional training to act in a reasonable and prudent manner within the identified scope of practice or within the guidelines identified by the state regulating agency

H. **Negligence**

  1. The omission to do something that a reasonable person would do, or doing something that a reasonable person would not do.

  2. Negligence can be mitigated by following practice standards, communicating effectively with the health care team, and accurate/timely documentation.

I. **Nursing Interventions:** Nurses who are able to recognize the rights and responsibilities in legal matters are better able to protect themselves against liability or loss of licensure.

! Point to Remember

One of the most vital and basic functions of a professional nurse is the duty to intervene when the safety or well-being of a client or another person is obviously at risk.

Information Technology

I Informatics

The use of information technology (IT) as a communication and information-gathering tool that supports clinical decision-making and scientifically based nursing practice.

A. Allows candidates to test for nursing licensure (NCLEX®) with rapid results

B. Permits verification of licensure online for nurses and other health care professionals

C. IT resources are used to gather data in a systematic way to support clinical decision-making and scientifically based nursing practice

D. Client Care: Electronic documentation, medication dispensing, and client education resources

E. Professional education (medications, diseases, procedures, treatments)

F. Client portals: Allows integration of electronic health, collaboration between clients and providers

II Data Security

A. Passwords are necessary to prevent improper access to computers and medication systems.

B. Only individuals who have a professional relationship with a client can access the client's personal health information, per HIPAA regulations.

C. Computer terminals must be logged off and locked when not in immediate use.

D. Monitor screens must be shielded or situated so that unauthorized individuals cannot see the information.

III Use of Technology in Health care

A. Documentation

B. Databases for teaching and learning

C. Electronic Health Record

D. Mobile applications

E. Telehealth/telemedicine

! Point to Remember

A nurse should not share computer passwords with another person, including coworkers and family members.

Nurses should instruct clients to review valid and credible websites. The author, institution, and credentials should be reviewed.

UNIT THREE

Community Health Nursing

The Nurse's Role in Community Nursing

I Community Assessment: Individuals, Families, and Aggregates

A comprehensive assessment clarifying the client problem by evaluating:

A. Biological factors

B. Social factors

C. Cultural factors

D. Physical factors

E. Environmental factors

F. Social systems

G. Financial constraints (The client's eligibility for service and situational constraints must also be considered.)

II Community Nurse Referrals

Assist in linking the community resource with the client to provide holistic care; must have thorough knowledge of resource individuals and organizations.

A. Use computerized records, databases, and telecommunication technologies for physical, audio, and visual data.

B. Responsible for coordination, providing continuity of care, and evaluating the outcome.

C. Examples of community nursing referrals

1. Psychological services

2. Support groups

3. Medical equipment providers

4. Meal delivery services

5. Transportation services

6. Life care planner

D. Examples of community health nurse practice settings

1. Home health nurse

2. Hospice nurse

3. Occupational health nurse

4. Parish nurse

5. School nurse

6. Case managers

III Community Health Nursing

Goal is to preserve, protect, promote, and maintain health of individuals, families, and groups in the community.

A. **Vulnerable groups**

1. Migrant workers and immigrants

2. People who are poor or homeless

3. People who experience violence or abuse

4. People who have substance use disorder

5. People who have severe mental illness

6. Older adults

7. Pregnant adolescents

8. Individuals who have communicable diseases

Disaster Planning

I Disaster

A serious disruption of the functioning of a community that causes widespread human, material, economic, or environmental losses that exceed the ability of the affected community or society to cope with using its own resources. Prevention, preparedness, response, and recovery are the four stages of disaster management.

A. **Internal disasters** are events in the health care facility that threaten to disrupt the care environment.

1. Structural (e.g., fire, loss of power)

2. Personnel-related (e.g., strike, high absenteeism)

B. **External disasters** are events outside the health care facility and may be human-made or natural.

1. Human-made disasters

   a. Transportation-related incidents (e.g., car, train, plane, and subway crashes)

   b. Terrorist attacks, including bombs (e.g., suicide bombs and dirty bombs) and bioterrorism

   c. Industrial accidents

   d. Chemical spills or toxic gas leaks

   e. Structural fires

2. Natural disasters

   a. Extreme weather conditions, including blizzards, ice storms, hurricanes, tornadoes, and floods

   b. Ecological disasters, including earthquakes, landslides, tsunamis, volcanoes, and forest fires

   c. Microbial disasters such as epidemics and pandemics

   d. A combined internal/external disaster situation can arise when an external disaster, such as a severe weather condition, causes mass casualties and prevents health care providers from getting to the facility, perhaps due to traffic or road conditions.

II Disaster Prevention

A. **Reducing risk from natural and human-made hazards**

1. Protecting buildings and infrastructure

2. Improving security and public health awareness

III Disaster Preparedness

A. **Occurs at the national, state, and local levels**

B. **Interagency cooperation within the community is essential in a disaster and requires:**

1. Community-wide planning for emergencies and/or hazards that may affect the local area.

2. Coordination between community emergency system and health care facilities.

3. Developing a local emergency communications plan and/or network.

4. Identification of potential emergency public shelters.

C. **Role of the nurse**

1. In the health care facility

   a. The Joint Commission mandates specific standards for hospital preparedness, including an Emergency Operation Plan (EOP).

   b. An EOP includes training for personnel, criteria for activation, and specific actions for various emergency/disaster scenarios.

   c. Disaster drills should be conducted at least twice annually; one involving community-wide resources and actual or simulated clients.

2. In the community

   a. Education provided to families about disaster planning

      1) A family disaster plan should include:

         a) What to do in an evacuation

         b) Plans for family pets

         c) Where to meet in case of an emergency

      2) A family disaster kit should include:

         a) A flashlight with extra batteries

         b) A battery-powered radio

         c) Nonperishable food that requires no cooking (along with a nonelectric can opener)

         d) One gallon of water per person

         e) Basic first-aid supplies

         f) Matches in a waterproof container

         g) Household liquid bleach for disinfection

         h) Emergency blanket and/or sleeping bag and pillow

         i) Rain gear

         j) Clothing and sturdy footwear

         k) Prescription and OTC medications

         l) Toiletries

         m) Important documents and money

3. **Nursing interventions**

   a. Collect data to identify risks in the community.

IV Disaster Response

A. **Emergency management system**

1. Provides public access to immediate health care (911)

2. Dispatch communication center

3. Trained first responders: emergency medical technicians

4. Transportation to medical resources: ground (ambulance) and/or air (helicopter)

B. **Declaration of a disaster**

1. **Disaster area**: Local officials request that the governor of the state take appropriate action under state law and the state's emergency plan and declare a disaster area.

2. **Federal disaster area**: The governor of the affected state requests declaration of a disaster area by the president to qualify the affected area for federal disaster relief.

3. **Internal disaster**: The nursing or administrative supervisor may declare an internal disaster in case of a facility-related issue.

C. **Disaster relief organizations**

1. Federal Emergency Management Agency (FEMA)

   a. FEMA is part of the U.S. Department of Homeland Security.

      1) Manages federal response and recovery efforts

2. American Red Cross

   a. Not a government agency, but authorized by the government to provide disaster relief

   b. The American Red Cross provides:

      1) Shelter and food to address basic human needs

      2) Health and mental services

      3) Food to emergency and relief workers

      4) Blood and blood products to disaster victims

   c. The American Red Cross also handles inquiries from concerned family members outside the disaster area.

3. Hazardous material response team (Hazmat)

   a. Hazardous materials may be radioactive, flammable, explosive, toxic, corrosive, or biohazardous, or may have other characteristics that make them hazardous in specific circumstances.

   b. Hazmat team members are specially trained to respond to these situations and wear protective equipment.

   c. In a toxic exposure disaster, Hazmat will coordinate the decontamination effort.

4. Other agencies include: U.S. Department of Homeland Security (DHS), Center for Disease Control (CDC), and Office of Emergency Management (OEM).

v Role of the Nurse

A. **Triage**: Process of prioritizing which clients should receive care first

   1. **Non-mass casualty situation**: The nurse prioritizes client care so that clients who have conditions of the highest acuity are evaluated and treated first. Emergency services are presented with a large number of casualties. However, they are still functional and able to provide care to victims on all three levels.

      a. **Emergent:** immediate threat to life; critically injured

      b. **Urgent:** major injuries that require immediate treatment

      c. **Nonurgent:** minor injuries that do not require immediate treatment; slightly injured

   2. **Mass casualty disaster triage**: The field and/or emergency services are presented with a number of casualties and/or ground conditions and are unable to treat everyone. The staff must provide the greatest good for the greatest number. Consists of four levels:

      a. **Emergent or Class I (red tag)**: immediate threat to life; do not delay treatment

      b. **Urgent or Class II (yellow tag)**: major injuries that require treatment; can delay treatment 30 min to 2 hr

      c. **Nonurgent or Class III (green tag)**: minor injuries that do not require immediate treatment, can delay treatment 2 to 4 hr

      d. **Expectant or Class IV (black tag)**: expected and allowed to die; prepare for morgue

---

MASS CASUALTY DISASTER TRIAGE

Select the appropriate triage category after a mass casualty disaster triage (red, yellow, green, black).

	RED / YELLOW	GREEN / BLACK
1. Airway obstruction	☐ RED ☐ YELLOW	☐ GREEN ☐ BLACK
2. "Walking wounded"	☐ RED ☐ YELLOW	☐ GREEN ☐ BLACK
3. Requires immediate attention	☐ RED ☐ YELLOW	☐ GREEN ☐ BLACK
4. Closed fracture	☐ RED ☐ YELLOW	☐ GREEN ☐ BLACK
5. Shock	☐ RED ☐ YELLOW	☐ GREEN ☐ BLACK
6. Expected and allowed to die	☐ RED ☐ YELLOW	☐ GREEN ☐ BLACK
7. Contusions	☐ RED ☐ YELLOW	☐ GREEN ☐ BLACK
8. Massive head trauma	☐ RED ☐ YELLOW	☐ GREEN ☐ BLACK
9. Need treatment within 30 min to 2 hr	☐ RED ☐ YELLOW	☐ GREEN ☐ BLACK
10. Cardiac arrest	☐ RED ☐ YELLOW	☐ GREEN ☐ BLACK
11. Open fracture with a distal pulse	☐ RED ☐ YELLOW	☐ GREEN ☐ BLACK
12. Treatment can be delayed more than 2 hr	☐ RED ☐ YELLOW	☐ GREEN ☐ BLACK

Answer Key: 1. Red; 2. Green; 3. Red; 4. Green; 5. Red; 6. Black; 7. Green; 8. Black; 9. Yellow; 10. Black; 11. Yellow; 12. Green

---

B. **Health care facility disaster plan**

   1. A nursing or administrative supervisor may implement the disaster plan due to extreme weather conditions or an anticipation of mass casualties.

   2. Plans to implement

      a. Establishment of an incident command center

      b. Premature discharge of clients who are stable from the facility

      c. Transfer of clients who are stable from the intensive care unit

      d. Postponement of scheduled admissions and elective operations

      e. Mobilization of personnel (call in off-duty individuals)

      f. Protection of personnel and visitors

      g. Evacuation plan

   3. Role of the charge nurse during a disaster

      a. Preparation of a discharge list that features clients who can safely and quickly be discharged, such as the most stable, non-bedridden clients (e.g., clients admitted for observation, scheduled for diagnostic tests, or those who can be cared for at home or at a rehab facility)

      b. Personnel sent to the command center, if required

      c. Off-duty personnel called in, if requested

      d. Disaster victims prepared for admittance

vi Disaster Recovery

Begins when danger no longer exists and the "stand down" order has been given.

A. **Crisis intervention**

   1. Mental health response team employs advanced crisis intervention techniques to help victims, survivors, and their families better handle the powerful emotional reactions associated with crises and disasters.

   2. Goals

      a. Reduce the intensity of an individual's emotional reaction.

      b. Assist individuals in recovering from the crisis.

      c. Help to prevent serious long-term problems from developing.

B. **Posttraumatic stress disorder (PTSD)**: A mental health condition that can develop following any traumatic or catastrophic life experience

   1. PTSD symptoms can develop in survivors of a disaster weeks, months, or even years following the catastrophic event.

C. **Critical incident stress debriefing and administrative review**
  1. Health care providers who respond to a highly stressful event that is extremely traumatic or overwhelming may experience significant stress reactions.
  2. The critical incident stress debriefing process is designed to prevent the development of posttraumatic stress among first responders and health care professionals.
     a. Defusing: discussion of feelings shortly after the disaster/critical incident (such as at the end of a shift)
     b. Formal debriefing: discussion some hours or days after the disaster/critical incident, in a large group setting, with mental health teams of peer support personnel serving as the leaders
  3. Administrative review to identify areas of the agency response plan that were effective and areas that need improvement

VII Agents of Bioterrorism

A. **Three categories (A, B, C) of priority based on ease of transmission and morbidity and mortality rates**
  1. **Category A:** highest priority and threat to national security because agents are easily transmitted and have high mortality rates. Include: smallpox, botulism, anthrax, tularemia, hemorrhagic viral fevers (e.g., Ebola), and plague.
  2. **Category B:** second-highest priority, agents are moderately easy to disseminate and have moderate morbidity rates and low mortality rates. Include: typhus fever, ricin toxin, diarrheagenic *E. coli*, and West Nile virus.
  3. **Category C:** third-highest priority, emerging pathogens that could be engineered for mass dissemination. Agents are easy to produce and have a potential for high morbidity and mortality rates. Include: hantavirus, influenza virus, tuberculosis, and rabies virus.

Culturally Competent Care

I Cultural Care

A. **Culture:** Knowledge, beliefs, values, and traditions that are shared by a group of people about life and the world, which passes to the next generation

B. **Cultural competence:** The ability to provide care that respects and integrates aspects of culture to meet client needs

C. **Cultural humility:** Continuing self-reflection and awareness of cultural biases, assumptions, and values; better knowing of one's self that results in better care

II Cultural Competence

There are twelve standards to serve as a guide for providing culturally competent care.

A. Social justice
B. Critical reflection
C. Knowledge of cultures
D. Culturally competent practice
E. Cultural competence in health care systems and organizations
F. Client advocacy and empowerment
G. Multicultural workforce
H. Education and training in culturally competent care
I. Cross-cultural communication
J. Cross-cultural leadership
K. Policy development
L. Evidence-based practice and research

III Cultural Assessment

Collect data to identify values, beliefs, meaning, and behavior of clients

A. What is the client's ethnic affiliation, and what is its importance in the client's daily life?
B. What languages does the client speak, write, read, or understand?
C. What dietary preferences or prohibitions does the client follow?
D. Are there rituals or customs that the client wishes to keep related to transitions such as birth and death?
E. Does the client want or need to have family involved in care?
F. Is the client using herbal or other traditional remedies?
G. What behaviors or views are important to the spirituality of the client?

IV Cultural Factors Affecting Health

A. **Time Orientation**

1. Past: Cultures that focus on past orientation look to the past to provide direction for current situations. Review weekly progress to assist clients with health promotion and disease prevention.

2. Present: Place greater value on quality of life and view present time as being more important than future time. Focus on immediate benefits versus long-term outcomes as an effective approach when discussing disease prevention.

3. Future: Delays immediate gratification until future goals are met. Focus on long-term goals.

B. **Language and Communication:** Verbal and Nonverbal

1. Speak in a low, moderate voice.

2. Discuss one topic at a time.

3. Eye contact and the use of touch varies among cultural groups.

4. Language and communication barriers may impact a client's utilization of health care.

5. Recognize nonverbal cures of poor understanding.

   a. Blank expression

   b. Inappropriate laughter

   c. Absence of questions

C. **Space:** Preferred Distance Between Individuals

1. Take cues from the client and be aware of spatial distance preferences.

2. Clients may move closer or farther away from the nurse depending on personal space preference.

D. **Beliefs and practices:** An individual's beliefs regarding health affects actions taken to treat and prevent disease.

1. Biomedical beliefs: Focus is on identifying a cause for every effect on the body. This is the basis for the current United States health system.

2. Naturalistic beliefs: Relates the individual as a part of nature or creation. An imbalance in nature is believed to cause disease.

3. Magico-religious beliefs: Illness and health are linked to supernatural forces. Some religions share this belief as faith healing.

4. Folk healer beliefs: Clients may seek help from a spiritual healer, folk doctor, or shaman.

V Nursing Interventions

A. Address the client by their last name, unless the client gives permission to use another name.

B. Recognize individual uniqueness and the diversity within cultures.

C. Respect the client's values, beliefs, and practices.

D. Remain sensitive to the client's spiritual beliefs.

1. Spirituality is a subjective concept that implies connectedness.

2. Spirituality may or may not include religion.

3. Addressing clients' spiritual needs is required for all health care facilities by the Joint Commission.

E. Provide a diet that is consistent with client's customs and preferences.

F. Allow family to be involved in care, if desired.

G. Review the client's herbal and/or alternative methods to provide client education and prevent interactions with currently prescribed medications or treatments.

H. Consider cultural factors that affect health when providing care, such as time orientation, language and communication, space, and beliefs and practices.

I. Provide a qualified interpreter if necessary.

VI National CLAS Standards

The U.S. Department of Health and Human Services has identified culturally and linguistically appropriate services standards (CLAS) to promote equitable care and improve quality of health services. CLAS standards include:

A. Offering language and communication assistance as needed at no charge to the individual and ensuring that they are informed regarding availability of services

B. Ensuring that only qualified people provide language assistance

C. Providing written materials in the languages of commonly-served populations

D. Ensuring continuous quality improvement and accountability in the implementation of CLAS standards

E. Partner with the local community to establish and implement services that ensure cultural and linguistic appropriateness

VII Using an Interpreter

The nurse should use a qualified interpreter when it is difficult for a nurse or client to understand the other's language.

A. Observe the client for nonverbal messages.

B. Address the client, as well as the interpreter.

C. Interpreters should have knowledge of health-related terminology.

D. Have the interpreter translate written materials into the client's primary language.

E. Consider client preferences when selecting the age and gender of an interpreter.

F. Federal government mandates require agencies to have a plan that will improve access to federal health care programs for individuals who have limited English proficiency.

G. Review the material with the client to ensure that nothing has been missed or misunderstood.

H. The use of family members as interpreters should be avoided because clients may need privacy in discussing sensitive matters. Family members can have difficulty understanding medical terminology.

RELIGIOUS/SPIRITUAL INFLUENCES ON HEALTH

	BIRTH PRACTICES	DEATH PRACTICES	DIETARY RESTRICTIONS	HEALTH PRACTICES
Buddhism	Believe in reincarnation. Contraception to prevent conception is acceptable.	Ensure a calm, peaceful environment. Chanting is common. Monk delivers last rites. Organ donation is encouraged. Cremation is common.	Vegetarian diet practiced by many. Avoidance of alcohol.	A quiet, peaceful environment allows client to rest and practice meditation and prayer. May refuse care on holy days.
Catholicism	Contraception, abortion, and sterilization are prohibited. Baptism is required.	Priest administers last rites. Organ donation is acceptable. Suicide may prevent burial in Catholic cemetery.	Some may abstain from eating meat on Ash Wednesday and on Fridays during Lent.	Most want to see a priest when hospitalized. May request communion or confession to aid in healing. May wear cross or medal or display religious statues.
Christian Science	Abortion is prohibited. A client may choose to give birth at home.	Unlikely to seek medical help to prolong life. Organ donation is discouraged.	Must abstain from alcohol.	Medications and blood products are avoided. Healing ministers practice spiritual healing and do not use medical or psychological techniques.
Hinduism	Contraception is acceptable. Abortion may be prohibited. Males are not circumcised. Child is not named until the tenth day of life.	Believe in reincarnation. Allowing a natural death is traditional. Client may want to lie on floor while dying. A thread is placed around the neck/wrist. Organ donation is acceptable. Prefer cremation.	Vegetarian diet is encouraged. Most abstain from beef and pork. Right hand is used for eating and left hand for toileting and hygiene. Several days a year are set aside for fasting.	Personal hygiene is very important. Future lives are influenced by how one faces illness, disability, and death.
Islam (Muslim)	Contraception is acceptable. Abortion is permitted in certain circumstances. A prayer is said into the infant's ear at birth. Circumcision is customary.	Client may want to confess sins prior to death. A dying client may wish to be placed facing Mecca (usually east). Organ donation and autopsy is acceptable by some. Devout Muslims may refuse both, fearing desecration of the dead. Rituals include traditional bathing with burial within 24 hr. Cremation is prohibited.	Food must be halal (lawful). Pork, alcohol, and some shellfish are prohibited. Ramadan is a period of fasting during the ninth lunar month. Halal (permitted) meats are from animals that have been slaughtered during a payer ritual. Haram (prohibited) foods include pork, gelatin, alcohol, and animals with fangs.	A client may wish to pray five times a day, facing Mecca, and may have a prayer rug. Privacy during prayer is important. Women are very modest and wear clothes that cover their entire body. Women may refuse/avoid male health care workers.

Religious and spiritual influences on health care may not reflect the beliefs and practices of individual clients. This material is presented for overall cultural competence and NCLEX preparation.

	BIRTH PRACTICES	DEATH PRACTICES	DIETARY RESTRICTIONS	HEALTH PRACTICES
Judaism	Abortion is permitted. Ritual circumcision of males is called a bris, performed on the eighth day of life. Orthodox Jewish males are not allowed in the delivery room.	An autopsy is discouraged. Organ donation is permitted. Someone stays with the body at all times. Ritual bathing and burial within 24 hr. Cremation is prohibited.	Food is required to be kosher. Milk and meat cannot be served at the same meal or prepared on the same dishes. Pork and shellfish prohibited. Fasting required on Yom Kippur. Lactose intolerance is common among Jews of European origin.	Saving a life overrides nearly all religious obligations. Prayers of well-being of the sick may be said. Anything that can be done to ease the client's suffering is encouraged. During the Sabbath, Orthodox Jews refrain from using electrical appliances.
The Church of Jesus Christ of Latter-day Saints (Mormon)	Contraception is at the discretion of the man and woman. Abortion is opposed except in certain maternal circumstances. Infants are not baptized.	Organ donation is permitted. An autopsy is permitted. Life continues beyond death.	Alcohol, coffee, and tea are prohibited. Fasting is required once a month.	May want to use herbal remedies in addition to medical care. When blessing the sick, a person is anointed with oil by two elders.
Seventh-Day Adventist	Abortion is acceptable in some circumstances. Opposed to infant baptism.	An autopsy is acceptable. Organ donation is acceptable.	Vegetarian diet is encouraged. Alcohol, coffee, and tea are prohibited.	Healing accomplished through medical intervention and divine healing. Prayer and anointing with oil may be performed.

Religious and spiritual influences on health care may not reflect the beliefs and practices of individual clients. This material is presented for overall cultural competence and NCLEX preparation.

UNIT FOUR

Pharmacology in Nursing

Calculations and Conversions

Basic medication dose conversion and calculation skills are essential to providing safe nursing care. Standard conversions are used to solve dosage calculation problems. Nurses are responsible for the administration of the correct amount of medication based on the type of medication being administered.

A. **Standard Conversion Factors**

1. 1 mg = 1,000 mcg
2. 1 g = 1,000 mg
3. 1 kg = 1,000 g
4. 1 kg = 2.2 lb
5. 60 mg = 1 grain
6. 30 mL = 1 oz
7. 1 L = 1,000 mL
8. 5 mL = 1 tsp
9. 15 mL = 1 tbsp
10. 1 tbsp = 3 tsp

B. **Temperature Conversions**

1. $37.0°C = 98.6°F$
2. $°C = (°F - 32) \times (5/9)$
3. $°F = (°C \times 9/5) + 32$

C. **Calculations for IV Administration**

1. Number of hours = total volume / mL/hr
2. gtt per min = total volume × gtt/mL in administration set / total number of minutes

D. **Calculations for Dosage**

1. Dosage on hand (H)/mL = Dosage desired (D)/mL

PRACTICE TEST QUESTIONS

1. A client has the following food for lunch: 12 oz ice chips, ½ cup tea, 1 cup coffee, and 300 mL milk. The client eats the ice chips, and drinks all of the tea, coffee, and half of the milk. What is the total intake for lunch?

2. A client has a prescription for 0.25 mg digoxin. The dose on hand is digoxin 0.5 mg tablets. How many tablets will the client receive?

3. A client's IV infusion rate is 125 mL/hr. How many hours will it take for a 1 L bag of IV fluid to infuse?

4. The IV rate is 100 mL/hr and the administration set is 15 drops/mL. How many drops per minute will deliver the required fluids?

5. A client has a prescription for heparin sodium 6,000 units IV. The vial contains 10,000 units/mL. How many milliliters of heparin will the nurse administer?

6. A nurse is preparing 300,000 units of procaine penicillin. The vial contains 1,500,000 units/2 mL. How many milliliters will the nurse administer?

7. A client weighs 136 lb and has a prescription for 0.5 mL of medication per kilogram of body weight. How many milliliters of medication will the client receive? (Round the answer to the nearest whole number.)

8. A client is receiving dextrose 5% in water at 50 mL/hr in one IV and D_5W 75 mL/hr in another IV. The client also receives IV piggyback medication every 12 hr prepared in 100 mL of fluid. What is the total amount of IV fluid the client will receive in 24 hr?

9. The IV administration set delivers 10 drops/mL. What is the rate of flow in drops/min for 1,000 mL dextrose 5% in water to infuse in 8 hr?

10. When measuring a client's output, the nurse records 300 mL of urine at 0800, 450 mL of liquid stool at 1130, 225 mL of urine at 1300, and 35 mL of emesis at 1430. What is the client's total output for this shift?

11. A client receiving an IV infusion has a prescription for 1,000 mL in 12 hr. Using a microdrip system that delivers 60 microdrops/mL, the nurse should regulate the infusion for how many drops per minute?

    A. 45

    B. 68

    C. 83

    D. 96

12. A client's temperature is 100° F. What is this temperature in degrees centigrade?

13. A nurse has available ondansetron 2 mg/mL. The prescription is to administer 4 mg. How many milliliters will the nurse administer?

14. A nurse is preparing an IV antibiotic in 100 mL dextrose 5% in water to infuse over 20 min. The infusion set is calibrated for 10 drops/mL. What drip rate should the nurse use?

Answer Key: 1. 690; 2. 0.5; 3. 8; 4. 25; 5. 0.6; 6. 0.4; 7. 31; 8. 3,200; 9. 21; 10. 1,010; 11. C (83); 12. 37.8; 13. 2 mL; 14. 50

Medication Therapies

I Medication Actions, Interactions, and Reactions

A. **Medication Properties (Pharmacokinetics):** The absorption, distribution, metabolism, and excretion of a medication; describes the onset of action, peak level, duration of action, and bioavailability

B. **Medication Interactions:** When a medication is given with another medication and alters the effect of either or both medications

C. **Adverse Reactions:** Negative effects experienced by a client as the result of a specific medication; can be hazardous, tolerated, or subside with continued use

II Pharmacotherapy Across the Life Span

A. **Medications and Pregnancy:** A majority of medications cross the placental barrier, thereby increasing the risk of teratogenicity. All medications should be given with extreme caution to ensure safety to the developing fetus.

B. **Medications and Breastfeeding:** Most medications taken by a client who is breastfeeding appear in breast milk. Medication levels tend to be the highest in the newborn immediately after the medication is administered to the client. Clients who are breastfeeding are advised to breastfeed before taking the medication. For additional guidelines, review Unit Seven: Mental Health Nursing.

C. **Medication in Children:** Pharmacokinetics are influenced by a child's age, size, and maturity of the targeted organ. To reduce the risk of toxicity, the following factors must be considered: safe calculation of the child's dosage (mg/kg/day), medication that is age-appropriate, monitoring of IV medications to prevent fluid overload (use smaller solution containers to avoid infusing too much fluid), and administration of inhalants using a metered-space device. For additional guidelines, review Unit Eight: Maternal and Newborn Nursing.

D. **Medication in Older Adult Clients:** Age-related changes affect therapeutic effects of medications in older adult clients. Older adult clients experience more adverse effects than younger adults due to aging body systems. Confusion, lethargy, falls, and weakness can be mistaken for senility, rather than adverse reactions. If the adverse reaction is not identified, unnecessary medication might be prescribed to treat complications caused by the medication. As the client continues to receive medications, the risk for toxicity increases, especially in cases of polypharmacy. Toxicity in older adult clients is a greater risk when taking diuretics, antihypertensives, digoxin, steroids, anticoagulants, hypnotics, and over-the-counter medications.

III Safe Medication Administration

A. **The RN is prepared to administer medications using the enteral, parenteral, and transcutaneous routes.**

   1. The PN is prepared to calculate and monitor IV flow rate.

   2. The PN is prepared to administer IV secondary medications.

B. **The PN must validate the client's**

   1. Allergies and adverse effects.

   2. Current medication regimen for potential interactions.

   3. Physiologic status compared to baseline assessment data.

C. **The PN follows the six rights of medication administration** (right client, right drug, right dose, right route, right time, right documentation) to protect the safety of the client and follow the scope of practice to maintain professional licensure.

IV Laboratory Profiles in Pharmacology

Laboratory testing can be indicated for specific medications. The nurse is accountable for collaborating with the provider in ensuring client safety when laboratory testing is prescribed.

A. **Therapeutic Drug Monitoring**

   1. Measures blood drug levels to determine effective medication dosages and prevent medication toxicity. The test can also be used to identify non-adherence with medication regimens.

   2. Blood testing is preferred because it provides information about current therapeutic levels, whereas urine levels reflect the presence of a drug over several days.

B. **Peak levels reflect the highest concentration.**

AVERAGE TIMES FOR DRAWING PEAK LEVELS

ROUTE OF ADMINISTRATION	TIME SPECIMEN IS DRAWN AFTER ADMINISTRATION
Oral intake	1 to 2 hr
Intramuscular	1 hr
Intravenous	30 min

C. **Trough levels** reflect the lowest concentration or residual level and are usually obtained within 15 min prior to administration of the next scheduled dose. The scheduled dose of medication should not be administered until the trough level is confirmed.

NOTE: The timing for drawing a peak and trough level varies based on the half-life (time required for the body to decrease the medication blood level by 50%) for the medication.

D. **Culture and Sensitivity:** Cultures are obtained to detect the presence of pathogens within the specimen collected. If a culture produces organisms, testing is performed in the laboratory to identify the appropriate antibiotic therapy (sensitivity). Begin antibiotic therapy after obtaining the lab sample.

NOTE: When prescribed, cultures should be obtained prior to initiating antibiotic therapy (definitive therapy). When cultures cannot be drawn prior, the provider will prescribe a broad-spectrum antibiotic (empirical therapy). Monitoring culture results is imperative to ensure proper antimicrobial treatment.

v Intravenous Therapy

Administration of fluids via an intravenous catheter (peripheral or central vein access) for the purpose of providing medication, fluid, electrolyte, or nutrient replacement

A. **Guidelines for Safe IV Administration**

1. Review medication guidelines for precautions related to IV administration for compatibility, rate of administration, necessity of infusion pump, and serious adverse reactions.
2. Never administer medications through tubing being used for blood administration.
3. Implement standard precautions and follow policies related to IV site changes.
4. Fluids should be infused within 24 hr (discard unused portion) to prevent infection.
5. Maintain patency of IV access.

B. **Types of IV Access**

1. Peripheral vein
2. Central venous catheters
   a. Peripherally inserted central catheter (PICC)
   b. Nontunneled percutaneous central venous catheter
   c. Tunneled central venous catheter
   d. Implanted port

C. **Prevent complications associated with IV infusion.**

COMPLICATIONS ASSOCIATED WITH IV INFUSION

COMPLICATION	NURSING INTERVENTIONS
Infiltration	**Prevention:** Use the smallest catheter for the prescribed therapy. Stabilize port access. Monitor blood return. **Treatment:** Stop infusion. Remove peripheral catheters. Apply cold compress. Elevate extremity. Insert new catheter in opposite extremity.
Extravasation	**Prevention:** Know vesicant potential before giving medication. **Treatment:** Stop infusion. Discontinue administration set. Aspirate medication if possible. Apply cold compress. Document condition of site (may photograph).
Phlebitis/ thrombophlebitis	**Prevention:** Rotate sites every 72 to 96 hr. Secure catheter. Use aseptic technique. For PICCs, avoid excessive activity with the extremity. **Treatment:** Stop infusion. Remove peripheral IV catheters. Apply heat compress. Insert new catheter in opposite extremity.
Hematoma	**Prevention:** Avoid veins not easily seen or palpated. Obtain hemostasis after insertion. **Treatment:** Remove IV device and apply light pressure for bleeding. Monitor for signs of phlebitis and treat.
Catheter embolus	**Prevention:** Do not reinsert stylet needle into catheter. **Treatment:** Immediately apply tourniquet high on extremity to limit venous flow. Prepare for removal under x-ray.

D. **Complications Associated with Central Venous Catheters**

COMPLICATIONS OF CENTRAL VENOUS CATHETERS

COMPLICATION	NURSING INTERVENTIONS
Pneumothorax (during insertion)	**Prevention:** Use ultrasound to locate veins. Avoid subclavian insertion when possible. **Treatment:** Administer oxygen. Assist provider with chest tube insertion.
Air embolism	**Prevention:** Have client lie flat when changing administration set or needleless connectors. Ask client to perform Valsalva maneuver if possible. **Treatment:** Place client in left lateral Trendelenburg. Administer oxygen.
Lumen occlusion	**Prevention:** Flush promptly with normal saline between, before, and after each medication. **Treatment:** Use 10 mL syringe with a pulsing motion.
Bloodstream infection	**Prevention:** Maintain sterile technique. **Treatment:** Change entire infusion system. Notify provider. Obtain cultures. Administer antibiotics.

E. **Complications Associated with PICC Lines**

COMPLICATIONS ASSOCIATED WITH PICC LINES

COMPLICATION	NURSING INTERVENTIONS
Catheter occlusions	Prevent kinks. Reposition arm. Confirm blood return. Flush catheter between medications. Administer approved antithrombolytic.
Catheter dislodges	Monitor blood return and for discomfort in jaw, chest, or ear. Contact provider.
Phlebitis	Apply low-degree heat. Discontinue if not resolved.
Catheter embolism	Secure catheter. Avoid pulling. Follow safe practices for catheter removal.
Infection	Use aseptic technique. Keep dressing clean and dry. Intervene immediately for any sign of infection.

vi Total Parenteral Nutrition (TPN)

Hypertonic solution containing dextrose, proteins, electrolytes, minerals, trace elements, and insulin prescribed according to the client's needs and administered via central venous device (PICC line, subclavian or internal jugular vein)

A. **Care and Maintenance of TPN**

1. Before administering, verify prescription and solution with another nurse.
2. Administer via infusion pump.
3. Monitor weight daily.
4. Monitor and record I&O, noting fluid balance.
5. Monitor serum glucose levels every 4 to 6 hr.
6. Monitor for signs of infection.
7. Change dressing every 48 to 72 hr per facility protocol.
8. Change IV tubing and fluid every 24 hr.
9. If TPN solution is unavailable, administer dextrose 10% in water to prevent hypoglycemia.

VII Antidote/Reversal Agents

A. **Acetaminophen:** acetylcysteine
B. **Benzodiazepine:** flumazenil
C. **Curare:** edrophonium
D. **Cyanide poisoning:** methylene blue
E. **Digitalis:** digoxin immune fab
F. **Ethylene poisoning:** fomepizole
G. **Heparin and enoxaparin:** protamine sulfate
H. **Iron:** deferoxamine
I. **Lead:** succimer
J. **Magnesium sulfate:** calcium gluconate 10%
K. **Narcotics:** naloxone
L. **Warfarin:** phytonadione (vitamin K)

VIII Therapeutic Drug Levels

A. **Aminophylline:** 10 to 20 mcg/mL
B. **Carbamazepine:** 5 to 12 mcg/mL
C. **Digoxin:** 0.8 to 2.0 ng/mL
D. **Gentamicin:** 5 to 10 mcg/mL
E. **Lidocaine:** 1.5 to 5.0 mcg/mL
F. **Lithium:** 0.4 to 1.4 mEq/L
G. **Magnesium sulfate:** 4 to 8 mg/dL
H. **Phenobarbital:** 10 to 40 mcg/mL
I. **Phenytoin:** 10 to 20 mcg/mL
J. **Salicylate:** 100 to 250 mcg/mL
K. **Theophylline:** 10 to 20 mcg/mL
L. **Tobramycin:** 5 to 10 mcg/mL
M. **Trough Drug Levels**
   1. Gentamicin: 1 to 2 mcg/mL
   2. Tobramycin: 1 to 2 mcg/mL
   3. Vancomycin: 15 to 20 mcg/mL

IX Toxic Drug Levels

A. **Acetaminophen:** greater than 250 mcg/mL
B. **Aminophylline:** greater than 20 mcg/mL
C. **Amitriptyline:** greater than 500 ng/mL
D. **Digoxin:** greater than 2.4 ng/mL
E. **Lidocaine:** greater than 5 mcg/mL
F. **Lithium:** greater than 2.0 mEq/L
G. **Magnesium sulfate:** greater than 9 mg/dL
H. **Methotrexate:** greater than 10 mcmol over 24 hr
I. **Phenobarbital:** greater than 40 mcg/mL
J. **Phenytoin:** greater than 30 mcg/mL
K. **Salicylate:** greater than 300 mcg/mL
L. **Theophylline:** greater than 20 mcg/mL

X Common Drug Class Suffixes

COMMON DRUG CLASS SUFFIXES

SUFFIX	MEDICATION CATEGORY
-dipine	Calcium channel blocker
-afil	Erectile dysfunction
-caine	Anesthetic
-pril	ACE inhibitor
-pam, -lam	Benzodiazepine
-statin	Antilipidemic
-asone, -solone	Corticosteroid
-olol	Beta blocker
-cillin	Penicillin
-ide	Oral hypoglycemic
-prazole	Proton pump inhibitor
-vir	Antiviral
-ase	Thrombolytic
-azine	Antiemetic
-phylline	Bronchodilator
-arin	Anticoagulant
-dine	Antiulcer
-zine	Antihistamine
-cycline	Antibiotic
-mycin	Aminoglycoside
-floxacin	Antibiotic
-tyline	Tricyclic antidepressant
-pram, -ine	SSRI

MEDICATION CATEGORIES

This worksheet will build on your overall knowledge of medications. Learning medications by categories will help you group medications and reduce the number to memorize. This list is not all-inclusive, but is a great place to start. NCLEX® will expect you to know entry-level pharmacology. Column one lists generic medication categories or classifications. In column two, write the commonly used suffix for the medication classification. In column three, write an example of a medication that would be included in the classification.

MEDICATION CATEGORY	SUFFIX	MEDICATION
1. ACE inhibitors	pril	Captopril
2. Antivirals	vir	
3. Antifungals	azole	
4. Antilipidemics	statin	
5. Angiotensin II receptor blockers (ARBs)	olol sartan	losartan
6. Beta blockers	olol	
7. Calcium-channel blockers	dipine	Nifedipine
8. Erectile dysfunction medications	afil	
9. Histamine₂ receptor antagonists	dine	
10. Proton pump inhibitors	prazole	

Answer Key for Suffixes: 1. –pril; 2. –vir; 3. –azole; 4. –statin; 5. –sartan; 6. –olol; 7. –dipine; 8. –afil; 9. –dine; 10. –prazole
Medications: Answers may vary.

SIDE EFFECTS AND ADVERSE REACTIONS

This worksheet will build upon your knowledge of medication side effects and adverse reactions. NCLEX will expect you to be able to manage clients experiencing side effects and adverse reactions to medications. Match the side effect or adverse reaction with the medication or classification. Each should only be used once.

____ 1. ACE inhibitors

____ 2. Benzodiazepines

____ 3. Beta blockers

____ 4. Ciprofloxacin

____ 5. Digoxin

____ 6. Doxycycline

____ 7. Furosemide

____ 8. Lithium

____ 9. Tobramycin

____ 10. Valacyclovir

A. Angioedema

B. Bronchospasm

C. Yellow tinge to vision

D. Hypokalemia

E. Tendon rupture

F. Tooth discoloration

G. Ototoxicity

H. Thrombotic thrombocytopenic purpura

I. Anterograde amnesia

J. Tremors

Answer Key: 1. A; 2. I; 3. B; 4. E; 5. C; 6. F; 7. D; 8. J; 9. G; 10. H

Medications for the Cardiovascular System

Antihypertensives

Treatment for clients who have hypertension includes lifestyle modification and medications.

A. **Nursing interventions for clients taking antihypertensive medications**

1. Monitor weight, vital signs, and hydration status.
2. Monitor blood pressure in supine, sitting, and standing positions.
3. Monitor laboratory profiles (renal function, coagulation).
4. Clients should take medication at the same time each day.
5. Clients should avoid hot tubs and saunas.
6. Do not discontinue medication abruptly.
7. Prevent orthostatic hypotension.

B. **Angiotensin-Converting Enzyme (ACE) Inhibitors and Angiotensin II Receptor Blockers (ARBs)**
1. **Action**
   a. ACE inhibitors block the conversion of angiotensin I to angiotensin II.
   b. ARBs selectively block the binding of angiotensin II to AT_1 receptors found in tissues.

ACE INHIBITORS	ARBS
Captopril	Losartan
Enalapril	Valsartan
Enalaprilat (IV route)	Irbesartan
Fosinopril	
Lisinopril	

2. **Therapeutic Use**: Hypertension, heart failure, MI, diabetic nephropathy
3. **Precautions/Interactions**
   a. Use with caution if diuretic therapy is in place.
   b. Monitor potassium levels.
4. **Side/Adverse Effects**
   a. Persistent nonproductive cough with ACE inhibitors
   b. Angioedema, hypotension
   c. Should not be used in second and third trimester of pregnancy
5. **Nursing Interventions and Client Education**
   a. Captopril should be taken 1 hr before meals.
   b. Monitor blood pressure.
   c. Monitor for angioedema and promptly administer epinephrine 0.5 mL of 1:1,000 solution subcutaneously.

C. **Calcium-Channel Blockers**
1. **Action:** Slows movement of calcium into smooth-muscle cells, resulting in arterial dilation and decreased blood pressure
2. **Medications**
   a. Nifedipine
   b. Verapamil
   c. Diltiazem
   d. Amlodipine
3. **Therapeutic Use**
   a. Angina, hypertension
   b. Verapamil and diltiazem can be used for atrial fibrillation, atrial flutter, or SVT.
4. **Precautions/Interactions**
   a. Use cautiously in clients taking digoxin and beta blockers.
   b. Contraindicated for clients who have heart failure, heart block, or bradycardia.
   c. Do not consume grapefruit juice (toxic effects).

5. **Side/Adverse Effects**
   a. Constipation
   b. Reflex tachycardia
   c. Peripheral edema
   d. Toxicity
6. **Nursing Interventions and Client Education**
   a. Do not crush or chew sustained-release tablets.
   b. Administer IV injection over 2 to 3 min.
   c. Slowly taper dose if discontinuing.
   d. Monitor heart rate and blood pressure.

D. **Alpha Adrenergic Blockers (Sympatholytics)**
1. **Action:** Selectively inhibit $alpha_1$ adrenergic receptors, resulting in peripheral arterial and venous dilation that lowers blood pressure
2. **Medications**
   a. Prazosin
   b. Doxazosin mesylate
3. **Therapeutic Use**
   a. Primary hypertension
   b. Doxazosin mesylate can be used in treatment of benign prostatic hypertrophy (BPH).
4. **Precautions/Interactions**
   a. Increased risk of hypotension and syncope if given with other antihypertensives, beta blockers, or diuretics.
   b. NSAIDs can decrease the effect of prazosin.
5. **Side/Adverse Effects**
   a. Dizziness
   b. Fainting
6. **Nursing Interventions and Client Education**
   a. Monitor heart rate and blood pressure.
   b. Take medication at bedtime to minimize effects of hypotension.
   c. Advise to notify prescriber immediately about adverse reactions.
   d. Consult prescriber before taking any OTC medications.

E. **Centrally Acting Alpha₂ Agonists**
1. **Action:** Stimulate alpha adrenergic receptors ($alpha_2$) in the brain to reduce peripheral vascular resistance, heart rate, and systolic and diastolic blood pressure
2. **Medications**
   a. Clonidine
   b. Guanfacine HCl
   c. Methyldopa
3. **Therapeutic Use**
   a. Primary hypertension (can be used in combination with diuretics or antihypertensives)
   b. Hypertensive crisis
   c. Severe cancer pain (parenteral administration via epidural)

4. **Precautions/Interactions**

   a. Contraindicated with anticoagulant therapy and hepatic failure.

   b. Do not administer to clients taking MAOIs.

   c. Do not administer methyldopa through IV line with barbiturates or sulfonamides.

   d. Use cautiously in clients who have CVA, MI, diabetes mellitus, major depression, or chronic kidney failure.

   e. Do not use during lactation.

5. **Side/Adverse Effects**

   a. Dry mouth

   b. Drowsiness and sedation (resolves over time)

   c. Rebound hypertension

   d. Black or sore tongue

   e. Leukopenia

6. **Nursing Interventions and Client Education**

   a. Monitor for adverse CNS effects.

   b. Monitor CBC, heart rate, and blood pressure.

   c. Monitor for weight gain or edema.

   d. Monitor closely for rebound hypertension when medication is discontinued (48 hr).

   e. Never skip a dose.

   f. Administer at bedtime to minimize effects of hypotension.

   g. Notify prescriber of any involuntary jerky movements, prolonged dizziness, rash, or yellowing of skin.

F. **Beta Adrenergic Blockers (Sympatholytics)**

1. **Action:** Inhibit stimulation of receptor sites, resulting in decreased cardiac excitability, cardiac output, myocardial oxygen demand; lower blood pressure by decreasing release of renin in the kidney

   NOTE: Beta$_1$ receptors are primarily in the cardiac and renal tissues. Beta$_2$ receptors are found primarily in the lungs, gastrointestinal tract, liver, uterus, vascular smooth muscle, and skeletal muscle.

2. **Medications:** Can be selective or nonselective

   a. Cardioselective Beta$_1$ Medications

      1) Metoprolol

      2) Atenolol

      3) Metoprolol succinate

   b. Nonselective (Beta$_1$ and Beta$_2$) Medications

      1) Propranolol

      2) Nadolol

      3) Labetalol

3. **Therapeutic Use**

   a. Primary hypertension

   b. Angina

   c. Tachydysrhythmias, heart failure, and MI

4. **Precautions/Interactions**

   a. Contraindicated in clients who have AV block and sinus bradycardia.

   b. Do not administer nonselective beta blockers to clients who have asthma, bronchospasm, or heart failure.

   c. Propranolol can mask effects of hypoglycemia in clients who have diabetes mellitus.

   d. Do not administer labetalol in the same IV line with furosemide.

5. **Side/Adverse Effects**

   a. Bradycardia

   b. Nasal stuffiness

   c. AV block

   d. Rebound myocardium excitation if stopped abruptly

   e. Bronchospasm

6. **Nursing Interventions and Client Education**

   a. Administer 1 to 2 times daily.

   b. Do not discontinue without consulting the provider.

   c. Do not crush (or chew) extended-release tablets.

   d. Hold medication and notify the provider for systolic blood pressure less than 100 mm Hg or heart rate less than 60/min.

   e. Monitor clients who have diabetes mellitus for indications of hypoglycemia.

G. **Vasodilators**

1. **Action:** Direct vasodilation of arteries and veins resulting in rapid reduction of blood pressure (decreased preload and afterload)

2. **Medications**

   a. Nitroglycerin

   b. Enalaprilat

   c. Nitroprusside

   d. Hydralazine

3. **Therapeutic Use**

   a. Hypertensive emergencies

4. **Precautions/Interactions**

   a. Clients who have hepatic or renal disease

   b. Older adult clients

   c. Electrolyte imbalances

5. **Side/Adverse Effects**

   a. Dizziness

   b. Headache

   c. Profound hypotension

   d. Cyanide toxicity

   e. Thiocyanate poisoning

6. **Nursing Interventions and Client Education**

   a. Nitroprusside cannot be mixed with any other medication.

   b. Apply protective cover to container.

   c. Discard unused fluid after 24 hr.

   d. Provide continuous ECG and blood pressure monitoring.

II Cardiac Glycosides

Used in the treatment of clients who have cardiac failure or ineffective pumping mechanism of the heart muscle.

A. **Action**

1. Increase the force and velocity of myocardial contractions to improve stroke volume and cardiac output.

2. Slow the conduction rate, allowing for increased ventricular filling.

B. **Medication**

1. Digoxin

C. **Therapeutic Uses**

1. Heart failure

2. Atrial fibrillation

D. **Precautions/Interactions**

1. Thiazide or loop diuretics increase risk of hypokalemia and precipitate digoxin toxicity.

2. ACE inhibitors and ARBs increase risk of hyperkalemia.

3. Verapamil increases risk of toxicity.

E. **Side/Adverse Effects**

1. Digoxin toxicity: GI effects (anorexia, nausea, vomiting, abdominal pain), CNS effects (fatigue, weakness, diplopia, blurred vision, yellow-green or white halos around objects)

F. **Nursing Interventions and Client Education**

1. Monitor apical pulse for 1 min prior to administration.

2. Notify provider for heart rate less than 60/min (adult), less than 70/min (child), or less than 90/min (infant).

3. Monitor for signs of digoxin toxicity, hypokalemia, and hypomagnesemia.

4. Notify the provider of any sudden increase in pulse rate that previously had been normal or low.

5. Maintain therapeutic digoxin level.

G. **Management of Digoxin Toxicity**

1. Discontinue digoxin and potassium-wasting medications.

2. Treat dysrhythmias with phenytoin (or lidocaine).

3. Treat bradycardia with atropine.

4. For overdose, administer digoxin immune fab to prevent absorption.

III Antianginal Medications

The use of organic nitrates, beta adrenergic-blocking agents, and calcium channel blockers to treat pain related to imbalances between myocardial oxygen supply and demand

A. **Organic Nitrates**

1. **Action**

   a. Relax peripheral vascular smooth muscles, resulting in dilation of arteries and veins, thus reducing venous blood return (reduced preload) to the heart, which leads to decreased oxygen demands on the heart

   b. Increase myocardial oxygen supply by dilating large coronary arteries and redistributing blood flow

2. **Medications**

   a. Nitroglycerin:
      1) Sublingual tablet
      2) Sustained release tablet
      3) Transdermal ointment
      4) Transdermal unit (patch)

B. **Therapeutic Use**

1. Acute angina attack

2. Prophylaxis of chronic stable or variant angina

C. **Precautions/Interactions**

1. Contraindicated in clients who have head injury

2. Hypotensive risk with antihypertensive medications

3. Contraindicated if taking erectile dysfunction medications—life-threatening hypotension

D. **Side/Adverse Effects**

1. Headache

2. Orthostatic hypotension

3. Reflex tachycardia

4. Tolerance

E. **Nursing Interventions and Client Education**

1. Nitroglycerin tablet

   a. Administer sublingual.

   b. Rest for 5 min. If pain is not relieved by the first tablet, call 911, then take a second tablet. May use up to three tablets taken 5 min apart. Keep Nitrostat in original dark container.

   c. Nitrolingual can be used prophylactically 5 to 10 min before exercise.

   d. Do not shake Nitrolingual canister (forms bubbles).

   e. Replace nitroglycerin tablets every 6 months.

   f. Wear medical alert identification.

2. Nitroglycerin transdermal ointment

   a. Wear gloves for administration.

   b. Do not massage or rub area.

   c. Apply to an area without hair (chest, flank, or upper arm is preferable).

   d. Cover the area where the patch is placed with a clear plastic wrap, and tape in place.

   e. Gradually reduce the dose and frequency of application over 4 to 6 weeks.

3. Nitroglycerin transdermal unit (patch)
   a. Skin irritation can alter medication absorption.
   b. Optimal locations for patch are the upper chest or side; pelvis; and inner, upper arm.
   c. Rotate skin sites.
   d. Patch is usually worn for 12 to 14 hr, then removed.

IV Antidysrhythmic Agents

A. **Action:** Antidysrhythmic agents are complex agents with multiple mechanisms of action. They are classified according to their effects on the electrical conduction system of the heart (Class I, II, III, IV).

B. **Medications**
   1. Adenosine: Slows conduction time through the AV node, interrupts AV node pathways to restore NSR.
   2. Amiodarone: Prolongs repolarization, relaxes smooth muscles, decreases vascular resistance.
   3. Atropine: Increases the heart rate by counteracting the muscarine-like actions of acetylcholine and other choline esters.

C. **Precautions/Interactions**
   1. Toxicity is a major concern due to additive effects.
   2. Caution is needed when used who has an AV block.
   3. Caution is needed when using anticholinergic medications.

ANTIDYSRHYTHMIC MEDICATIONS

Adenosine

THERAPEUTIC USE	Convert SVT to sinus rhythm
SIDE/ADVERSE EFFECTS	Flushing, nausea Bronchospasm, prolonged asystole
NURSING INTERVENTIONS	Rapid IV push (1 to 2 seconds). Flush immediately with normal saline.

Amiodarone

THERAPEUTIC USE	Ventricular fibrillation Unstable ventricular tachycardia
SIDE/ADVERSE EFFECTS	Bradycardia Cardiogenic shock Pulmonary disorders
NURSING INTERVENTIONS	Incompatible with heparin. Can be given in PO maintenance dose. Monitor for respiratory complications.

Atropine

THERAPEUTIC USE	Bradycardia Known exposure to chemical nerve agent Reduce secretions
SIDE/ADVERSE EFFECTS	No contraindications when used for life-threatening emergency
NURSING INTERVENTIONS	Monitor for dry mouth, blurred vision, photophobia, urinary retention, and constipation.

V Antilipemic Medications

A. **Action:** Aid in lowering low-density lipoprotein (LDL) levels and increasing high-density lipoprotein (HDL) levels. Therapy includes diet, exercise, and weight control.

B. **Therapeutic Uses**
   1. Primary hypercholesterolemia
   2. Prevention of coronary events
   3. Protection against MI and stroke in clients who have diabetes mellitus

C. **Precautions/Interactions**
   1. Should be discontinued during pregnancy.
   2. Use with caution in renal dysfunction.

D. **Side/Adverse Effects**
   1. Muscle aches
   2. Hepatotoxicity
   3. Rhabdomyolysis
   4. Peripheral neuropathy

E. **Nursing Interventions and Client Education**
   1. Take medication in the evening (cholesterol synthesis increases).
   2. Monitor liver and renal function laboratory profiles.
   3. Low-fat, high-fiber diet.
   4. Note dietary precautions with specific classes.

F. **Statin Medications**
   1. **Action:** Interfere with hepatic enzyme HMG-CoA to reduce formation of cholesterol precursors
   2. **Medications**
      a. Atorvastatin
      b. Simvastatin
      c. Lovastatin
      d. Pravastatin sodium
      e. Rosuvastatin
      f. Fluvastatin
   3. **Precautions/Interactions**
      a. Prolonged bleeding in clients taking warfarin
      b. Multiple drug interactions: digoxin, warfarin, thyroid hormones, thiazide diuretics, phenobarbital, NSAIDs, tetracycline, beta-blocking agents, gemfibrozil, glipizide, glyburide, oral contraceptives, phenytoin
   4. **Nursing Interventions and Client Education**
      a. Do not administer with grapefruit juice.

G. **Cholesterol Absorption Inhibitor**
   1. **Action:** Inhibits the absorption of cholesterol secreted in the bile and from food. Often used in combination with other antilipemic medications.
   2. **Medications**
      a. Ezetimibe
   3. **Nursing Interventions and Client Education**
      a. Take 2 hr before or 4 hr after other antilipemics.
      b. Risk of liver damage increased when combined with statins.

Medications for the Respiratory System

Medications used to treat chronic inflammatory conditions caused by asthma, bronchitis, and emphysema

A. **Treatment for chronic respiratory disorders often includes multiple drug therapies.** When administered as inhalation therapies, the following guidelines should be implemented.

1. Advise clients to take the beta₂ agonist before the inhaled glucocorticoid to increase steroid absorption.

2. Reinforce instructions on procedures for inhalation.

   a. Remove the mouthpiece cap.

   b. If appropriate for the medication, shake container.

   c. Stand up or sit upright. Exhale deeply.

   d. Place the mouthpiece between teeth, and close lips tightly around the inhaler.

   e. While breathing in, press down on the inhaler to activate and release the medication. Continue breathing in slowly for several more seconds. (Slow, long, steady inhalation is better than quick short breaths.)

   f. Hold breath for 5 to 10 seconds.

   g. Breathe in/out normally.

3. Examine mouth for irritation.

4. Perform frequent oral care.

I Beta₂ Adrenergic Agonists

A. **Action:** Promote bronchodilation by activating beta₂ receptors in bronchial smooth muscle

BETA₂ ADRENERGIC AGONISTS MEDICATIONS

Albuterol

ROUTE/ONSET	Inhaled (short-acting) 5 to 15 min
USE	Acute bronchospasm

Formoterol, salmeterol

ROUTE/ONSET	Inhaled (long-acting) Formoterol: Onset 1 to 3 min; Duration 10 hr Salmeterol: Onset 10 to 20 min; Duration 12 hr
USE	Long-term control of asthma

Terbutaline

ROUTE/ONSET	Oral (long-acting)
USE	Long-term control of asthma

B. **Precautions/Interactions**

1. Contraindicated for clients who have tachydysrhythmias.

2. Caution: Diabetes mellitus, hyperthyroidism, heart disease, hypertension, angina.

3. Beta blockers reduce effects.

4. MAOIs increase effects.

C. **Side/Adverse Effects**

1. Tachycardia, palpitations

2. Tremors

D. **Nursing Interventions and Client Education**

1. Caution against using salmeterol more frequently than every 12 hr.

II Methylxanthines

A. **Action:** Relaxation of bronchial smooth muscle, resulting in bronchodilation

B. **Medications**

1. Aminophylline

2. Theophylline

C. **Therapeutic Uses**

1. Relief of bronchospasm

2. Long-term control of asthma

D. **Precautions/Interactions**

1. Contraindicated with active peptic ulcer disease.

2. Caution: Diabetes mellitus, hyperthyroidism, heart disease, hypertension, angina.

3. Do not mix parenteral form with other medications.

4. Phenobarbital and phenytoin decrease theophylline levels.

5. Caffeine, furosemide, cimetidine, fluoroquinolones, acetaminophen, and phenylbutazone falsely elevate therapeutic levels.

E. **Side/Adverse Effects**

1. Irritability and restlessness

2. Toxic effects: tachycardia, tachypnea, seizures

F. **Nursing Interventions and Client Education**

1. Monitor therapeutic levels for aminophylline and theophylline.

2. Avoid caffeine intake.

3. Monitor for signs of toxicity.

4. Smoking will decrease effects.

5. Alcohol abuse will increase effects.

G. **Treatment of Toxicity**

1. Stop parenteral infusion.

2. Activated charcoal decreases absorption in oral overdose.

3. Lidocaine for dysrhythmias.

4. Diazepam to control seizures.

III Inhaled Anticholinergics

A. **Action:** Muscarinic receptor blocker resulting in bronchodilation

B. **Medications**
   1. Ipratropium
   2. Tiotropium

C. **Therapeutic Uses**
   1. Prevent bronchospasm
   2. Manage allergen- or exercise-induced asthma
   3. COPD

D. **Precautions/Interactions**
   1. Contraindicated for clients who have peanut allergy (contains soy lecithin).
   2. Use extreme caution with narrow-angle glaucoma and BPH.
   3. Do not use for treatment of acute bronchospasms.

E. **Side/Adverse Effects**
   1. Dry mouth and eyes
   2. Urinary retention

F. **Nursing Interventions and Client Education**
   1. Maximum effects can take up to 2 weeks.
   2. Shake inhaler well before administration.
   3. When using two different inhaled medications, wait 5 min between.
   4. If administered via nebulizer, use within 1 hr of reconstitution.

IV Glucocorticoids

A. **Action:** Prevent inflammatory response by suppression of airway mucus production, immune responses, and adrenal function

GLUCOCORTICOID MEDICATIONS

Oral	Inhalation	Intravenous
Prednisone	Beclomethasone dipropionate	Hydrocortisone sodium succinate
Prednisolone	Budesonide	Methylprednisolone sodium succinate
Betamethasone	Fluticasone propionate	Betamethasone sodium phosphate
	Triamcinolone acetonide	

B. **Respiratory Therapeutic Uses**
   1. Short-term
      a. IV agents: Status asthmaticus
      b. Oral: Treatment of symptoms following an acute asthma attack
   2. Long-term
      a. Inhaled: Prophylaxis of asthma
      b. Oral: Treatment of chronic asthma

C. **Precautions/Interactions**
   1. Clients who have diabetes mellitus can require higher doses.
   2. Never stop medication abruptly.

D. **Side/Adverse Effects**
   1. Euphoria, insomnia, psychotic behavior
   2. Hyperglycemia
   3. Peptic ulcer
   4. Fluid retention
   5. Withdrawal symptoms
   6. Increased appetite

E. **Nursing Interventions and Client Education**
   1. Monitor client activity and behavior.
   2. Administer medication with meals.
   3. Reinforce teaching of symptoms to report.
   4. Do not take with NSAIDs.
   5. Reinforce teaching about gradual reduction of dose to prevent Addisonian crisis.

V Leukotriene Modifiers

A. **Action:** Prevent effects of leukotriene, resulting in decreased inflammation, bronchoconstriction, airway edema, and mucus production

B. **Medications**
   1. Montelukast
   2. Zileuton
   3. Zafirlukast

C. **Therapeutic Uses**
   1. Long-term management of asthma in adults and children
      a. Montelukast can be given to clients 1 year and older.
      b. Zileuton can be given to clients 12 years and older.
      c. Zafirlukast can be given to clients 5 years and older.
   2. Prevention of exercise-induced bronchospasm

D. **Precautions/Interactions**
   1. Do not use for acute asthma attack.
   2. Zileuton or zafirlukast: High risk of liver disease, increased warfarin effects, and theophylline toxicity.
   3. Phenobarbital decreases circulating levels of montelukast.
   4. Chewable tablets contain phenylalanine.

E. **Side/Adverse Effects**
   1. Elevated liver enzymes (zileuton or zafirlukast)
   2. Warfarin and theophylline toxicity (zileuton or zafirlukast)
   3. Can increase levels of beta blockers leading to hypotension and bradycardia (propranolol)

F. **Nursing Interventions and Client Education**
   1. Never abruptly substitute for corticosteroid therapy.
   2. Reinforce teaching to take daily in the evening.
   3. Do not decrease or stop taking other prescribed asthma medications until instructed.
   4. If using oral granules, pour directly into mouth or mix with cold soft foods (never liquids).
   5. Use open packets within 15 min of taking medication.

VI Antitussives, Expectorants, Mucolytics

DRUG ACTIONS AND THERAPEUTIC USE BY CLASS

Antitussives: hydrocodone, codeine

ACTION	Suppress cough through action in the CNS
THERAPEUTIC USE	Chronic nonproductive cough

Expectorants: guaifenesin

ACTION	Promote increased mucous secretion to increase cough production
THERAPEUTIC USE	Often combined with other agents to manage respiratory disorders

Mucolytics: acetylcysteine, hypertonic saline

ACTION	Enhance the flow of secretions in the respiratory tract
THERAPEUTIC USE	Acute and chronic pulmonary disorders with copious secretions
	Cystic fibrosis
	Antidote for acetaminophen poisoning

A. **Precautions/Interactions**
  1. Only saline solutions should be used in children younger than 2 years.
  2. Opioid antitussives have potential for abuse.
  3. Caution with OTC medications (potentiate effects).

B. **Side/Adverse Effects**
  1. Drowsiness
  2. Dizziness
  3. Aspiration and bronchospasm risk with mucolytics
  4. Constipation

C. **Nursing Interventions and Client Education**
  1. Monitor cough frequency, effort, and ability to expectorate.
  2. Monitor character and tenacity of secretions.
  3. Auscultate for adventitious lung sounds.
  4. Reinforce why multiple therapies are needed.
  5. Promote fluid intake.

VII Decongestants, Antihistamines

DRUG ACTIONS AND THERAPEUTIC USE BY CLASS

Decongestants: phenylephrine, pseudoephedrine, naphazoline

ACTION	Stimulate alpha$_1$ adrenergic receptors, causing reduced inflammation of nasal membranes
THERAPEUTIC USE	Allergic rhinitis
	Sinusitis
	Common cold

Antihistamines: diphenhydramine, loratadine, cetirizine, fexofenadine, desloratadine

ACTION	Decrease allergic response by competing for histamine receptor sites
THERAPEUTIC USE	Relieve/prevent hypersensitivity reactions

A. **Precautions/Interactions**
  1. Use cautiously in clients who have hypertension, glaucoma, peptic ulcer disease, or urinary retention.
  2. Children can have symptoms of excitation, hallucinations, incoordination, and seizures.
  3. Avoid alcohol intake.
  4. Products containing pseudoephedrine should not be used longer than 7 days.

B. **Side/Adverse Effects**
  1. Anticholinergic effects
  2. Drowsiness

C. **Nursing Interventions and Client Education**
  1. Monitor for hypokalemia.
  2. Monitor blood pressure.
  3. Reinforce teaching to manage anticholinergic effects.
  4. Advise to take at night.

Medications for the Endocrine System

I Oral Hypoglycemics

Used in conjunction with diet and exercise to control glucose levels in clients who have type 2 diabetes mellitus

A. **Precautions/Interactions**
  1. Caution in clients who have renal, hepatic, or cardiac disorders.
  2. Generally avoided during pregnancy and lactation. Tell clients to discuss with the prescriber.

ORAL HYPOGLYCEMIC MEDICATIONS

Alpha-glucosidase inhibitors: acarbose, miglitol

ACTION	Slows carbohydrate absorption and digestion
PRECAUTIONS/INDICATIONS	Contraindicated in clients who have intestinal disease due to increased gas formation

Biguanides: metformin

ACTION	Reduces gluconeogenesis
	Makes muscle tissue more sensitive to insulin
PRECAUTIONS/INDICATIONS	Withhold 48 hr prior to and 48 hr after a test with contrast media
	Contraindicated in clients who have severe infection, shock, or hypoxic conditions

Gliptins: sitagliptin

ACTION	Promotes release of insulin
	Lowers glucagon secretion
	Slows gastric emptying
PRECAUTIONS/INDICATIONS	Caution with impaired renal function; dose will be reduced

ORAL HYPOGLYCEMIC MEDICATIONS (CONTINUED)

Meglitinides: repaglinide, nateglinide

ACTION	Stimulates beta cells to release insulin
PRECAUTIONS/ INDICATIONS	Short-acting
	Administer before each meal
	Risk of hypoglycemia

Sulfonylureas: glipizide, glyburide

ACTION	Promotes release of insulin from the pancreas
PRECAUTIONS/ INDICATIONS	Extreme high risk of hypoglycemia in clients who have renal, hepatic, or adrenal disorders
	Can cause disulfiram-like reaction with alcohol ingestion

Thiazolidinediones: rosiglitazone, pioglitazone

ACTION	Decreases cellular insulin resistance
PRECAUTIONS/ INDICATIONS	Exacerbation of heart failure

B. **Nursing Interventions and Client Education**

1. Reinforce teaching of signs and management for hypoglycemia, especially with sulfonylureas.
2. Encourage diet and exercise to follow American Diabetes Association (ADA) recommendations.
3. Monitor glycosylated hemoglobin (HbA1C).
4. Refer to a diabetes nurse educator.

II Insulin

Various forms of insulin are available to manage diabetes. The medications vary in onset, peak, and duration.

FORMS OF INSULIN

	ONSET	PEAK	DURATION
Rapid-acting: Lispro	15 to 30 min	0.5 to 2.5 hr	3 to 6 hr
Short-acting: Regular	0.5 to 1 hr	1 to 5 hr	6 to 10 hr
Intermediate: NPH	1 to 2 hr	6 to 14 hr	16 to 24 hr
Long-acting: Insulin glargine	70 min	None	24 hr

A. **Therapeutic Uses**

1. Glycemic control of diabetes mellitus (type 1, type 2, gestational) to prevent complications
2. Clients taking oral hypoglycemic agents can require insulin therapy when:
   a. Undergoing diagnostic tests; NPO status
   b. Pregnant
   c. Severe kidney or liver disease is present
   d. Oral agents are inefficient
   e. Treatment of hyperkalemia

B. **Precautions/Interactions**

1. When mixing regular with NPH insulin, draw up regular first.
2. Do not mix other insulins with lispro, glargine, or combination 70/30.
3. Only regular insulin is given IV (only in normal saline).
4. Administer glargine at bedtime.

C. **Side/Adverse Effects**

1. Hypoglycemia/hyperglycemia
2. Lipodystrophy

D. **Nursing Interventions and Client Education**

1. Monitor serum glucose levels before meals and at bedtime or patterned schedule–specific to client.
2. Roll vial of insulin (except regular) to mix; do not shake.
3. Rotate injection sites to prevent lipodystrophy.
4. Reinforce teaching about signs and management for hypo/hyperglycemia.
5. Encourage diet and exercise to follow ADA recommendations.
6. Monitor HbA1c.
7. Refer to diabetes nurse educator.

III Glycemic Agent

A. **Action:** Initiates regulatory processes to promote breakdown of glycogen to glucose in the liver, resulting in increased serum glucose levels

B. **Medications**

1. Glucagon

C. **Therapeutic Uses**

1. Emergency treatment of severe hypoglycemia

D. **Precautions/Interactions**

1. Do not mix with sodium chloride or dextrose solutions.

E. **Side/Adverse Effects**

1. Nausea and vomiting
2. Rebound hypoglycemia

F. **Nursing Interventions and Client Education**

1. Administer medication for unresponsive clients.
2. Monitor blood glucose levels.
3. Self-monitor for early signs of hypoglycemia.
4. Wear medical alert ID.
5. Advise clients to teach family members how to administer medication.
6. Provide carbohydrates when clients awaken from hypoglycemic reaction.

IV Thyroid Hormone

A. **Action:** Stimulates metabolism of all body systems by accelerating the rate of cellular oxygenation

B. **Medications**
1. Levothyroxine/T_4

C. **Therapeutic Uses**
1. Hypothyroidism
2. Emergency treatment of myxedema coma

D. **Precautions/Interactions**
1. Overmedication can result in signs of hyperthyroidism.

E. **Side/Adverse Effects**
1. Tachycardia
2. Restlessness
3. Diarrhea
4. Weight loss
5. Decreased bone density
6. Heat intolerance
7. Insomnia

F. **Nursing Interventions and Client Education**
1. Monitor cardiac system.
2. Therapy is initiated with low doses. Advance to higher dosages while monitoring laboratory values.
3. Monitor T_4 and TSH levels.
4. Take in early morning.

V Thyroid Hormone Antagonist

A. **Action:** Inhibits synthesis of thyroid hormone

B. **Medication**
1. Methimazole

C. **Therapeutic Uses**
1. Hyperthyroidism
2. Preoperative thyroidectomy
3. Thyrotoxic crisis
4. Thyroid storm

D. **Precautions/Interactions**
1. Administer with caution to clients who have bone marrow depression, hepatic disease, or bleeding disorders.
2. Discontinue prior to radioactive iodine uptake testing.
3. Contraindicated with breastfeeding.

E. **Side/Adverse Effects**
1. Skin rash, pruritus
2. Abnormal hair loss
3. GI upset
4. Paresthesias
5. Periorbital edema
6. Joint and muscle pain
7. Jaundice
8. Agranulocytosis
9. Thrombocytopenia

F. **Nursing Interventions and Client Education**
1. Administer with food at the same time each day.
2. Increase fluids to 3 L/day.
3. Avoid OTC products containing iodine.
4. Take medication as prescribed.
5. If discontinuing, dose must be tapered off.
6. Monitor clients for therapeutic response (weight gain; decreased pulse, blood pressure, and T_4 levels).
7. Monitor clients for signs of overdose and signs of hypothyroid (periorbital edema, cold intolerance, mental depression).

VI Anterior Pituitary/Growth Hormones

A. **Action:** Increase production of insulin-like growth factor throughout the body

B. **Medications**
1. Somatropin

C. **Therapeutic Use**
1. Treat growth hormone deficiencies
2. Turner's syndrome

D. **Precautions/Interactions**
1. Contraindicated in clients who are severely obese.
2. Therapy must be discontinued prior to epiphyseal closure.
3. Avoid concurrent use of glucocorticoids.

E. **Side/Adverse Effects**
1. Hyperglycemia
2. Hypothyroidism

F. **Nursing Interventions and Client Education**
1. Monitor growth patterns.
2. Reconstitute medication per manufacturer instructions.
3. Administer subcutaneous per protocol.
4. Dose is individualized.

VII Posterior Pituitary Hormones/ Antidiuretic Hormones

A. **Action:** Promote reabsorption of water with the kidneys; vasoconstriction of vascular smooth muscle

B. **Medications**
1. Desmopressin (DDAVP): oral, intranasal, subcutaneous, IV
2. Vasopressin: intranasal, subcutaneous, IV

C. **Therapeutic Uses**
1. Diabetes insipidus
2. Cardiac arrest
3. Nocturnal enuresis
4. Hemophilia (Desmopressin)

D. **Precautions/Interactions**
1. Contraindicated in clients who have chronic nephritis or high risk for myocardial infarction

E. Side/Adverse Effects

1. Hyponatremia
2. Seizures
3. Coma

F. Nursing Interventions and Client Education

1. Monitor urine specific gravity.
2. Monitor blood pressure.
3. Monitor urinary output.
4. Prevent hyponatremia due to water intoxication.
5. Reinforce teaching regarding use of nasal spray.

VIII Adrenal Hormone Replacement

A. Action: Anti-inflammatory, suppresses immune response

B. Medications

1. Dexamethasone
2. Hydrocortisone sodium succinate
3. Fludrocortisone acetate
4. Prednisone

C. Therapeutic Uses

1. Acute and chronic replacement for adrenocortical insufficiency (Addison's disease)
2. Inflammation, allergic reactions, cancer

D. Precautions/Interactions

1. Contraindicated in clients who have systemic fungal infection.
2. Caution in clients who have hypertension, gastric ulcers, diabetes, osteoporosis.
3. Requires higher doses in acute illness or extreme stress.

E. Side/Adverse Effects

1. Adrenal suppression when administered for inflammation, allergic reactions
2. Infection
3. Hyperglycemia
4. Osteoporosis
5. GI bleeding
6. Fluid retention

F. Nursing Interventions and Client Education

1. Do not skip doses.
2. Monitor blood pressure.
3. Monitor fluid and electrolyte (F&E) balance, weight, and output.
4. Monitor for signs of bleeding and GI discomfort.
5. Reinforce teaching to take calcium supplements and maintain vitamin D levels.
6. Give with food.
7. Taper off dose regimen when discontinuing medication.
8. Provide immunoprotection.

Medications for the Hematologic System

I Blood and Blood Products

A. Examples

1. Whole blood
2. Packed red blood cells (PRBCs)
3. Platelet concentrations

ADMINISTRATION OF BLOOD PRODUCTS

Whole blood

TIME COMPLETED	2 to 4 hr	
ACTION/ THERAPEUTIC USE	Replace volume > Hemorrhage > Surgery > Trauma	> Burns > Shock
MONITOR FOR REACTION	Acute hemolytic Febrile Anaphylactic	Mild allergic Hypervolemia Sepsis

Packed RBCs

TIME COMPLETED	2 to 4 hr	
ACTION/ THERAPEUTIC USE	Increase available RBC Severe anemia Hemoglobinopathies	Hemolytic anemia Erythroblastosis fetalis
MONITOR FOR REACTION	Acute hemolytic Febrile Anaphylactic	Mild allergic Sepsis

Platelets

TIME COMPLETED	15 to 30 min	
ACTION/ THERAPEUTIC USE	Increase platelet count Active bleeding Thrombocytopenia	Aplastic anemia Bone marrow suppression
MONITOR FOR REACTION	Febrile	Sepsis

Fresh frozen plasma (FFP)

TIME COMPLETED	30 to 60 min	
ACTION/ THERAPEUTIC USE	Replace clotting factors > Hemorrhage > Burns > Shock	> Thrombotic thrombocytopenic purpura (TTP) > Reverse effects of warfarin
MONITOR FOR REACTION	Acute hemolytic Febrile Anaphylactic	Mild allergic Hypervolemia Sepsis

Pheresed granulocytes

TIME COMPLETED	45 to 60 min	
ACTION/ THERAPEUTIC USE	Severe neutropenia Neonatal sepsis	Neutrophil dysfunction
MONITOR FOR REACTION	Acute hemolytic Febrile Anaphylactic	Mild allergic Hypervolemia Sepsis

Albumin

TIME COMPLETED	5% (1 to 10 mL/min)	25% (4 mL/min)
ACTION/ THERAPEUTIC USE	Expand volume via oncotic changes Hypovolemia Hypoalbuminemia	Burns Severe nephrosis Hemolytic disease of the newborn
MONITOR FOR REACTION	Risk for hypervolemia and pulmonary edema	

B. **Nursing Interventions and Client Education**

1. Client ID, name, and blood type must be verified by two nurses.

2. Prior to administration, measure baseline vital signs, including temperature.

3. Establish IV access, 18- to 20-gauge catheter.

4. Must have 0.9% sodium chloride primed tubing.

5. For the first 15 min, stay with the client and infuse slowly, monitoring for any reaction. If a reaction occurs, perform the following interventions.

   a. Stop blood immediately and take vital signs.

   b. Infuse 0.9% sodium chloride.

   c. Notify the provider.

   d. Follow facility policy (send urine sample, CBC, and bag and tubing to laboratory for analysis).

6. Complete infusion of product within 4 hr.

II Hematopoietic Growth Factors

A. **Action:** Stimulate the bone marrow to synthesize the specific blood cells.

MEDICATIONS FOR HEMATOPOIETIC GROWTH FACTORS

Epoetin alfa

THERAPEUTIC USES	Stimulate RBC production Anemia related to: Chronic kidney disease Retrovir therapy Chemotherapy
SIDE/ADVERSE EFFECTS	Hypertension
NURSING INTERVENTIONS	Subcutaneous or IV Do not agitate vial. Monitor hematocrit and hemoglobin.

Filgrastim, injection
Pegfilgrastim, IV over 2 to 4 hr

THERAPEUTIC USES	Stimulate WBC production Neutropenia related to cancer
SIDE/ADVERSE EFFECTS	Bone pain Leukocytosis
NURSING INTERVENTIONS	Subcutaneous or IV Do not agitate vial. Monitor CBC.

Oprelvekin

THERAPEUTIC USES	Stimulate platelet production Thrombocytopenia related to cancer
SIDE/ADVERSE EFFECTS	Fluid retention Blurred vision Cardiac dysrhythmia
NURSING INTERVENTIONS	Administer within 6 to 24 hr after chemotherapy. Subcutaneous

III Iron Preparations

A. **Action:** Treat iron deficiency

B. **Medications**

1. Oral

   a. Ferrous sulfate

   b. Ferrous gluconate

   c. Ferrous fumarate

   d. Dilute liquid preparations with juice or water and administer with a plastic straw or medication dosing syringe (avoid contact with teeth).

   e. Encourage orange juice fortified with vitamin C. (Vitamin C facilitates absorption.)

   f. Avoid antacids, coffee, tea, dairy products, and whole-grain breads concurrently and for 1 hr after administration due to decreased absorption.

   g. Monitor for constipation and gastrointestinal upset.

2. Parenteral

   a. Iron dextran

   b. Used for clients unable to take oral medication

   c. Intramuscular

      1) Use a large-bore needle (19- to 20-gauge, 3-inch).

      2) Change needle after drawing up from vial.

      3) Z-track (ventrogluteal preferable), never in deltoid muscle.

      4) Do not massage injection site.

   d. IV (preferred over IM)

      1) Administer a small test dose (25 mg over 5 min). Observe patient for 15 min then slowly administer additional preparation.

      2) Use manufacturer's recommendation for specific product.

IV Anticoagulant

A. **Action:** Modify coagulation by altering the clotting cascade or dissolving an existing clot

1. Parenteral

   a. Modify or inhibit clotting or cellular properties to prevent clot formation (heparin)

   b. Prevent conversion of prothrombin to thrombin by inactivating coagulation enzymes (low molecular weight heparin: enoxaparin)

2. Oral

   a. Prevent synthesis of coagulation factors VII, IX, X, and prothrombin (warfarin)

   b. Inhibiting thrombin formation (dabigatran)

   c. Inhibit factor Xa (rivaroxaban)

B. **Medications and Therapeutic uses**

1. Parenteral

   a. Stroke

   b. Pulmonary embolism

   c. Deep-vein thrombosis

   d. Cardiac catheterization

   e. MI

   f. DIC

2. Oral (warfarin)

   a. Venous thrombosis

   b. Prevent thrombus formation for clients who have atrial fibrillation or prosthetic heart valves

   c. Prevent recurrent MI

   d. Prevent transient ischemic attacks (TIAs)

3. Oral (dabigatran etexilate)

   a. Reduce risk of stroke/embolism for clients who have nonvalvular atrial fibrillation

4. Oral (rivaroxaban)

   a. Reduce risk of stroke/embolism for clients who have nonvalvular atrial fibrillation

   b. Prevent deep-vein thrombosis (DVT) and pulmonary emboli (PE) in clients undergoing total hip or knee arthroplasty

C. **Precautions/Interactions**

1. Parenteral

   a. Administer subcutaneous or IV.

   b. Incompatible with many medications (any bicarbonate base).

   c. Avoid NSAIDs, aspirin, and medications containing salicylates.

2. Oral (warfarin)

   a. Not safe for use during pregnancy (category X).

   b. Contraindications: Thrombocytopenia, vitamin K deficiency, liver disease, alcohol use disorder.

   c. Decreased effects with phenobarbital, carbamazepine phenytoin, and oral contraceptives.

   d. Food sources high in vitamin K can decrease effects.

3. Oral (dabigatran)

   a. Caution if changing anticoagulation medication.

   b. Discontinue 1 to 2 days prior to surgical procedures.

4. Oral (rivaroxaban)

   a. No antidote for severe bleeding (prepare to administer activated charcoal to prevent further absorption).

   b. Wait 6 hr before restarting after removal of epidural catheters.

D. **Side Effects/Interactions**

1. Parenteral

   a. Hemorrhage

   b. Heparin-induced thrombocytopenia

   c. Toxicity/overdose

2. Oral (warfarin)

   a. Hemorrhage

   b. Toxicity/overdose

3. Oral (dabigatran, rivaroxaban)

   a. Bleeding

   b. GI discomfort (dabigatran)

   c. Bleeding, bruising, headache, or eye pain (rivaroxaban)

E. **Nursing Interventions/Client Education**

1. Parenteral

   a. Heparin: Monitor aPTT every 4 to 6 hr for IV administration.

   b. Monitor for signs of bleeding.

   c. Safety precautions to prevent bleeding.

   d. Administer subcutaneous heparin to abdomen, 2 inches from umbilicus. (Do not aspirate or massage.)

   e. Rotate injection sites and observe for bleeding or hematoma.

   f. Administer protamine sulfate for heparin toxicity (1 mg neutralizes 100 units of heparin).

2. Oral (warfarin)

   a. Administer once daily.

   b. Monitor INR or PT.

   c. Bleeding risk remains up to 5 days after discontinued therapy.

   d. Avoid NSAIDs and medications with aspirin.

   e. Wear medical alert bracelet.

   f. Client can self-monitor for PT/INR using a coagulation monitor.

   g. Reinforce measures to prevent injury and bleeding.

   h. Administer vitamin K for warfarin toxicity.

   i. Garlic, ginger, ginkgo (may increase bleeding) and ginseng (may decrease effectiveness).

   j. Avoid alcohol.

3. Oral (dabigatran, rivaroxaban)

   a. Take medication daily and avoid skipping doses.

   b. If a dose is missed, it should not be taken within 6 hr of the next scheduled dose.

   c. Tablets should not be crushed, broken, or chewed.

   d. Avoid NSAIDs and medications with aspirin.

   e. Reinforce teaching to monitor for signs of bleeding and report to provider

   f. Reinforce teaching to monitor for signs of GI bleeding.

v Antiplatelet Medications

A. **Action:** Prevent platelets from aggregating (clumping together) by inhibiting enzymes and factors that normally promote clotting

B. **Medications**
1. Aspirin
2. Abciximab
3. Clopidogrel
4. Ticlopidine
5. Pentoxifylline
6. Dipyridamole

C. **Therapeutic Uses**
1. Prevention of acute myocardial infarction or acute coronary syndromes
2. Prevention of stroke
3. Intermittent claudication

D. **Precautions/Interactions**
1. Contraindicated in thrombocytopenia
2. Caution with peptic ulcer disease

E. **Side/Adverse Effects**
1. Prolonged bleeding
2. Gastric bleeding
3. Thrombocytopenia

F. **Nursing Interventions and Client Education**
1. Monitor for signs of prolonged bleeding.
2. Reinforce teaching to report tarry stool, ecchymosis.

vi Thrombolytic Medications

A. **Action:** Dissolve clots that have already formed by converting plasminogen to plasmin, which destroys fibrinogen and other clotting factors

B. **Medications**
1. Alteplase
2. Tenecteplase
3. Reteplase

C. **Therapeutic Uses**
1. Acute myocardial infarction
2. DVT
3. PE
4. Ischemic stroke (alteplase)

D. **Precautions/Interactions**
1. Contraindicated for intracranial hemorrhage, active internal bleeding, aortic dissection, brain tumors.
2. Use caution when using in clients who have severe hypertension.
3. Concurrent use of anticoagulants or antiplatelet medications increases risk for bleeding.

E. **Side/Adverse Effects**
1. Serious bleeding risks from recent wounds, puncture sites, weakened vessels
2. Hypotension
3. Possible anaphylactic reaction

F. **Nursing Interventions and Client Education**
1. Administration must take place within 4 to 6 hr of symptom onset.
2. Continuous monitoring is required.
3. Clients will begin anticoagulant therapy to prevent repeated thrombotic event.

SECTION 7

Medications for the Gastrointestinal System

i Antacids

A. **Action:** Neutralize gastric acid and inactivate pepsin

MEDICATIONS FOR THE GASTROINTESTINAL SYSTEM

	SIDE/ADVERSE EFFECTS
Aluminum hydroxide	Constipation
	Hypophosphatemia
Magnesium hydroxide (milk of magnesia)	Diarrhea
	Renal impairment
	Hypermagnesemia
Sodium bicarbonate	Constipation

B. **Therapeutic Uses**
1. Peptic ulcer disease
2. GERD

C. **Precautions/Interactions**
1. Prolonged use can result in hypophosphatemia.
2. Can decrease absorption of some medications.

D. **Nursing Interventions and Client Education**
1. Clients who have renal impairment should only use aluminum-based preparations.
2. Other medications should be taken 1 hr before or after antacids.
3. Older adult clients who have poor nutritional status are at high risk of hypophosphatemia.
4. Do not self-prescribe antacid use for longer than 2 weeks.

II Antisecretory/Blocking Agents

A. **Action:** Prevent or block selected receptors within the stomach

B. **Medications**

1. **Proton Pump Inhibitors (PPI)**
   a. Omeprazole
   b. Lansoprazole
   c. Rabeprazole sodium
   d. Esomeprazole

2. Histamine$_2$ Receptor Antagonists (H$_2$ Blockers)
   a. Cimetidine
   b. Nizatidine
   c. Famotidine

C. **Therapeutic Uses**

1. Gastric and duodenal ulcers
2. GERD
3. Zollinger-Ellison syndrome

D. **Precautions/Interactions**

1. Contraindicated during lactation.
2. Use with caution if client has COPD.

E. **Side Effects/Adverse Effects**

1. Can increase the risk for osteoporosis with long-term use, pneumonia in clients who have COPD, and acid rebound (PPI)
2. Decreased libido/impotence (H$_2$ blocker)
3. Lethargy, depression, confusion (H$_2$ blocker)

F. **Nursing Interventions and Client Education**

1. Reinforce teaching to seek appropriate care. (Many take OTC preparations.)
2. Review medication regimen and reinforce teaching about precautions related to time of administration as required.
3. Do not crush, chew, or break tablets.
4. Notify prescriber of any sign of GI bleeding.
5. Modify diet as prescribed.

III Mucosal Protectants

A. **Sucralfate**

1. **Action:** Adheres to injured gastric ulcers upon contact with gastric acids; protective action for up to 6 hr; no systemic effects

B. **Therapeutic Use**

1. Gastric and duodenal ulcers
2. GERD

C. **Precautions/Interactions**

1. Chronic kidney failure

D. **Nursing Interventions and Client Education**

1. Administer on an empty stomach at least 1 hr before meals.
2. Do not administer within 30 min of antacids.

IV Antiemetics

A. **Action:** Multiple classifications of medications that affect the GI tract or the "vomiting center" of the brain to reduce nausea/vomiting

B. **Therapeutic Uses**

1. Postoperative
2. Chemotherapy
3. Nausea/vomiting associated with disease process

ANTIEMETIC MEDICATIONS

Promethazine

SIDE/ADVERSE EFFECTS	Drowsiness
	Anticholinergic effects
	Severe respiratory depression in children younger than 2 years
	EPS
	Potentiates effects when given with narcotics
PRECAUTIONS/ INTERACTIONS	Cardiovascular and hepatic disease
NURSING INTERVENTIONS	Monitor vital signs
	Safety precautions
	IM—large muscle

Metoclopramide

SIDE/ADVERSE EFFECTS	Drowsiness
	Diarrhea
	Restlessness
	EPS
	Tardive dyskinesia
PRECAUTIONS/ INTERACTIONS	Seizures, cardiovascular disease, pheochromocytoma
NURSING INTERVENTIONS	Reinforce teaching about rapid GI emptying.
	Discontinue with signs of EPS.

Ondansetron

SIDE/ADVERSE EFFECTS	Headache
	EPS
NURSING INTERVENTIONS	Administer tablets 30 min prior to chemotherapy and 1 to 2 hr before radiation.
PRECAUTIONS/ INTERACTIONS	Risk for dysrhythmia
	Do not administer to clients who have prolonged QT interval.

Scopolamine

SIDE/ADVERSE EFFECTS	Blurred vision
	Sedation
	Anticholinergic effects
PRECAUTIONS/ INTERACTIONS	Increased mydriatic effect causes increased ocular pressure
	Use with caution for clients who have glaucoma.
NURSING INTERVENTIONS	Apply transdermal patches behind ear.
	Use lubricating eye drops.

v Antidiarrheals

A. **Action:** Activate opioid receptors in the GI tract to decrease intestinal motility and to increase the absorption of fluid and sodium in the intestine

B. **Medications**
   1. Diphenoxylate plus atropine
   2. Loperamide
   3. Paregoric

C. **Therapeutic Uses**
   1. Management of diarrhea

D. **Precautions/Interactions**
   1. Increased risk of megacolon for clients who have IBS
   2. Contraindicated in clients who have COPD (paregoric)

E. **Side/Adverse Effects**
   1. Constipation
   2. Drowsiness
   3. Dry mouth
   4. Blurred vision

F. **Nursing Interventions and Client Education**
   1. Monitor F&E.
   2. Avoid caffeine intake (increases GI motility).

vi Stool Softeners/Laxatives

A. **Action:** Facilitates peristalsis and bowel movements

STOOL SOFTENER/LAXATIVE MEDICATIONS

	THERAPEUTIC USES
Psyllium	Decrease diarrhea (bulk-forming)
Docusate sodium	Relieve constipation (surfactant)
Bisacodyl	Preprocedure colon evacuation (stimulant)
Magnesium hydroxide	Prevent painful elimination (low-dose osmotic)
	Promote rapid evacuation (high-dose osmotic)

B. **Precautions/Interactions**
   1. Contraindicated in clients who have fecal impaction, bowel obstruction.
   2. Most laxatives are contraindicated in clients who have ulcerative colitis and diverticulitis (psyllium may be used).

C. **Side/Adverse Effects**
   1. F&E imbalances
   2. GI irritation
   3. Can lead to toxic levels of magnesium
   4. Fluid retention (laxatives with sodium)

D. **Nursing Interventions and Client Education**
   1. Contraindicated with fecal impaction, bowel obstruction, and acute surgical abdomen.
   2. Encourage regular exercise and promote regular bowel elimination.
   3. Monitor for chronic laxative use/abuse.
   4. Provide adequate fluid and fiber intake to avoid obstruction.

Medications for the Urinary System

i Diuretics

A. **Action:** Increase the amount of fluid excretion via the renal system

DIURETIC MEDICATIONS

Loop	Thiazide	Potassium-Sparing
Furosemide	Hydrochlorothiazide	Spironolactone
Bumetanide	Chlorothiazide	Triamterene

B. **Therapeutic Use**
   1. Pulmonary edema caused by heart failure
   2. Edema unresponsive to other diuretics
   3. Hypertension unresponsive to other diuretics

C. **Precautions/Interactions**
   1. Use cautiously in clients who have diabetes mellitus.
   2. Contraindicated in pregnancy.
   3. NSAIDs reduce diuretic effect.

D. **Side/Adverse Effects**
   1. Loop and thiazide diuretics
      a. Hypovolemia
      b. Ototoxicity (loop diuretics)
      c. Hypokalemia
      d. Hyponatremia
      e. Hyperglycemia
      f. Digoxin toxicity
      g. Lithium toxicity
   2. Potassium-sparing diuretics
      a. Hyperkalemia
      b. Endocrine effects (impotence, menstrual irregularities)

E. **Nursing Interventions and Client Education**
   1. Monitor I&O.
   2. Monitor vital signs.
   3. Monitor for F&E imbalances.
   4. Administer early morning to prevent nocturia.
   5. When taking loop/thiazide diuretics, increase intake of foods high in potassium.
   6. When taking potassium-sparing diuretics, avoid foods high in potassium, such as salt substitutes.

II Osmotic Diuretics

A. **Action:** Pull fluid back into the vascular and extravascular space by increasing serum osmolality to promote osmotic changes

B. **Medication**

1. Mannitol

C. **Therapeutic Uses**

1. Prevent kidney failure related to hypovolemia

2. Decrease intracranial pressure related to cerebral edema

3. Decrease intraocular pressure

D. **Precautions/Interactions**

1. Use with caution in heart failure.

E. **Side/Adverse Effects**

1. Pulmonary edema

2. F&E imbalances

3. Thirst, dry mouth

F. **Nursing Interventions and Client Education**

1. Monitor daily weight, I&O, and electrolytes.

2. Monitor for signs of hypovolemia.

3. Monitor neurological status.

III Alpha Adrenergic Blockers for Urinary Hesitancy

A. **Tamsulosin**

1. **Action:** Inhibits smooth muscle contraction in the prostate, which improves the rate of urine flow for clients who have BPH

2. **Precautions/Interactions**

   a. Rule out bladder cancer prior to administering tamsulosin.

   b. Combined use with cimetidine can facilitate toxicity.

   c. Use cautiously with medications causing hypotension (such as sildenafil)

B. **Bethanechol**

1. **Action:** Increases detrusor muscle tone to allow strong start to voiding for clients who have postoperative urinary hesitancy

2. **Precautions/Interactions**

   a. Contraindicated for clients who have urinary tract obstruction.

   b. Contraindicated for clients who have hypotension or decreased cardiac output. Can cause bradycardia.

ALPHA ADRENERGIC BLOCKERS

Tamsulosin

SIDE/ADVERSE EFFECTS	Can cause decreased libido, headache, and dizziness
NURSING INTERVENTIONS AND CLIENT EDUCATION	Take 30 min after meal at same time each day. If dose is missed for several days, restart at the lowest dose. Can cause orthostatic hypotension

Bethanechol

SIDE/ADVERSE EFFECTS	Excessive salivation, abdominal cramps, diarrhea
NURSING INTERVENTIONS	Administer on empty stomach

IV Anticholinergic Medications for Overactive Bladder

A. **Action:** Antispasmodic actions to decrease detrusor muscle spasms and contractions

B. **Medications**

1. Oxybutynin

2. Tolterodine

3. Darifenacin

4. Solifenacin

5. Trospium

6. Fesoterodine

C. **Therapeutic Use**

1. Urinary incontinence

2. Urinary urgency and frequency

D. **Precautions/Interactions**

1. Do not use for clients who have intestinal obstruction.

2. Use with other anticholinergics can increase anticholinergic effects.

3. Risk for cognitive impairment in older clients.

E. **Side/Adverse Effects**

1. Anticholinergic symptoms

2. Drowsiness

3. Dyspepsia

F. **Nursing Interventions and Client Education**

1. Manage anticholinergic side effects.

2. Report constipation lasting longer than 3 days.

V Sexual Dysfunction

A. **Action:** Enhances the effect of nitric oxide to promote relaxation of penile muscles, allowing increased blood flow to produce an erection

B. **Medications**

1. Sildenafil
2. Tadalafil
3. Vardenafil

C. **Therapeutic Uses**

1. Erectile dysfunction
2. Less commonly used in the treatment of pulmonary arterial hypertension

D. **Precautions/Interactions**

1. Contraindicated for clients taking nitrate drugs, alpha blockers for BPH, or antihypertensives
2. Contraindicated for clients who have history of stroke, hypo/hypertension, or heart failure

E. **Side/Adverse Effects**

1. Hypotension
2. Priapism (erection lasting longer than 4 hr)
3. Vision impairment
4. Hearing loss
5. Headache
6. Flushing

F. **Nursing Interventions and Client Education**

1. Administer 1 hr before sexual activity. Do not use more than once daily.
2. Notify the provider of all medications currently taken, including herbal preparations.
3. Avoid intake of any organic nitrates.
4. Stop taking medication and notify the prescriber immediately for an erection lasting longer than 4 hr or any loss of vision.

Medications for the Immune System

I Immunizations

A. **Action:** Stimulate production of antibodies to prevent illness

CHILDHOOD IMMUNIZATIONS*

TYPE	SIDE/ADVERSE EFFECTS**	CONTRAINDICATION
DTaP, Tdap	Fever Irritability Seizures	Occurrence of seizures within 3 days of vaccine
Hib	Low-grade fever	Age younger than 6 weeks
Rotavirus	Irritability, diarrhea, vomiting, and intussusception	History of intussusception Maximum age for the final dose is 8 months, 0 days
IPV	Anaphylactic reaction to neomycin, streptomycin, or polymyxin B	
MMR	Joint pain Anaphylaxis Thrombocytopenia	Allergy to eggs, gelatin, or neomycin Immunocompromised, pregnancy
Varicella	Vesicles on skin Pruritus	Pregnancy Allergy to gelatin and neomycin Immunocompromised
Seasonal influenza	Fever	Nasal spray contraindicated for children younger than 2 years, adults older than 50 years, and clients who are immunocompromised History of Guillain-Barré
Hepatitis A, B	Anaphylaxis	Hep A: pregnancy Hep B: allergy to yeast
Meningococcal vaccine		History of Guillain-Barré
HPV (up to age 26)		Pregnancy Allergy to yeast

*Schedule is determined by the Centers for Disease Control and Prevention.
**Risk in addition to localized inflammation

ADULT IMMUNIZATIONS (18 YEARS AND OLDER)*

TYPE	SCHEDULE
Tetanus booster	Every 10 years
MMR	One or two doses at ages 19 to 49
Varicella	Two doses if no history of disease
Pneumococcal (PPSV)	Once after age 65
	Recommended for immunocompromised, COPD, living in long-term care facility
Hepatitis A	Two doses for high-risk clients
Hepatitis B	Three doses for high-risk clients
Seasonal influenza	Annually
Meningococcal vaccine	Students entering college
	Adults older than 56 years
	Repeat every 5 years for high-risk clients
Herpes zoster	Over age 60

*Schedule is determined by the Centers for Disease Control and Prevention.

B. **Nursing Interventions and Client Education**
  1. Consult CDC guidelines for schedule of administration.
  2. Reinforce teaching about the purpose of immunizations and keeping records.
  3. Avoid administration of aspirin for management of adverse effects in children.
  4. Reinforce teaching regarding side/adverse effects and management.

II Antimicrobials

A. **Action:** Inhibit growth, destroy, or otherwise control replication of microbes

MULTIGENERATION ANTIBIOTICS

Aminoglycosides

MEDICATIONS	Amikacin	Gentamicin sulfate	Streptomycin
THERAPEUTIC USE	Septicemia, meningitis, pneumonia		
PRECAUTIONS	High risk for ototoxicity, nephrotoxicity		
	Monitor creatinine and BUN.		
	Monitor trough levels.		

Cephalosporins

MEDICATIONS	Cephalexin	Cefaclor	Cefotaxime
THERAPEUTIC USE	Upper respiratory, skin, urinary infections		
	Used as prophylaxis for clients at risk		
PRECAUTIONS	Cross-sensitivity with penicillins		
	Monitor for signs of Clostridium difficile.		

Fluoroquinolones

MEDICATIONS	Ciprofloxacin	Levofloxacin
THERAPEUTIC USE	Bronchitis, chlamydia, gonorrhea, PID, UTI, pneumonia, prostatitis, sinusitis	
PRECAUTIONS	Caution with hepatic, renal, or seizure disorders	

MULTIGENERATION ANTIBIOTICS (CONTINUED)

Macrolides

MEDICATIONS	Azithromycin
	Clarithromycin
	Erythromycin
THERAPEUTIC USE	Upper respiratory infections, sinusitis, Legionnaires' disease, whooping cough, acute diphtheria, chlamydia
PRECAUTIONS	Used for clients who have penicillin allergy
	Administer with meals.

Nitrofurantoin

THERAPEUTIC USE	UTI
PRECAUTIONS	Broad-spectrum
	Contraindicated in renal dysfunction
	Urine will have brown discoloration.

Penicillins

MEDICATIONS	Amoxicillin
	Ampicillin
THERAPEUTIC USE	Pneumonia, upper respiratory infections, septicemia, endocarditis, rheumatic fever, GYN infections
PRECAUTIONS	Hypersensitivity with possible anaphylaxis

Sulfonamides

MEDICATIONS	Trimethoprim/sulfamethoxazole
THERAPEUTIC USE	UTI, bronchitis, otitis media
PRECAUTIONS	Consume at least 3 L/day of fluid.
	Use backup contraceptives.
	Avoid sun exposure.

Tetracyclines

MEDICATIONS	Doxycycline calcium
	Tetracycline HCl
THERAPEUTIC USE	Fungal, bacterial, protozoal, rickettsial infections
PRECAUTIONS	Consume at least 3 L/day of fluid.
	Use backup contraceptives.
	Avoid sun exposure.
	Permanent tooth discoloration if given to children younger than 8 years

Glycopeptide

MEDICATION	Vancomycin
THERAPEUTIC USE	MRSA, bacterial, C. difficile infections
PRECAUTIONS	Contraindication: Allergy to corn
	Caution: Ototoxicity, nephrotoxicity
	Administer over 1 hr IV to prevent red man syndrome.
	Monitor trough levels.

SPECIAL CLASSES OF ANTIMICROBIALS

Antifungal

MEDICATIONS	Fluconazole
THERAPEUTIC USE	Candidiasis infections
PRECAUTIONS	Monitor hepatic and renal function. Refrigerate suspensions. Increased risk of bleeding for clients taking anticoagulants

Antimalarials

MEDICATIONS	Hydroxychloroquine Quinine sulfate
THERAPEUTIC USE	Prevent malarial attacks, rheumatoid arthritis Systemic lupus
PRECAUTIONS	Increased risk of psoriasis Monitor for drug-induced retinopathy.

Antiprotozoal

MEDICATIONS	Metronidazole
THERAPEUTIC USE	Trichomoniasis and giardiasis, *Clostridium difficile*, amoebic dysentery, PID, vaginosis
PRECAUTIONS	Take with food. Do not consume alcohol during therapy or 48 hr after completion of regimen.

Antituberculars

MEDICATIONS	Isoniazid (INH) Rifampin
THERAPEUTIC USE	Prevention and treatment of TB Latent TB INH: 6 to 9 months Active TB: multiple therapy up to 24 months
PRECAUTIONS	Risk of neuropathies and hepatotoxicity Consume foods high in vitamin B_6. Avoid foods with tyramine (INH). Increased risk of phenytoin toxicity (INH). Avoid alcohol. Discoloration of urine, saliva, sweat, and tears (rifampin)

Antiretrovirals

MEDICATIONS	Acyclovir Valacyclovir HCl Zidovudine
THERAPEUTIC USE	Genital herpes, shingles, HIV
PRECAUTIONS	Acyclovir and valacyclovir: Administer with food. Increase fluid intake. Begin therapy with first onset of symptoms.

B. **Nursing Interventions and Client Education**

1. Identify history of medication allergies and treatment.
2. Monitor for signs of medication reaction.
3. Monitor for signs of secondary infections.
4. Administer medications at appropriate time intervals to maintain therapeutic effects.
5. If C&S is prescribed, perform test before initiating therapy.
6. Complete the entire medication regimen.

SECTION 10

Medications for the Musculoskeletal System

Bisphosphonates

A. **Action:** Decrease the number and action of osteoclasts, resulting in bone resorption

B. **Medications**

1. Alendronate: daily or weekly
2. Risedronate: daily, weekly, monthly
3. Ibandronate: monthly or every 3 months
4. Zoledronate: IV annually

C. **Therapeutic Use**

1. Prevention and treatment of osteoporosis
2. Paget's disease
3. Hypercalcemia related to malignancy

D. **Precautions/Interactions**

1. Contraindicated during lactation.
2. Clients who have esophageal stricture or difficulty swallowing may only use zoledronate.
3. Absorption is decreased when taken with calcium supplements, antacids, orange juice, and caffeine.

E. **Side/Adverse Effects**

1. Musculoskeletal pain
2. Esophagitis and GI discomfort
3. Jaw pain (zoledronate)
4. Atrial fibrillation (zoledronate)

F. **Nursing Interventions and Client Education**

1. Administer medication in the morning on an empty stomach.
2. Consume at least 8 oz water (not carbonated).
3. Remain upright (sitting or standing) for 30 min after taking medication.
4. Consume adequate amounts of vitamin D.

II Antirheumatics

A. **Action:** Provide symptomatic relief and delay in disease progression by inhibiting or modulating inflammatory processes.

ANTIRHEUMATIC DRUG CATEGORIES

Disease-modifying antirheumatic drugs (DMARDs)

MEDICATIONS	Methotrexate
	Hydroxychloroquine
	Etanercept
	Infliximab
	Adalimumab
ACTION	Interrupt complex immune responses, preventing disease progression

Glucocorticoids

MEDICATIONS	Prednisone
	Prednisolone
ACTION	Decrease inflammation by suppressing leukocytes and fibroblasts, and reversing capillary permeability

NSAIDs

MEDICATIONS	Ibuprofen
	Indomethacin
	Naproxen
	Celecoxib
ACTION	Inhibit prostaglandin synthesis, resulting in decreased inflammatory responses

III DMARDs

A. **Therapeutic Use**
1. Slow joint degeneration and progression of rheumatoid arthritis

B. **Precautions/Interactions**
1. Methotrexate: Contraindicated in pregnancy, kidney or liver failure, psoriasis, alcohol use disorder, or hematologic dyscrasias.

C. **Side/Adverse Effects**
1. Methotrexate: Increased risk of infection, bone marrow suppression, and GI ulceration
2. Hydroxychloroquine: Retinal damage (blindness)

D. **Nursing Interventions and Client Education**
1. Reinforce teaching about measures to prevent infection.
2. Monitor liver function tests.
3. Use reliable contraception.
4. Initial effects can take 3 to 6 weeks, and full therapeutic effects can take several months.
5. Administer with food.
6. Reinforce teaching about the critical importance of retinal examination every 6 months for clients taking hydroxychloroquine.

IV Glucocorticoids

A. **Therapeutic Use**
1. Provide symptomatic relief of inflammation and pain.

B. **Precautions/Interactions**
1. Contraindicated in systemic fungal infection.
2. Do not administer live virus vaccines during therapy.
3. Should only be used for a short duration.

C. **Side/Adverse Effects**
1. Risk of infection
2. Osteoporosis
3. Adrenal suppression
4. Fluid retention
5. GI discomfort
6. Hyperglycemia
7. Hypokalemia

D. **Nursing Interventions and Client Education**
1. Do not skip doses.
2. Monitor blood pressure.
3. Monitor F&E balance and weight.
4. Monitor for signs of bleeding, GI discomfort.
5. Reinforce teaching to take calcium supplements and maintain vitamin D levels.
6. Give with food.
7. Never stop abruptly.
8. Provide immunoprotection.

V NSAIDs

A. **Therapeutic Use**
1. Provide rapid, symptomatic relief of inflammation and pain

B. **Precautions/Interactions**
1. Hypersensitivity to aspirin or other NSAIDs
2. Can increase the risk of MI and stroke (nonaspirin NSAIDS)

C. **Side/Adverse Effects**
1. GI discomfort
2. GI ulceration
3. Renal impairment
4. Photosensitivity

D. **Nursing Interventions and Client Education**
1. Administer with food and an 8 oz glass of water.
2. Avoid lying down for 30 min after administration.
3. Use only as needed for symptoms to reduce risk of GI ulceration.
4. Use sunscreen.

VI Antigout

ANTIGOUT MEDICATIONS

Allopurinol

ACTION	Inhibits uric acid production
THERAPEUTIC USE	Chronic gouty arthritis

Colchicine

ACTION	Inhibits processes to prevent leukocytes from invading joints
THERAPEUTIC USE	Acute gouty arthritis

A. **Precautions/Interactions**
1. Use caution in clients who have renal, cardiac, or gastrointestinal dysfunction.
2. Should not be combined with theophylline.

B. **Side/Adverse Effects**
1. GI distress
2. Rash and fever (discontinue immediately)
3. Decreases the metabolism of warfarin

C. **Nursing Interventions and Client Education**
1. Avoid foods high in purines to reduce uric acid.
2. Monitor CBC and uric acid levels.
3. Avoid aspirin.
4. Administer with meals.

SECTION 11

Medications for the Nervous System

I Antianxiety Medications

A. **Action:** Increase the efficacy of GABA to reduce anxiety

B. **Medications**
1. Benzodiazepines
   a. Alprazolam
   b. Chlordiazepoxide
   c. Diazepam
   d. Lorazepam
2. Buspirone
3. Antidepressants
   a. Venlafaxine
   b. Duloxetine
   c. Paroxetine
   d. Escitalopram

C. **Therapeutic Use**
1. Generalized anxiety disorder and panic disorder
2. Insomnia
3. Alcohol withdrawal
4. Induction of anesthesia

D. **Precautions/Interactions**
1. Benzodiazepines are used with caution in clients who have substance use disorder and liver disease.
2. Venlafaxine, an SNRI, is contraindicated for clients taking MAOIs.

E. **Side/Adverse Effects**
1. CNS depression
2. Paradoxical response (insomnia, excitation, euphoria)
3. Withdrawal symptoms (not with buspirone)
4. Risk of abuse and potential for overdose (benzodiazepines)

F. **Nursing Interventions and Client Education**
1. Monitor vital signs.
2. Never abruptly discontinue medication.
3. Monitor for side/adverse effects.
4. Avoid alcohol.

II Antidepressants

A. **Action**
1. SSRIs inhibit serotonin reuptake.
2. SNRIs block reuptake of norepinephrine, as well as serotonin, with effects similar to the SSRIs.
3. Tricyclic blocks reuptake of norepinephrine and serotonin.
4. MAOI increases norepinephrine, dopamine, and serotonin by blocking MAO–A.

ANTIDEPRESSANT CLASSES

SSRIs and SNRIs

	SSRIs	SNRIs
MEDICATIONS	> Citalopram > Fluoxetine > Paroxetine > Sertraline	> Duloxetine > Venlafaxine
PRECAUTIONS/ INTERACTIONS	Avoid alcohol. Do not discontinue abruptly. Monitor for serotonin syndrome (agitation, confusion, hallucinations) within first 72 hr.	
SIDE/ADVERSE EFFECTS	Weight gain Sexual dysfunction Fatigue Drowsiness	

Tricyclic

MEDICATIONS	Amitriptyline Imipramine
PRECAUTIONS/ INTERACTIONS	Do not administer with MAOIs or St. John's wort. Must avoid alcohol. Contraindicated for clients who have seizure disorders
SIDE/ADVERSE EFFECTS	Anticholinergic effects Orthostatic hypotension Cardiac dysrhythmias Decreased seizure threshold

ANTIDEPRESSANT CLASSES (CONTINUED)

MAOI

MEDICATIONS	Isocarboxazid
	Tranylcypromine
	Phenelzine
PRECAUTIONS/ INTERACTIONS	Avoid foods containing tyramine.
	Antihypertensives have additive hypotensive effect.
	Contraindicated with SSRIs, tricyclics, heart failure, CVA, and renal insufficiency
SIDE/ADVERSE EFFECTS	CNS stimulation
	Orthostatic hypotension
	Hypertensive crisis with intake of tyramine, SSRIs, and tricyclics

B. **Nursing Interventions and Client Education**

1. Monitor clients for suicide risk.
2. Take on daily basis and never miss a dose.
3. Reinforce teaching about therapeutic effects and time of onset.
4. Avoid discontinuing drug abruptly.
5. Take SSRIs in the morning to minimize sleep disturbances.
6. Provide clients taking MAOIs a list of foods containing tyramine.
7. Avoid taking other medications without consulting the provider.

III Bipolar Disorder Medications

A. **Action:** Produce neurochemical changes in the brain to control acute mania, depression, and incidence of suicide
B. **Medication**
   1. Lithium carbonate
C. **Therapeutic Uses**
   1. Bipolar disorder
   2. Alcohol use disorder
   3. Bulimia
   4. Schizophrenia
D. **Precautions/Interactions**
   1. Use cautiously in clients who have renal dysfunction, heart disease, hyponatremia, and dehydration.
      a. NSAIDs will increase lithium levels.
      b. Monitor serum sodium levels.
E. **Side/Adverse Effects**
   1. GI distress
   2. Fine hand tremors
   3. Polyuria
   4. Hypothyroidism
   5. Renal toxicity

F. **Nursing Interventions and Client Education**

1. Monitor therapeutic levels.
2. Monitor serum sodium levels.
3. Therapeutic effects begin in 7 to 14 days.
4. Doses must be administered 1 to 3 times daily per provider prescription.
5. Provide nutritional counseling to include food sources for sodium.
6. Administer with food to decrease GI distress.

IV Antipsychotic Medications

A. **Action:** Block dopamine, acetylcholine, histamine, and norepinephrine receptors in the brain and periphery
B. **Medications**
   1. Typical
      a. Chlorpromazine
      b. Fluphenazine
      c. Haloperidol
      d. Thiothixene
   2. Atypical (less severe side/adverse effects)
      a. Aripiprazole
      b. Clozapine
      c. Olanzapine
      d. Paliperidone
      e. Quetiapine
      f. Ziprasidone
C. **Therapeutic Use**
   1. Acute and chronic psychosis
   2. Schizophrenia
   3. Manic phase of bipolar disorders
   4. Tourette syndrome
   5. Delusional and schizoaffective disorders
   6. Dementia
D. **Precautions/Interactions**
   1. Contraindicated for clients who have severe depression, Parkinson's disease, prolactin-dependent cancer, and severe hypotension.
   2. Use with caution in clients who have glaucoma, paralytic ileus, prostate enlargement, or seizure disorder.
E. **Side/Adverse Effects**
   1. Typical
      a. Sedation
      b. Extrapyramidal effects
      c. Anticholinergic effects
      d. Tardive dyskinesia
      e. Agranulocytosis
      f. Neuroleptic malignant syndrome
      g. Seizures

2. Atypical
   a. Agranulocytosis
   b. Weight gain
   c. Diabetes
   d. Dyslipidemia
   e. Orthostatic hypotension
   f. Extrapyramidal effects

F. **Nursing Interventions and Client Education**
   1. Monitor for side effects within 5 hr to 5 days of administration.
   2. Advise clients of potential side effects.
   3. Monitor CBC.
   4. Encourage fluids.
   5. Stop medication for signs of neuroleptic malignant syndrome.

V Attention Deficit Hyperactivity Disorder Medications

A. **Action:** Increase attention span; reduce impulsive behavior and hyperactivity
   1. Stimulants increase levels of norepinephrine, serotonin, and dopamine into the CNS.
   2. Nonstimulants increase levels of norepinephrine into the CNS.

ADHD CLASSES

Stimulants

MEDICATION	Dextroamphetamine and amphetamine Methylphenidate
SIDE EFFECTS	Insomnia Headache Suppressed appetite Abdominal pain
NURSING INTERVENTIONS AND CLIENT EDUCATION	Administer in early morning. Give with or after meals. Do not abruptly discontinue. Monitor for signs of abuse. Monitor for signs of agitation.

Nonstimulants

MEDICATION	Atomoxetine Guanfacine can be used in treatment of Asperger syndrome
SIDE EFFECTS	GI upset Insomnia Mood swings
NURSING INTERVENTIONS AND CLIENT EDUCATION	Take medication daily. Do not crush or chew. Immediately report worsening of anxiety or agitation. Do not take with MAOIs.

VI Sedative/Hypnotic Medications

A. **Action:** Slow neuronal activity in the brain to induce sedation/sleep

B. **Medications**
   1. Benzodiazepines
      a. Lorazepam
      b. Temazepam
   2. Benzodiazepine-like medications
      a. Zolpidem
      b. Eszopiclone

C. **Therapeutic Use**
   1. Short-term insomnia
   2. Difficulty falling or staying asleep

D. **Precautions/Interactions**
   1. Use cautiously in clients who have severe mental depression.
   2. Avoid combined use with alcohol and medications that depress CNS function.

E. **Side/Adverse Effects**
   1. Amnesia
   2. Respiratory depression
   3. Daytime drowsiness and dizziness

F. **Nursing Interventions and Client Education**
   1. Take immediately before bedtime because medication has abrupt onset of sleep.
   2. Avoid alcohol.
   3. Warn client and caregivers of potential for sleep activities without recall; notify prescriber immediately.

VII Abstinence Maintenance Medications

A. **Disulfiram**
   1. **Action:** Interferes with hepatic oxidation of alcohol, resulting in elevation of blood acetaldehyde levels
   2. **Therapeutic Use**
      a. Adjunct to maintain sobriety in treatment of alcohol use disorder
   3. **Precautions/Interactions**
      a. INH increases the risk of adverse CNS effects for clients taking disulfiram.
      b. Ingestion of large amounts of alcohol can cause respiratory depression, dysrhythmias, and cardiac arrest.
      c. Adjust medication doses of warfarin and phenytoin.
   4. **Side/Adverse Effects**
      a. Drowsiness
      b. Headache
      c. Metallic taste
      d. Hepatotoxicity

5. **Nursing Interventions and Client Education**
   a. Wait 12 hr between time of last alcohol intake and starting medication.
   b. Consumption of alcohol while taking disulfiram will result in flushing, throbbing in head and neck, respiratory difficulty, nausea, copious vomiting, sweating, thirst, chest pain, palpitation, dyspnea, hyperventilation, tachycardia, hypotension, syncope, marked uneasiness, weakness, vertigo, blurred vision, and confusion.
   c. Undesirable effects last 30 min to several hours when alcohol is consumed.
   d. Effects of disulfiram can stay in the body for weeks after therapy is discontinued.
   e. Therapy can last months to years.

B. **Methadone**
1. **Action:** Binds with opiate receptors in CNS to produce analgesic and euphoric effects
2. **Therapeutic Use**
   a. Prevents withdrawal symptoms in clients who were addicted to opiate drugs
3. **Precautions/Interactions**
   a. Do not use in clients who have severe asthma, chronic respiratory disease, or history of head injury.
   b. Avoid in clients who have QT syndrome.
4. **Side/Adverse Effects**
   a. Sedation
   b. Respiratory depression
   c. Paradoxical CNS excitation
5. **Nursing Interventions and Client Education**
   a. Monitor clients for signs of drug tolerance and psychological dependence.
   b. Monitor for respiratory depression.
   c. Methadone must be slowly reduced to produce detoxification.
   d. Client must be monitored through treatment center.

VIII Chronic Neurological Disorders

A. **Cholinesterase Inhibitors**
1. **Action:** Prevent cholinesterase from inactivating acetylcholine, resulting in improved transmission of nerve impulses
2. **Medications**
   a. Neostigmine
   b. Ambenonium
   c. Edrophonium
3. **Therapeutic Use**
   a. Myasthenia gravis
4. **Precautions/Interactions**
   a. Do not administer if heart rate is less than 60/min.

5. **Side/Adverse Effects**
   a. Slow heart rate
   b. Chest pain, weak pulse, increased sweating, and dizziness
   c. Client feeling like he or she might pass out
   d. Weak or shallow breathing
   e. Urinating more than usual
   f. Seizures
   g. Trouble swallowing
6. **Nursing Interventions and Client Education**
   a. Dose must be individualized.
   b. Keep an individual diary to record side effects.
   c. Wear a medical alert bracelet.
   d. Monitor for cholinergic crisis.

B. **Anti-Parkinson's**
1. **Action:** Increase dopamine to minimize tremors and rigidity
2. **Medications**
   a. Benztropine
   b. Carbidopa/levodopa
   c. Levodopa
3. **Therapeutic Use**
   a. Parkinson's disease
4. **Precautions/Interactions**
   a. Do not use levodopa within 2 weeks of MAOI use.
   b. Pyridoxine (vitamin B_6) decreases effects of levodopa.
   c. Benztropine is contraindicated in clients who have narrow-angle glaucoma.
   d. Discontinue 6 to 8 hr before anesthesia.
5. **Side/Adverse Effects**
   a. Muscle twitching (especially eyelid spasms)
   b. Headache
   c. Dizziness
   d. Dark urine
   e. Orthostatic hypotension
6. **Nursing Interventions and Client Education**
   a. Advise family members to assist with medication regimen.
   b. Notify prescriber if sudden loss of the medication effects occurs.
   c. Maximum therapeutic effects can take 4 to 6 weeks.
   d. Monitor closely for signs of adverse reactions.
   e. Avoid high-protein meals and snacks.
   f. Keep medication away from heat, light, and moisture. If pills become darkened, they have lost potency and must be discarded.

c. **Antiseizure**

1. **Action:** Slows rates of neuronal activity in the brain by blocking specific channels responsible for neuron firing, which results in an elevation of the seizure threshold

2. **Medications**
   a. Carbamazepine
   b. Gabapentin
   c. Phenobarbital
   d. Phenytoin
   e. Valproic acid

3. **Therapeutic Use**
   a. Prevent or control seizure activity

ANTISEIZURE MEDICATIONS

Carbamazepine

PRECAUTIONS/ INTERACTIONS	Contraindicated in clients who have bone marrow suppression or bleeding disorders
	Decreases the effectiveness of oral contraceptives and warfarin
SIDE/ADVERSE EFFECTS	Anemia, leukopenia, Stevens-Johnson syndrome

Gabapentin

PRECAUTIONS/ INTERACTIONS	Do not abruptly discontinue.
SIDE/ADVERSE EFFECTS	Headaches, weight gain, nausea
	Report CNS depression, seizures, visual changes, and unusual bruising.

Phenobarbital

PRECAUTIONS/ INTERACTIONS	Contraindicated in history of substance use disorder
SIDE/ADVERSE EFFECTS	Drowsiness, hypotension, respiratory depression

Phenytoin

PRECAUTIONS/ INTERACTIONS	Causes increased excretion of digoxin, warfarin, oral contraceptives
SIDE/ADVERSE EFFECTS	Gingival hypertrophy, diplopia, drowsiness, hirsutism

Valproic acid

PRECAUTIONS/ INTERACTIONS	Contraindicated in liver disease, pregnancy
SIDE/ADVERSE EFFECTS	Hepatotoxicity, teratogenic effects, pancreatitis

4. **Nursing Interventions and Client Education**
   a. Monitor for therapeutic effects.
   b. Monitor clients taking phenytoin for toxic effects, including serum levels for toxicity.
   c. Reinforce teaching regarding the importance of adherence. Medication is a treatment, not a cure.
   d. Individualize treatment regimen.
   e. Reinforce teaching regarding side/adverse effects.
   f. For status epilepticus: diazepam or lorazepam IV push followed by IV phenytoin or fosphenytoin.

D. **Ophthalmologic Medications (Antiglaucoma)**

1. **Action:** Reduction of aqueous humor

2. **Medications**
   a. Levobunolol
   b. Timolol
   c. Pilocarpine
   d. Latanoprost

3. **Precautions/Interactions**
   a. Caution in clients taking oral beta blocker or calcium channel blocker

4. **Side/Adverse Effects**
   a. Systemic effect of beta blockers: bradycardia, heart failure, bronchospasm
   b. Brown discoloration of the iris (latanoprost)
   c. Retinal detachment (pilocarpine)

5. **Nursing Interventions and Client Education**
   a. Use sterile technique when handling applicator portion of the container.
   b. Hold gentle pressure on the nasolacrimal duct for 30 to 60 seconds immediately after instilling drops.
   c. Monitor pulse rate/rhythm for clients taking oral beta or calcium-channel blocker.

SECTION 12

Medications for Pain and Inflammation

I NSAIDs

See Section 10: Medications for the Musculoskeletal System.

II Acetaminophen

A. **Action:** Slows production of prostaglandins in the CNS

B. **Therapeutic Use**
   1. Analgesic
   2. Antipyretic

C. **Precautions/Interactions**
   1. Use caution in clients who consume three or more alcoholic beverages per day.
   2. Concurrent use of rifampin, INH, carbamazepine, and barbiturates can increase hepatotoxic effects.
   3. Slows the metabolism of warfarin.

D. **Side/Adverse Effects**
   1. Nausea and vomiting
   2. Long-term therapy: hemolytic anemia, leukopenia, neutropenia, and thrombocytopenia

E. **Nursing Interventions and Client Education**
1. Monitor liver function.
2. Monitor kidney function.
3. Be aware of OTC sources of acetaminophen.
4. Take as prescribed, and do not exceed 3,000 mg/24 hr.
5. Reinforce teaching about the risk of hepatotoxicity.
6. Administration to children should be based on age, not to exceed five doses per day (read labels carefully).
7. Treat acetaminophen overdose with acetylcysteine.

III Opioid Analgesics

A. **Action:** Bind with opiate receptors in the CNS to alter the perception of and emotional response to pain

B. **Medications**
1. Fentanyl
2. Hydromorphone
3. Morphine sulfate
4. Meperidine
5. Codeine, oxycodone

C. **Therapeutic Use**
1. Relief of moderate to severe pain
2. Sedation

D. **Precautions/Interactions**
1. Meperidine is preferred for clients who have biliary associated pain.
2. Monitor for potentiation of effects when given with barbiturates, benzodiazepines, phenothiazines, hypnotics, and sedatives.

E. **Side/Adverse Effects**
1. Orthostatic hypotension
2. Constipation
3. Urinary retention
4. Blurred vision
5. Respiratory depression
6. Abstinence syndrome

F. **Nursing Interventions and Client Education**
1. Monitor vital signs.
2. Monitor for respiratory depression.
3. Reinforce teaching regarding administration with PCA pump.
4. Administer naloxone for clients who have respiratory depression.
5. Prevent constipation.
6. Monitor for urinary retention.

Medications for the Reproductive System

I Contraception

A. **Consider the following when providing client education and support regarding contraception.** Factors that influence choice of a contraceptive include the following.
1. Age and health status, including risk for STI
2. Religion and culture
3. Plans for future conception
4. Frequency of intercourse
5. Number of sexual partners
6. Personal concerns about availability, spontaneity, ease of use

CONTRACEPTION METHODS

Rhythm method

CONSIDERATIONS FOR USE	Develop "fertile awareness" by noting > Cervical mucus changes > Menstrual cycle pattern > Basal temperature
CLIENT EDUCATION	Do not have sexual intercourse during "fertile periods." Low reliability for preventing pregnancy

Oral contraceptives

CONSIDERATIONS FOR USE	Pill is taken daily. Adverse effects: breast tenderness, bleeding, nausea/vomiting
CLIENT EDUCATION	Antibiotic therapy, phenytoin, and rifampin reduce effectiveness. Avoid smoking.

Ethinyl estradiol and norelgestromin (contraceptive patch)

CONSIDERATIONS FOR USE	Replace patch each week for 3 weeks.
CLIENT EDUCATION	Apply patch to buttocks, abdomen, upper torso, or upper/outer arm. Period will begin on week 4 (no patch).

Medroxyprogesterone

CONSIDERATIONS FOR USE	Injection is administered every 3 months during menstrual cycle.
CLIENT EDUCATION	Use backup form of birth control for 7 days after first injection. Fertility returns approximately 1 year after stopping.

Emergency contraception

CONSIDERATIONS FOR USE	A larger-than-normal dose of oral contraceptive Taken no later than 72 hr after unprotected sex Second dose is repeated 12 hr later. Antiemetics can be needed.
CLIENT EDUCATION	Discuss options with provider. Should not be used as the primary method of birth control

CONTRACEPTION METHODS (CONTINUED)

Etonogestrel, ethinyl estradiol vaginal ring

CONSIDERATIONS FOR USE	Placed deep into the vagina once every 3 weeks
CLIENT EDUCATION	One size fits most clients.
	If it falls out, rinse in warm water and replace within 3 hr.
	Remove ring during week 4. Menses should begin.

Intrauterine device (IUD)

CONSIDERATIONS FOR USE	Contraindicated for clients who have diabetes or history of PID
	Risk of infection
	Can have cramping and heavier periods
CLIENT EDUCATION	Hormonal IUD effective for up to 5 years
	Copper IUD effective for up to 10 years
	Monitor for signs of infection.
	Verify string is present.

Cervical diaphragm

CONSIDERATIONS FOR USE	Use with spermicide.
	Fit by prescriber
	Refitted after childbirth or weight gain/loss
CLIENT EDUCATION	Insert 6 hr prior to and leave in for 6 hr after intercourse.
	Can be inserted up to 6 hr prior to intercourse; must be left in 6 hr after intercourse
	Refit size with weight change of 10 lb or greater and following childbirth.

Condom

CONSIDERATIONS FOR USE	Use with spermicide.
CLIENT EDUCATION	Protects against STIs
	Apply and remove correctly.
	Use only water-soluble lubricants.

Spermicides

CONSIDERATIONS FOR USE	Available as: > Cream > Foam > Gel > Suppository > Film
CLIENT EDUCATION	Use with barrier method.
	Can insert up to 1 hr before intercourse

B. Nursing Interventions and Client Education

1. Discuss conception and contraceptive plans with clients to include reliability, benefits, and risks.
2. Maintain regular health screening visits.
3. Reinforce teaching about measures to prevent PID, STIs.
4. Contraceptive decisions can change over the life span.
5. Unreliable forms of birth control include coitus interruptus (withdrawal), douching, and breastfeeding.

II Oxytocic

A. Cervical "Ripening"

1. **Action:** Prostaglandins cause cervical softening in preparation for cervical dilation and effacement.
2. **Medication**
   a. Dinoprostone cervical gel
   b. Misoprostol (unlabeled use)
3. **Precautions/Interactions**
   a. Contraindicated in clients who have acute PID, history of pelvic surgery, abnormal fetal position
4. **Side/Adverse Effects**
   a. Nausea
   b. Headache
   c. Tremor, tension
   d. Feeling of warmth in the vaginal area
   e. Elevated temperature
5. **Nursing Interventions and Client Education**
   a. Maintain client on bed rest for at least 2 hr (30 min for gel) after insertion.
   b. Monitor and record maternal vital signs and fetal heart rate.
   c. Monitor for uterine contractions.
   d. Oxytocin augmentation can be initiated as needed.
   e. Major adverse effect is tachysystole.

B. Oxytocin

1. **Action:** Stimulates uterine contractions for the purpose of induction or augmentation of labor and prevents postpartum hemorrhage.
2. **Therapeutic Use**
   a. Antepartum for contraction stress test (CST)
   b. Intrapartum for induction or augmentation of labor
   c. Postpartum to promote uterine tone
3. **Precautions/Interactions**
   a. Contraindicated with placental abnormalities, fetal malpresentation, previous uterine surgery, and fetal distress
   b. Bishop Score of 6 and greater when planning induction
4. **Side/Adverse Effects**
   a. Intense uterine contractions
   b. Uterine hyperstimulation
   c. Uterine rupture
   d. Water intoxication
5. **Nursing Interventions and Client Education**
   a. Administer as secondary infusion via infusion pump for induction or augmentation.
   b. Continuously monitor uterine contractions and fetal heart rate.
   c. Discontinue oxytocin with any signs of uterine hyperstimulation or signs of maternal or fetal distress.
   d. Administer oxygen via face mask 10 L for signs of hyperstimulation.
   e. When used in postpartum, monitor for uterine bleeding.

III Methylergonovine

A. **Action:** Acts directly on the uterine muscle to stimulate forceful contractions

B. **Therapeutic Use**

1. Postpartum hemorrhage

C. **Precautions/Interactions**

1. Use with extreme caution in clients who have hypertension, preeclampsia, heart disease, venoatrial shunts, mitral valve stenosis, sepsis, cardiovascular, hepatic or renal impairment.

D. **Side/Adverse Effects**

1. Potent vasoconstriction

2. Hypertension

3. Headache

E. **Nursing Interventions and Client Education**

1. Continuously monitor blood pressure.

2. Monitor uterine bleeding and uterine tone.

IV Tocolytics

A. **Action:** Act on uterine muscle to cease contractions

B. **Therapeutic Use**

1. Stop preterm labor

TOCOLYTIC MEDICATIONS

Terbutaline sulfate

SIDE/ADVERSE EFFECTS	Nervousness	Hyperglycemia
	Tremulousness	Severe palpitations
	Headache	Chest pain
	Nausea and vomiting	Pulmonary edema
NURSING INTERVENTIONS	Monitor contractions and FHR.	
	Monitor vital signs.	
	Do not administer if pulse rate is greater than 130/min or client has chest pain.	
	Administer beta-blocking agent as antidote.	

Nifedipine

SIDE/ADVERSE EFFECTS	Hypotension	Nausea
	Headache	Flushing
NURSING INTERVENTIONS	Monitor blood pressure.	
	Avoid concurrent use with magnesium sulfate.	
	Monitor contractions and FHR.	
	Prevent complication with hypotension.	

Magnesium sulfate

SIDE/ADVERSE EFFECTS	Warmth	Diminished DTRs
	Flushing	Decreased urine output
	Respiratory depression	Pulmonary edema
NURSING INTERVENTIONS	Monitor vital signs and DTRs.	
	Monitor magnesium levels (therapeutic range: 4 to 8 mg/dL).	
	Administer via infusion pump in diluted form.	
	Use indwelling catheter to monitor urinary elimination.	
	Administer calcium gluconate 10% for signs of toxicity.	

V Antenatal Steroids—Betamethasone

A. **Action:** Stimulate production of surfactant in fetus between 24 and 34 weeks gestation.

B. **Therapeutic Use**

1. Promote fetal lung maturity in preterm labor when delivery is likely.

C. **Side/Adverse Effects**

1. Fluid retention

2. Elevated blood pressure

3. Maternal hyperglycemia and transient increase in WBC

D. **Nursing Interventions and Client Education**

1. Administer two doses (usually IM) 24 hr apart (repeat doses not recommended).

2. Provide emotional support to the family.

VI Medications for the Postpartum Client

A. **Rho(D) Immune Globulin**

1. **Action:** Suppresses the stimulation of active immunity by Rh-positive foreign red blood cells that enter the maternal circulation at the time of delivery

2. **Therapeutic Use**

   a. Rh factor incompatibility to prevent sensitization for subsequent pregnancies

3. **Precautions**

   a. Confirm that the client is Rh-negative.

   b. Never administer the IGIM full-dose or microdose products intravenously.

   c. Never administer to a neonate.

4. **Nursing Interventions and Client Education**

   a. Rho(D) immune globulin is administered within 72 hr after birth, if indicated (client is Rh-negative, neonate is Rh-positive, and Coombs' test is negative).

   b. Rho(D) immune globulin is also administered as an injection prophylactically at 28 weeks gestation and after any event where fetal cells can mix with maternal blood.

      1) Miscarriage

      2) Ectopic pregnancy

      3) Induced abortion

      4) Amniocentesis

      5) Chorionic villus sampling (CVS)

      6) Abdominal trauma

B. **Varicella Vaccine**

1. Clients who are not immune to varicella should be immunized in the postpartum period.

2. Use reliable form of contraception and avoid pregnancy for 3 months.

Complementary and Alternative Therapies

I Safety and Efficacy

A. **The Dietary Supplement Health and Education Act limits the U.S. Food and Drug Administration's (FDA) control over dietary supplements.**

1. Many herbal drug companies make claims based on their own studies, indicating health benefits from using herbal drugs.

   a. These studies are not approved by the FDA.

   b. Labels on the herbal medications must include a disclaimer stating that the FDA has not approved the product for safety and effectiveness.

2. Herbal medications can interact with other medicines and produce serious adverse effects.

II Saw palmetto (*Serenoa repens*)

A. **Purported Use**

1. Treat and prevent BPH

B. **Side/Adverse Effects**

1. Headache

2. Altered platelet function

C. **Herb/Medication Interactions**

1. Additive effect with anticoagulants

D. **Studies**

1. Several well-conducted studies support the use of saw palmetto for reducing symptoms of BPH.

E. **Nursing Considerations**

1. Allow 4 to 6 weeks to see effects.

2. Discontinue use prior to surgery.

III Valerian root

A. **Purported Uses**

1. Insomnia

2. Migraines

3. Menstrual cramps

B. **Side/Adverse Effects**

1. Drowsiness

2. Headache, nervousness with prolonged use

C. **Herb/Medication Interactions**

1. Additive effect with barbiturates and benzodiazepines

D. **Studies**

1. Several studies support the use of valerian for mild to moderate sleep disorders and mild anxiety.

E. **Nursing Interventions**

1. Advise clients against driving or operating machinery.

2. Advise clients against long-term use.

3. Discontinue valerian at least 1 week prior to surgery.

IV St. John's wort (*Hypericum perforatum*)

A. **Purported Uses**

1. Depression

2. Seasonal affective disorder

3. Anxiety

B. **Side/Adverse Effects**

1. Headache

2. Sleep disturbances

3. Phototoxicity (long-term use)

4. Constipation

C. **Herb/Medication Interactions**

1. Many interactions with other medications

   a. Oral contraceptives

   b. Cyclosporine

   c. Warfarin

   d. Reduced antiretroviral effects

   e. Digoxin

   f. Calcium channel blockers

   g. Antidepressants

D. **Studies**

1. Several well-conducted studies support the use of St. John's wort for mild to moderate depression.

E. **Nursing Considerations**

1. St. John's wort has many medication interactions and should not be taken with other medications.

2. Should not be used to treat severe depression.

3. Should only be used with medical guidance.

V Echinacea (*Echinacea purpurea*)

A. **Purported Uses**

1. Prevent and treat the common cold

2. Stimulate the immune system

3. Promote wound healing

B. **Side/Adverse Effects**

1. Fever and nausea (rare)

2. Anaphylaxis in susceptible individuals

C. **Herb/Medication Interactions**

1. Can reduce the effects of immunosuppressants

2. Can increase serum levels of alprazolam, calcium-channel blockers, and protease inhibitors

D. **Studies**

1. Well-conducted studies have conflicted as to the effectiveness of echinacea in the treatment of the common cold.

E. **Nursing Considerations**

1. Long-term use can cause immunosuppression.

VI Garlic

A. **Purported Uses**

1. Block LDL cholesterol and raise HDL cholesterol; lower triglycerides

2. Suppress platelet aggregation and disrupts coagulation

3. Act as a vasodilator (can lower blood pressure)

B. **Herb/Medication Interactions**

1. Increased risk of bleeding in clients taking NSAIDs, warfarin, and heparin

2. Decreases levels of saquinavir (a medication for HIV treatment) and cyclosporine

C. **Nursing Interventions**

1. Question clients about concurrent use of NSAIDs, heparin, and warfarin.

2. Have clients who are taking antiplatelet or anticoagulant medication, cyclosporine, or saquinavir contact the provider prior to taking garlic as a supplement.

VII Ginger root

A. **Purported Uses**

1. Relieve vertigo and nausea

2. Increase intestinal motility

3. Increase gastric mucous production

4. Decrease GI spasms

5. Produce an anti-inflammatory effect

6. Suppress platelet aggregation

7. Treat morning sickness, motion sickness, nausea from surgery

8. Decrease pain and stiffness of rheumatoid arthritis

B. **Herb/Medication Interactions**

1. Use cautiously in clients who are pregnant because high doses can cause uterine contractions

2. Interacts with medications that interfere with coagulation (NSAIDs, warfarin, and heparin)

3. Can increase hypoglycemic effects of diabetes

C. **Nursing Interventions**

1. Question clients about concurrent use with NSAIDs, heparin, and warfarin.

2. Monitor for hypoglycemia if the client takes insulin or other medication for diabetes.

VIII Ginkgo (*Ginkgo biloba*)

A. **Purported Uses**

1. Improve cerebral circulation to treat dementia and memory loss

2. Decrease pain with walking in clients who have PAD

B. **Side/Adverse Effects**

1. Dizziness

2. Stomach upset

3. Vertigo

C. **Herb/Medication Interactions**

1. Can increase the effects of MAOIs, anticoagulants, and antiplatelet aggregates

2. Can reduce the effectiveness of insulin

D. **Studies**

1. Studies conflict as to the effectiveness of ginkgo in all purported uses.

E. **Nursing Interventions**

1. Discontinue 2 weeks prior to surgery.

2. Can cause seizures with overdose.

3. Keep out of the reach of children.

IX Glucosamine (2-Amino-2-deoxyglucose)

A. **Purported Uses**

1. Relieve osteoarthritis

2. Promote joint health

B. **Side/Adverse Effects**

1. Nausea

2. Heartburn

C. **Herb/Medication Interactions**

1. Can increase resistance to antidiabetic agents and insulin

2. Can increase risk of bleeding. Use cautiously with clients taking anticoagulants

D. **Studies**

1. Several studies support the use of glucosamine in reducing the symptoms of osteoarthritis in the knees.

E. **Nursing Interventions**

1. Use glucosamine with caution in clients who have a shellfish allergy.

2. Monitor glucose frequently in clients who have diabetes mellitus.

3. Allow extended time to see the effects of glucosamine.

4. Used often in combination with chondroitin.

X Omega-3 fatty acids

A. **Purported Uses**

1. Improve hypertriglyceridemia

2. Help maintain cardiac health

B. **Side/Adverse Effects**

1. Nausea

2. Diarrhea

C. **Herb/Medication Interactions**

1. Can increase risk of vitamin A or D overdose

D. **Studies**

1. Several well-conducted studies support the use of omega-3 fatty acids in reducing blood triglyceride levels, preventing cardiovascular disease in clients who have a history of a heart attack, and slightly reducing blood pressure.

2. Studies support improvement in symptoms of bipolar disorder.

E. **Nursing Considerations**

1. Omega-3 fatty acids are found in fish oils, nuts, and vegetable oils.

2. Some fish contain methylmercury and polychlorinated biphenyls (PCBs) that can be harmful in large amounts, especially in clients who are pregnant or nursing.

XI Melatonin

A. **Purported Use**
   1. Treat insomnia and jet lag

B. **Side/Adverse Effects**
   1. Morning grogginess
   2. Lower body temperature
   3. Vivid dreams

C. **Herb/Medication Interactions**
   1. Beta blockers
   2. Warfarin
   3. Steroids

D. **Studies**
   1. Several studies support antioxidant effects.

E. **Nursing Considerations**
   1. Pregnant or nursing clients should not take melatonin.

XII Nursing Considerations for Herbal Medications

A. **Ask the client specifically about herbal medications, vitamins, or other supplements during the client interview.**

B. **Over-the-counter medications are often not considered medications by the client.**

C. **Nursing Interventions**
   1. Herbal medications and supplements are not regulated by the FDA, often interact with other medications, and can cause serious adverse effects.
   2. It is important to use herbal medications and supplements cautiously and with medical supervision.
   3. Discourage use in pregnant and nursing clients, infants, young children, and older adult clients who have cardiovascular or liver disease.

HERBS AND PURPORTED USES

Match the following herbs with their purported use.

1. Treat and prevent benign prostatic hypertrophy
2. Manage migraines, insomnia, and menstrual cramps
3. Treat depression, seasonal affective disorder, and anxiety
4. Prevent and treat the common cold, and stimulate the immune system
5. Improve cerebral circulation
6. Relieve osteoarthritis and promote joint health
7. Improve hypertriglyceridemia and maintain cardiac health
8. Manage insomnia and jet lag
9. Relieve vertigo and nausea

A. Glucosamine
B. Echinacea
C. Ginkgo
D. Omega-3 fatty acids
E. Ginger root
F. Saw palmetto
G. St. John's wort
H. Valerian root
I. Melatonin

Answer Key: 1. F; 2. H; 3. G; 4. B; 5. C; 6. A; 7. D; 8. I; 9. E

UNIT FIVE

Fundamentals for Nursing

Client Safety

ı Falls

A significant number of reported facility accidents are related to falls. The nurse is accountable for implementation of essential actions to reduce the risk associated with falls.

A. **Contributing Factors**

1. Identify characteristics that increase risk for falls.
   a. Age greater than 65 years
   b. Impaired mobility
   c. Cognitive and sensory impairment
   d. Bowel and bladder dysfunction
   e. Adverse effects of medications
   f. History of falls

B. **Nursing Interventions**

1. Collaborate with the health care team to complete a fall risk assessment upon admission and update as needed. An individualized plan of care should be completed based on the fall risk assessment. See the worksheet at the end of the Fundamentals section to complete a fall risk assessment.
2. Communicate identified risks with the health care team.
3. Assign clients at risk for falls to a room close to the nurses' station and monitor frequently.
4. Provide the client with nonskid footwear.
5. Keep the floor free of clutter, and maintain an unobstructed path to the bathroom.
6. Orient the client to the setting (grab bars, call light), including how to locate and use all necessary items.
7. Maintain the bed in a low position.
8. Instruct clients who are unsteady to use the call light for assistance before ambulating.
9. Answer call lights promptly to prevent clients who are at risk from trying to ambulate independently.
10. Provide adequate lighting (such as a nightlight for trips to the bathroom).
11. Determine the client's ability to use assistive devices (walkers, canes). Keep all items within reach.
12. Use chair or bed sensors for clients who are at risk of getting up unattended.
13. Lock wheels on beds, wheelchairs, and gurneys to prevent rolling during transfers or stops.
14. Report and document all incidents per the facility's policy.

ıı Restraints

A. **Current client safety standards focus on reducing the need for client restraints.** The type or technique of restraint or seclusion used must be the least restrictive intervention that will be effective to protect the client, staff members, or others from harm.

B. **Definition:** Restraints include human, mechanical, chemical, or physical devices that restrict freedom of movement or diminish the client's access to parts of the body.

C. **Nursing Interventions**

1. Implement nonpharmacological measures (distraction, frequent observation, diversion activities).
2. Prior to application, review manufacturer's instructions for correct application.
3. Notify the provider immediately when restraints are implemented.
4. Remove the restraints and monitor client every 2 hr.
5. Monitor neurovascular and neurosensory status every 2 hr.
6. Leave the restraint loose enough to prevent injury.
7. Always tie the restraint to the bed frame (using loose knots that are easily removed).
8. Collaborate with the health care team and determine need for continued use. Providers may renew the prescription with a maximum of 24 hr of consecutive use.
9. Document the following.
   a. Behaviors making restraint necessary
   b. Alternatives attempted and the client's behavior while in restraints
   c. Type and location of the restraint, and time applied
   d. Frequency and type of care (range of motion, removal, data collection of skin and neurovascular status)
10. Restraints and/or seclusion should **never**
    a. Interfere with treatment.
    b. Be used for staff convenience, client punishment, or for clients who are physically or emotionally unstable.

ııı Seizure Precautions

Seizures can have a sudden onset and include loss of consciousness, violent tonic–clonic movements, or risk of injury to the client (head injury, aspiration, falls).

A. **Nursing Interventions**

1. Collect data about seizure history, noting frequency, presence of auras, and sequence of events.
2. Identify precipitating factors that can exacerbate or lead to seizures.
3. Review medication history. If routine lab work is required (such as phenytoin), when was last level drawn?
4. Place rescue equipment (oxygen, oral airway, suction equipment) at the client's bedside.
5. Establish IV or saline lock access for clients at high risk.
6. Inspect the client's environment for items that may cause injury in the event of a seizure. Remove any unnecessary items from the immediate environment.
7. At the onset of a seizure, position the client for safety. Remain with the client.
8. If sitting or standing, ease the client to the floor. Protect the client's head. If the client is in bed, raise the side rails and pad for safety.
9. Roll the client to the side with the head flexed slightly forward.
10. Do not put anything in the client's mouth.
11. Loosen restrictive clothing.
12. Administer medications.
13. Document precipitating behaviors or events and a description of the event (movements, loss of consciousness, loss of continence, injuries, mention of aura, postictal state).
14. Report the seizure to the provider.

Environmental Safety

I Fire

All staff must be instructed in fire response procedures.

A. Nursing Interventions

1. Know the facility's fire drill and evacuation plan.
2. Keep emergency numbers near or on the phone at all times.
3. Know the location of all fire alarms, extinguishers, and exits, including oxygen shut-off valves.
4. Follow the fire response sequence in the facility (**RACE**).
   a. **R – Rescue:** Protect and evacuate clients in immediate danger.
   b. **A – Alarm:** Activate the alarm and report the fire.
   c. **C – Contain:** Close doors or windows.
   d. **E – Extinguish:** Use correct fire extinguisher to eliminate the fire.
      1) **Class A:** Paper, wood, cloth, or trash
      2) **Class B:** Flammable liquids and gases
      3) **Class C:** Electrical fires
5. Extinguish properly (**PASS**).
   a. **P – Pull**
   b. **A – Aim**
   c. **S – Squeeze**
   d. **S – Sweep**
6. Considerations for home health setting
   a. Post "no smoking" signs.
   b. Monitor for risks (oxygen therapy, smoking, electrical equipment).
   c. Reinforce teaching with clients to develop a plan of action in the event of a fire, including a route of exit and a location where family members will meet.
   d. Reinforce teaching with clients to keep fire extinguisher accessible.
   e. Review "Stop, Drop, and Roll."

II Equipment

All staff should be alert for potential safety hazards.

A. Nursing Interventions

1. Electrical equipment must be grounded.
2. Do not overcrowd outlets.
3. The use of extension cords is not permitted in any client care areas.
4. Only use equipment for its intended purpose.
5. Regularly inspect equipment for frayed cords.
6. Disconnect all equipment prior to cleaning.

III Chemical Agents and Radiation

Nurses must review institutional guidelines and follow all safety guidelines.

A. Nursing Interventions

1. Determine type and amount of radiation used.
2. Place a sign on door: "Caution: Radioactive Material."
3. Wear monitoring badge to record amount of exposure.
4. Wear appropriate protective equipment.
5. Dispose of items removed from the room in appropriate containers.
6. Never handle any type of radioactive agent with bare hands.

Ergonomics and Client Positioning

I Lifting and Transfer of Clients

Implement safe care using proper body mechanics when lifting, positioning, transporting, or assisting a client to reduce the risk of injury. Obtain proper training before using any mechanical lift device, and always follow manufacturers' recommendations for use.

A. Nursing Interventions

1. Collect data about mobility and strength.
2. Tell clients to assist when possible.
3. Use mechanical lift and assistive devices.
4. Avoid twisting the thoracic spine or bending at the waist.
5. Use major muscle groups, and tighten abdominal muscles.

II Client Transfer and Positioning

Maintain safe practices with client transfer and ensure proper positioning of clients to maintain good body alignment.

A. Nursing Interventions

1. Transferring clients from bed to chair or chair to bed
   a. Reinforce teaching with the client on how to assist when possible.
   b. Lower the bed to the lowest setting.
   c. Position the bed or chair so that the client is moving toward the strong side.
   d. Assist the client to stand, then pivot.
2. Repositioning clients in bed
   a. Raise the bed to waist level.
   b. Lower side rails.
   c. Use slide boards or draw sheets.
   d. Have the client fold his arms across his chest while lifting the head off of the bed.
   e. Proceed in one smooth movement.
   f. Collaborate with other staff members for assistance.

Position: Semi-Fowler's

DESCRIPTION	Head of bed elevated to 30°
INDICATIONS	Gastric feedings; head injury; increased intracranial pressure; respiratory illness; postoperative following cranial surgery or cataract removal

Position: Fowler's

DESCRIPTION	Head of bed elevated to 45° to 60°
INDICATIONS	Postoperative following abdominal surgery, thyroidectomy, or cataract removal; respiratory illness or cardiac problems with dyspnea; bleeding esophageal varices

Position: High-Fowler's

DESCRIPTION	Head of bed elevated to 90°
INDICATIONS	Respiratory illness with dyspnea; emphysema; status asthmaticus; pneumothorax; cardiac problems with dyspnea; feeding; hiatal hernia; during and after meals; insertion of nasogastric tube

Position: Supine

DESCRIPTION	Lying on back, head, and shoulders; slightly elevated with a small pillow
INDICATIONS	Spinal cord injury (no pillow)

Position: Prone

DESCRIPTION	Lying on abdomen, legs extended, and head turned to the side
INDICATIONS	Client who is immobilized or unconscious; postoperative following lumbar puncture 6 to 12 hr; following myelogram 12 to 24 hr (oil-based dye); postoperative following tonsillectomy and adenoidectomy

Position: Lateral (side-lying)

DESCRIPTION	Lying on side with most of the body weight borne by the lateral aspect of the lower ilium
INDICATIONS	Postoperative following abdominal surgery, tonsillectomy, and adenoidectomy; client who is unconscious; seizures (head to side); postoperative pyloric stenosis of the lower scapula and the lateral (right side); postoperative following liver biopsy (right side); rectal irrigations

Position: Sims' (semi-prone)

DESCRIPTION	Lying on left side with most of the body weight borne by the anterior aspect of the ilium, humerus, and clavicle
INDICATIONS	Client who is unconscious; enema administration

Position: Lithotomy

DESCRIPTION	Lying on the back with hips and knees flexed at right angles and feet in stirrups
INDICATIONS	Perineal, rectal, and vaginal procedures

Position: Trendelenburg

DESCRIPTION	Head and body lowered while feet are elevated
INDICATIONS	Some surgeries; during labor if umbilical cord pressure is trying to be relieved

Position: Modified Trendelenburg

DESCRIPTION	Supine with the legs elevated
INDICATIONS	Shock

Position: Reverse Trendelenburg

DESCRIPTION	Head elevated while feet are lowered
INDICATIONS	Cervical traction; feeding clients restricted to supine position, such as postoperative following cardiac catheterization

Position: Elevate one or more extremities

DESCRIPTION	Elevate legs/feet or arms/hands by adjusting or supporting with pillows
INDICATIONS	Thrombophlebitis; application of cast; edema, postoperative following procedure on extremity

Position: Dorsal Recumbent

DESCRIPTION	Supine with knees flexed
INDICATIONS	Urinary catheterization of female; abdominal data collection; abdominal wound evisceration

SECTION 4

Assistive Devices for Ambulation

Definition: Used to provide an extension of the upper extremities to help transmit body weight and provide support for the client (canes, crutches, walkers)

A. **Collaborative Care**

1. Nursing Interventions
   a. Determine mobility status and ability to bear weight per provider's prescription.
   b. Identify for the need of a safety belt.
   c. Tell the client to wear shoes with nonslip soles.
   d. Identify risk of orthostatic hypotension.
   e. Provide safe environment free of clutter.

B. **Client Education and Referral**

1. Avoid rapid position changes to prevent orthostatic hypotension.
2. Inspect rubber tips on the device for wear and replace as needed.
3. Physical therapy consult.

C. **Crutches**

1. Verify correct fit of crutches: Approximately 3 finger widths between the axilla and top of the crutch.
2. Position hands on hand grips with elbows flexed at 30°. (Do not bear weight on axilla.)

D. **Crutches: Non-weight-bearing**

1. Beginning in the tripod position, maintain weight on the "unaffected" (weight-bearing) extremity.
2. Advance both crutches and the affected extremity.
3. Move the unaffected weight-bearing foot/leg forward (beyond the crutches).
4. Advance both crutches, and then the affected extremity.
5. Continue sequence, making steps of equal length.

E. **Crutches: Weight-bearing**

1. Move crutches forward about one step's length.
2. Move affected leg forward, level with the crutch tips.
3. Move the unaffected leg forward.
4. Continue sequence, making steps of equal length.

BASIC TRIPOD POSITION

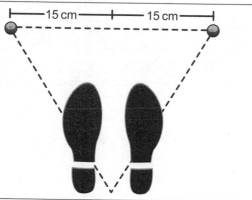

A. FOUR-POINT ALTERNATING GAIT	B. THREE-POINT GAIT	C. TWO-POINT GAIT
Order of foot/crutch movement is shown with solid foot and crutch tips.	Unaffected leg bears weight. Weight-bearing indicated with solid foot and crutch tips.	Weight partially distributed on each foot. Weight-bearing indicated with solid foot and crutch tips.

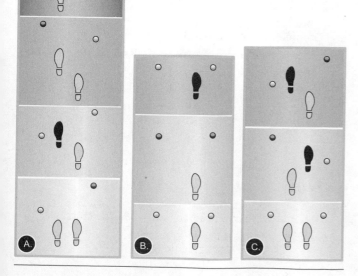

F. **Walking up stairs**

1. Hold onto rail with one hand, and crutches with the other hand.
2. Push down on the stair rail and the crutches, and step up with the unaffected leg.
3. If not allowed to place weight on the affected leg, hop up with the unaffected leg.
4. Bring the affected leg and the crutches up beside the unaffected leg.
5. Remember that the unaffected leg goes up first and the crutches move with the affected leg.

G. **Walking down stairs**

1. Place the affected leg and the crutches down on the step below. Support weight by leaning on the crutches and the stair rail.
2. Bring the unaffected leg down.
3. Remember that the affected leg goes down first and the crutches move with the affected leg.

H. **Cane**

1. For correct size, have the client wear shoes. The length is measured from the greater trochanter to the floor.
2. Cane is used on the unaffected (stronger) side to provide support to the opposite lower limb.
3. Move the cane forward 6 to 10 inches. Then move the weaker leg forward. Finally advance the stronger leg past the cane.
4. Another method of cane walking includes having the client move the affected extremity and cane at the same time.

I. **Walker**

1. For correct size, have the client wear shoes. The client's wrists are even with the hand grips on the walker when arms are dangling downward.
2. Advance the walker approximately 12 inches.
3. Advance with the affected lower limb.
4. Move unaffected limb forward.
5. Identify appropriateness of a rolling walker if walker is being used for support due to overall weakness. A rolling walker is not appropriate for a client who has Parkinson's disease due to shuffling gait.

Infection Control

All members of the health care team are accountable for adhering to measures to reduce the growth and transmission of infectious agents. According the Centers for Disease Control and Prevention (CDC), hand hygiene is the single most important practice in preventing health care associated infections (HAIs).

CHAIN OF INFECTION

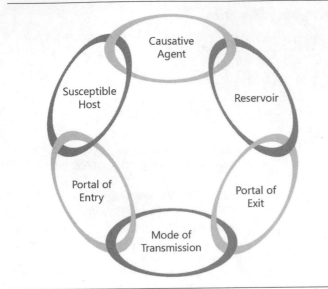

I Medical Asepsis (Clean Technique)

Precise practices to reduce the number, growth, and spread of micro-organisms

A. Nursing Interventions

1. Perform hand hygiene frequently.
2. Use personal protective equipment (PPE) as indicated.
3. Do not place items on the floor of client's room.
4. Do not shake linens.
5. Clean least soiled area first.
6. Place moist items in plastic bags.
7. Educate the client and caregivers.

II Surgical Asepsis (Sterile Technique)

Precise practices to eliminate all micro-organisms from an object or area (surgical technique)

A. Nursing Interventions

1. Avoid coughing, sneezing, and talking directly over the field.
2. Only dry, sterile items touch the field. (1-inch border is nonsterile.)
3. Keep all objects above the waist and within vision. (Do not turn back to sterile field.)
4. Wash hands and don sterile gloves to perform procedure.

III Isolation Guidelines

A group of actions that include hand hygiene and the use of barrier precautions intended to reduce the transmission of infectious organisms

IV Standard Precautions (Tier One)

Applies to all body fluids, nonintact skin, and mucous membranes. Standard precautions should be implemented for all clients.

A. **PPE:** As needed to prevent contact with body fluids—gloves, mask, gown, and goggles

B. **Nursing Interventions**

1. Implement standard precautions for all clients.
2. Determine need for client-specific, disease-specific precautions.
3. Provide education to health care team, clients, and visitors.
4. Report communicable diseases per CDC policy.
5. Handle all blood and body fluids as if contaminated.
6. Use PPE to reduce risk of transmission.
   a. Gown and gloves when touching blood or body fluids, nonintact skin, mucous membranes, or contaminated materials.
   b. Masks and face and eye protection when anticipating splashing of body fluids.
   c. Dispose of PPE in the client's room.
7. Consider room placement for client safety.
   a. Private room is needed only if the client is unable to maintain hygiene.
   b. Cohort (client must have same organism)
      1) Avoid placing clients on isolation precautions in the same room with clients who are immunocompromised, have open wounds, or have anticipated prolonged lengths of stay.
      2) Ensure clients are located more than 3 feet from each other. (Use privacy curtain between beds to minimize opportunities for direct contact.)
      3) Change protective attire and perform hand hygiene between contact with clients in the same room, regardless of disease status.
8. Clean equipment according to facility policy.
9. Discard all needles and sharps in the appropriate containers. Do not recap.
10. Place contaminated linens in the appropriate receptacle per the facility's policy.
11. Clean spills with a solution of bleach and water (1:10 dilution).

v Transmission-Based Precautions (Tier Two)

Transmission-based precautions are used in addition to standard precautions for clients who are known or suspected to be infected or colonized with infectious organisms.

A. **Airborne Precautions**

1. Diseases known to be transmitted by air for infectious agents smaller than 5 mcg (measles, varicella, pulmonary or laryngeal tuberculosis)

2. **PPE: Mask** (N95 respirator for known or suspected TB)

   a. **Nursing Interventions** (in addition to standard precautions)

      1) Provide private room with monitored negative airflow (air exchange and air discharge through HEPA filter).

      2) Keep door closed.

      3) Respiratory protection:

         a) The nurse must be fit-tested for N95 respirator.

         b) Apply a small-particle mask (surgical mask) to the client if leaving room for medical necessity.

B. **Droplet Precautions**

1. Prevent the transmission of pathogens spread through close contact with mucous membranes or respiratory secretions.

2. Protect against droplets larger than 5 mcg (streptococcal pharyngitis, pneumonia, scarlet fever, rubella, pertussis, mumps, mycoplasma pneumonia, meningococcal pneumonia/sepsis, pneumonic plague).

3. **PPE: Mask**

   a. **Nursing Interventions** (in addition to standard precautions)

      1) Private room is preferred; may cohort with client who has infection with same organism.

      2) Keep door closed.

      3) Mask is required when personnel is within 3 feet of the client.

C. **Contact Precautions** (includes enteric precautions)

1. Prevent transmission of infectious agents that are spread by direct or indirect contact with the client or the client's environment. These precautions are applied in the presence of wound drainage, fecal incontinence, or other bodily discharges that suggest an increased potential for environmental contamination and risk of transmission.

2. **PPE: Gloves, gown; as-needed use of mask and goggles**

   a. **Nursing Interventions** (in addition to standard precautions)

      1) Private room is preferred; may cohort with client who has infection with same organism

      2) Gloves and gown worn by caregivers and visitors

      3) Disposal of infectious dressing material into nonporous bag

      4) Dedicated equipment for the client or disinfect after each use

      5) Client to leave room only for essential clinical reasons

3. **Protective Isolation**

   a. Used to protect clients who have an increased susceptibility to infections, are receiving chemotherapy, or are immunosuppressed or neutropenic

   b. **Nursing Interventions**

      1) Follow standard precautions.

      2) Institute maximum protection, which can include the use of sterile linens, food, and other supplies.

      3) Minimize exposure to micro-organisms found on the outer layers of fresh flowers, fruits, and vegetables.

      4) Wear sterile gloves and gown/mask when in contact with the client.

      5) Maximum protection will require ventilated/positive-pressure room.

ORDER OF PPE APPLICATION	ORDER OF PPE REMOVAL
GOES UP THE BODY, THEN TO HANDS	REMOVAL IS IN ALPHABETICAL ORDER
Gown: Cover body from the bottom of the neck to the knees and wrists. Fasten securely behind the neck and at waist.	**Gloves:** Extend arms and slowly peel one glove downward, turning it inside out. With the ungloved hand, slide a finger under the inside portion of the remaining glove, turning inside out, and discard.
Mask: Secure with ties or elastic. Pinch the flexible bridge to secure at nose. Must extend below and under the chin.	**Goggles/face shield:** Grasp the ear pieces or headband only to remove.
Goggles/face shield: Verify fit is secure to prevent slipping.	**Gown:** Unfasten neck, then waist ties. Pull gown forward away from the body, folding it inside out and rolling it into a bundle for disposal.
Gloves: Use correct size for a snug fit. Must extend upward to completely cover the wrist portion of the gown.	**Mask:** Remove by only touching ties. Take care not to touch the front of the mask.

AIDS/HIV*

PRECAUTIONS	Standard
DURATION OF PRECAUTIONS	Duration of illness
RESERVOIR	Blood and body fluids, including breast milk
NURSING CONSIDERATIONS	PPE if in contact with potentially contaminated materials Transmission in health care settings is rare with adherence to proper sterilization and disinfection guidelines.

Chickenpox (varicella)*

PRECAUTIONS	Standard/airborne/contact
DURATION OF PRECAUTIONS	Until lesions crust over
RESERVOIR	Lesions, respiratory secretions
NURSING CONSIDERATIONS	Persons who are pregnant or have not had chickenpox or the vaccine should not care for the client.

Clostridium difficile

PRECAUTIONS	Standard/contact (enteric precautions)
DURATION OF PRECAUTIONS	Duration of illness
RESERVOIR	Feces
NURSING CONSIDERATIONS	Staff and visitors must don PPE upon entry to the room. Private room preferred. May cohort, but must provide a dedicated toilet for each client. Maintain precautions for duration of diarrhea.

Hepatitis A*

PRECAUTIONS	Standard/contact if client has fecal incontinence
DURATION OF PRECAUTIONS	Until 7 days after onset of jaundice
RESERVOIR	Feces
NURSING CONSIDERATIONS	Contact precautions used, particularly for clients wearing diapers or who are incontinent Can be spread up to 2 weeks before symptomatic

Hepatitis B*

PRECAUTIONS	Standard
DURATION OF PRECAUTIONS	Duration of illness
RESERVOIR	Blood and body fluids infected with hepatitis B virus
NURSING CONSIDERATIONS	Contact precautions for blood and body fluids Follow disinfection and sterilization guidelines for reusable equipment.

*Disease that must be reported to the CDC.

Hepatitis C*

PRECAUTIONS	Standard Additional precautions specific to hemodialysis unit
DURATION OF PRECAUTIONS	Duration of illness
RESERVOIR	Blood and body fluids infected with hepatitis C virus
NURSING CONSIDERATIONS	Contact precautions for blood and body fluids Follow disinfection and sterilization guidelines for reusable equipment.

Herpes simplex (recurrent oral, skin, genital)

PRECAUTIONS	Standard/contact
DURATION OF PRECAUTIONS	Until lesions crust over
RESERVOIR	Fluid from lesions
NURSING CONSIDERATIONS	Horizontal transmission from contact with skin and secretions Vertical transmission from mother to child in utero or childbirth

Herpes zoster (shingles) – disseminated or localized in clients who are immunocompromised

PRECAUTIONS	Standard/airborne/contact
DURATION OF PRECAUTIONS	Duration of illness or with visible lesions
RESERVOIR	Lesions
NURSING CONSIDERATIONS	Persons who have not had chickenpox or the vaccine should not provide care.

Measles (Rubeola virus)*

PRECAUTIONS	Standard/airborne
DURATION OF PRECAUTIONS	Duration of illness
RESERVOIR	Respiratory secretions
NURSING CONSIDERATIONS	Virus can live on infected surfaces for up to 2 hr. Contagious from 4 days before to 4 days after the rash appears. Nonimmune individuals must be excluded from areas of outbreak (school, hospital, childcare) until 21 days after onset of rash in diagnosed case of measles, unless they receive postexposure prophylaxis.

Meningococcal disease*

PRECAUTIONS	Standard/droplet
DURATION OF PRECAUTIONS	Until 24 hr therapy continuous
RESERVOIR	Respiratory secretions
NURSING CONSIDERATIONS	Postexposure prophylaxis is recommended to control outbreaks.

*Disease that must be reported to the CDC.

Methicillin-resistant Staphylococcus aureus (MRSA)

PRECAUTIONS	Standard/contact
DURATION OF PRECAUTIONS	Duration of illness
RESERVOIR	Body fluids and sites contaminated with MRSA
NURSING CONSIDERATIONS	Spread by direct contact with wound Can lead to complicated infections, sepsis, and pneumonia

Pneumonia

PRECAUTIONS	Standard/droplet
DURATION OF PRECAUTIONS	Until culture is negative
RESERVOIR	Respiratory secretions
NURSING CONSIDERATIONS	Consider organism-specific precautions as indicated. Streptococcus pnuemoniae, invasive disease must be reported to CDC.

Respiratory syncytial virus

PRECAUTIONS	Standard/contact/droplet
DURATION OF PRECAUTIONS	Duration of illness
RESERVOIR	Respiratory secretions
NURSING CONSIDERATIONS	Contact/droplet precautions Palivizumab for high-risk infants Follow established guidelines for administration of ribavirin.

Rotavirus

PRECAUTIONS	Standard/contact
DURATION OF PRECAUTIONS	Duration of illness
RESERVOIR	Feces
NURSING CONSIDERATIONS	Rotovirus vaccine effective in preventing severe disease in infants and young children. Continue enteric precautions for 3 days after illness subsides.

Rubella*

PRECAUTIONS	Standard/droplet
DURATION OF PRECAUTIONS	7 days after onset of rash
RESERVOIR	Respiratory secretions
NURSING CONSIDERATIONS	Nonimmune pregnant persons should not care for these clients.

*Disease that must be reported to the CDC.

Salmonellosis*

PRECAUTIONS	Standard/contact precautions
DURATION OF PRECAUTIONS	Duration of illness
RESERVOIR	Feces
NURSING CONSIDERATIONS	Increased risk of contamination while caring for children who are wearing diapers or incontinent

Shigellosis (dysentery)*

PRECAUTIONS	Standard/contact precautions
DURATION OF PRECAUTIONS	Duration of illness
RESERVOIR	Feces
NURSING CONSIDERATIONS	Contact precautions used, particularly for children who are wearing diapers or incontinent

Staphylococcus aureus (infection or colonization)

PRECAUTIONS	Standard/contact precautions
DURATION OF PRECAUTIONS	Duration of illness
RESERVOIR	Body fluids and sites contaminated with MRSA
NURSING CONSIDERATIONS	High-risk clients include those who have immunocompromised status, chronic disease, recent surgery, IV, or indwelling catheter. Risk for antibiotic resistance

Tuberculosis (TB) (pulmonary)*

PRECAUTIONS	Standard/airborne precautions
DURATION OF PRECAUTIONS	Until three sputum smears are negative on consecutive days or TB is ruled out
RESERVOIR	Airborne respiratory droplet nuclei
NURSING CONSIDERATIONS	N95 mask Client wears surgical mask when transported outside of negative-airflow room.

Vancomycin-resistant enterococci (VRE) (infection or colonization)*

PRECAUTIONS	Standard/contact precautions
DURATION OF PRECAUTIONS	Until three negative cultures from infectious site (1 week apart)
RESERVOIR	Intestines, female genital tract, and environment (normal flora)
NURSING CONSIDERATIONS	Most infections occur in hospital Can be spread by touching surfaces (such as equipment) that contain VRE

*Disease that must be reported to the CDC.

! Point to Remember

If moving clients to other areas of the facility, have the client wear a surgical mask if they have an airborne or droplet infection. Assure all draining wounds are covered.

Health Promotion and Disease Prevention

Nurses contribute greatly to the health of clients and population groups using health promotion and disease prevention strategies. Nursing care of the client incorporates knowledge of early detection of disease and actions to promote optimal health.

I Health Promotion

Includes client education, health risk data collection, wellness data collection, lifestyle and behavior changes, and environmental control programs

HEALTH PROMOTION AND DISEASE PREVENTION

PREVENTIVE CARE	EXAMPLES OF PREVENTION ACTIVITIES
Primary prevention: Focus is on promoting health and preventing disease.	Immunization programs Child car seat education Nutrition and fitness activities Health education programs
Secondary prevention: Focus is on early identification of illness, providing treatment, and conducting activities geared to prevent a worsening health status.	Communicable disease screening and case finding Early detection and treatment of hypertension Exercise programs for older adults who are frail
Tertiary prevention: Focus is on preventing long-term consequences of chronic illness or disability and supporting optimal functioning.	Prevention of pressure ulcers as a complication of spinal cord injury Promoting independence for a client following stroke

II Disease Prevention

A. **Nursing Interventions**

1. Identify risk factors.
2. Remind clients to follow standards for recommended screenings.
3. Identify lifestyle risk behaviors requiring modification.
4. Encourage clients to continue health-promoting behaviors.
5. Reinforce teaching about preventive immunizations.

SCREENING GUIDELINES*

TEST	FEMALE	MALE
Routine physical	20 to 40 years Annually	20 to 40 years Every 3 to 5 years Annually at age 40
Dental assessments	Every 6 months	Every 6 months
Blood pressure	Begin age 20 Minimum every 2 years Annually if higher than 120/80 mm Hg	Begin age 20 Minimum every 2 years Annually if higher than 120/80 mm Hg
Body mass index (BMI)	Begin age 20 Each health care visit	Begin age 20 Each health care visit
Blood cholesterol	Begin age 20 Minimum every 5 years (if no risk factors)	Begin age 20 Minimum every 5 years (if no risk factors)
Blood glucose	Begin age 45 Minimum every 3 years	Begin age 45 Minimum every 3 years
Colorectal screening	Fecal occult blood annually begin age 50 AND Flexible sigmoidoscopy every 5 years*, or Colonoscopy every 10 years, or Double-contrast barium enema every 5 years*, or CT colonography (virtual colonoscopy) every 5 years **NOTE:** Frequency may increase based upon results.	Fecal occult blood annually begin age 50 AND Flexible sigmoidoscopy every 5 years*, or Colonoscopy every 10 years, or Double-contrast barium enema every 5 years*, or CT colonography (virtual colonoscopy) every 5 years **NOTE:** Frequency may increase based upon results.
Pap test	Ages 21 to 65 years: Papanicolaou test (Pap smear) every 3 years; at age 30, may decrease Pap screening to every 5 years if human papilloma virus screening performed, as well. No testing is needed after age 65 if previous testing was normal and not high risk for cervical cancer.	n/a
Clinical breast exam	Begin at age 20, every 3 years Begin at age 40, yearly	n/a
Mammogram	Begin age 40, yearly Ages 55 and older may choose to have mammogram every 1 to 2 years.	n/a
Prostate-specific antigen test and digital rectal exam	n/a	Annual digital rectal examination (DRE) and prostate specific antigen (PSA) blood test
Testicular exam	n/a	Begin age 15 Monthly testicular self-exam, clinical testicular exam at each routine visit

*American Diabetes Association, American Heart Association, American Cancer Society, and National Institutes of Health, CDC

FALL RISK ACTIVITY

A 70-year-old client is admitted with infected diabetic ulceration of the right foot and possible fracture of the left arm after a fall at home. History reveals 36 pack-year history of smoking (stopped after MI), IDDM for 22 years, MI with CABG x three 2 years ago, and HTN. Current medications include insulin isophane, clopidogrel, metoprolol, furosemide, potassium chloride, zolpidem, and hydrocodone/acetaminophen PRN. **Based on the scenario, perform a fall assessment using the Morse Fall Scale below.**

Morse Fall Scale

		SCORE
1. History of falling; immediate or within 3 months	No = 0 Yes = 25	
2. Secondary diagnosis	No = 0 Yes = 15	
3. Ambulatory aid	None, bed rest, nurse = 0 Crutches, cane, walker = 15 Furniture = 30	
4. IV/heparin Lock	No = 0 Yes = 20	
5. Gait/transferring	Normal, bed rest, immobile = 0 Weak = 10 Impaired = 20	
6. Mental status	Oriented to own ability = 0 Forgets limitations = 15	
	TOTAL:	

Risk Level

According to the score, look at the risk level on chart below. Before viewing the interventions as instructed on the chart, identify five nursing actions you should implement for the client to minimize risk of falls.

1. _____

2. _____

3. _____

4. _____

5. _____

RISK LEVEL	MFS SCORE	ACTION
No Risk	0 to 24	None
Low Risk	25 to 50	See *Standard Fall Prevention Interventions* on following page
High Risk	51 or greater	See *High-Risk Fall Prevention Interventions* on following page

Source: http://www.ahrq.gov/sites/default/files/publications/files/fallpxtoolkit.pdf

Answer key on next page.

STANDARD FALL PREVENTION INTERVENTIONS

Clients who are scored as low-risk on the **Morse Fall Scale** (score of 25 to 50) will have the following interventions implemented by the nursing staff.

› Direct Care
  » Determine fall risk upon admission, change in status, transfer to another unit, and discharge.
  » Assign the client to a bed that enables the client to exit the bed toward the client's stronger side whenever possible.
  » Monitor coordination and balance before assisting with transfer and mobility activities.
  » Implement bowel and bladder programs to decrease urgency and incontinence.
  » Use treaded socks for all clients.
› All Staff
  » Approach the client toward the unaffected side to maximize participation in care.
  » Transfer the client toward the stronger side.
› Education
  » Actively engage the client and family in all aspects of fall prevention program.
  » Reinforce teaching about all activities prior to initiating assistive devices.
  » Reinforce teaching for the use of grab bars.
  » Reinforce teaching about medication time/dose, side/adverse effects, and interactions with food/medications.
› Equipment
  » Lock all movable equipment before transferring clients.
  » Individualize equipment specific to client needs.
› Environment
  » Place client care articles within reach.
  » Provide a physically safe environment. (Eliminate spills, clutter, electrical cords, and unnecessary equipment.
  » Provide adequate lighting.

HIGH-RISK FALL PREVENTION INTERVENTIONS

These interventions are designed to be implemented for clients who have multiple fall risk factors and those who have fallen. These interventions are designed to reduce severity of injuries due to falls, as well as to prevent falls from reoccurring, supplementing standard fall prevention interventions.

› Equipment
  » Bed and/or chair alarms
  » Alarms at exits
  » Nurse call and communication systems
  » Low beds
  » Raised-edge mattress
  » Video camera surveillance
  » Nonskid floor mat
› Environment
  » Clear from all hazards
› Education
  » Exercise
  » Nutrition
  » Home safety
  » Plan for emergency fall notification procedure

Answers to Fall Prevention Activity Answers

1. 25; 2. 15; 3. 0; 4. 0; 5. 0; Total: 40

Risk Level: Low Risk (answers may be any of the below)

1. Place call light in reach.
2. Place bed in low position.
3. Use nonskid footwear.
4. Assist the client with transfers/ambulation.
5. Determine the need for ambulation devices.
6. Provide adequate lighting, including night lights.
7. Promptly enter to assist the client when called
8. Monitor blood glucose before meals and at bedtime
9. Monitor for possible orthostatic hypotension after pain medications.
10. Monitor sensations in lower extremities due to impaired circulation

UNIT SIX

Adult Medical Surgical Nursing

UNIT SIX ADULT MEDICAL SURGICAL NURSING

Fluids and Electrolytes

I Fluids and Electrolytes

Nurses should review the client's health history and laboratory data and perform clinical assessment. Many health problems can cause changes in balance of fluids and electrolytes. The nurse should be prepared to manage the client who has imbalances.

A. Body Fluids

1. Adults: 50% to 60% of total body weight is water
2. Infants: 75% to 80% of total body weight is water
3. Two-thirds of body fluid is intracellular (ICF)
4. One-third of body fluid is extracellular (ECF)

NOTE: 1 kg (2.2 lb) of body weight is approximate to 1 L of fluid.

II Fluid Imbalance

A. Fluid Volume Deficit (FVD)

1. Fluid intake is less than needed to meet body requirements. The most common type is isotonic dehydration.
2. Contributing Factors
   a. Excess GI and/or renal loss
   b. Diaphoresis
   c. Fever
   d. Long-term NPO status
   e. Hemorrhage
   f. Insufficient intake
   g. Burns
   h. Diuretic therapy
   i. Aging: Older adults have less body water and decreased thirst sensation
3. Manifestations
   a. Weight loss
   b. Dry mucous membranes
   c. Increased heart rate and respirations
   d. Thready pulse
   e. Capillary refill less than 3 seconds
   f. Weakness, fatigue
   g. Orthostatic hypotension
   h. Poor skin turgor
   i. **LATE SIGNS:** Oliguria, decreased central venous pressure (CVP) flattened neck veins
4. Diagnostic Procedures
   a. Serum electrolytes, BUN, creatinine, Hct (can be high due to hemoconcentration)
   b. Urine: Specific gravity and osmolarity

5. Collaborative Care
   a. **Nursing Interventions**
      1) Monitor vital signs, pulse quality and amplitude.
      2) Monitor skin turgor. In older adults, check skin over sternum or forehead.
      3) Maintain strict I&O. Output should be at least 0.5 mL/kg/hr.
      4) Weigh the client daily.
      5) Monitor laboratory data.
      6) Correct underlying cause.
      7) Fluid replacement
         a) Increase oral fluid intake. Initiate oral rehydration solution.
         b) Maintain IV fluids for severe dehydration as prescribed.
         c) Monitor response to therapy.
      8) Initiate fall precautions.
   b. Medications
      1) Electrolyte replacement
      2) Intravenous fluids

INTRAVENOUS FLUIDS

Isotonic

INDICATION	Treatment of vascular system fluid deficit
CHARACTERISTICS	Concentration equal to plasma Prevent fluid shift between compartments
SOLUTIONS	Normal saline (0.9% NS) Lactated Ringer's (LR) 5% dextrose in water (D_5W)

Hypotonic

INDICATION	Treatment of intracellular dehydration
CHARACTERISTICS	Lower osmolality than the ECF Shift fluid from ECF to ICF
SOLUTIONS	0.45% normal saline (0.45% NS) 2.5% dextrose in 0.45% saline ($D_{2.5}$45% NS)

Hypertonic

INDICATION	Used only when serum osmolality is critically low
CHARACTERISTICS	Osmolality higher than the ECF Shift fluid from ICF to ECF
SOLUTIONS	10% dextrose in water ($D_{10}W$) 50% dextrose in water ($D_{50}W$) 5% dextrose in 0.9% saline (D_5NS) 5% dextrose in 0.45% saline (D_5W in 0.45% NaCl) 5% dextrose in lactated Ringer's (D_5LR)

B. **Fluid Volume Excess (FVE)**

1. Fluid intake or retention is greater than the body's needs.

2. Contributing Factors

   a. Kidney failure (late phase)

   b. Heart failure

   c. Cirrhosis

   d. Interstitial to plasma fluid shifts (hypertonic fluids, burns)

   e. Excessive water intake

   f. Long-term corticosteroid therapy

3. Manifestations

   a. Cough, dyspnea, crackles

   b. Increased blood pressure

   c. Tachypnea and tachycardia

   d. Bounding pulse

   e. Weight gain (1 L water = 1 kg weight)

   f. Jugular vein distention

   g. Increased central venous pressure

   h. Pitting edema

4. Diagnostic Procedures (can be decreased due to hemodilution)

   a. Serum: Electrolytes, BUN, creatinine, Hct

   b. Urine: Specific gravity and osmolarity

   c. Chest x-ray if respiratory complications present

5. Collaborative Care

   a. **Nursing Interventions**

      1) Monitor respiratory rate, symmetry, and effort.

      2) Monitor breath sounds for signs of pulmonary edema.

      3) Monitor for edema. Measure pitting edema on scale of 1+ (minimal) to 4+ (severe). Monitor dependent edema by measuring circumference of extremities.

      4) Monitor for ascites, and measure abdominal girth.

      5) Weigh the client daily.

      6) Maintain strict I&O.

      7) Monitor vital signs.

      8) Administer diuretics (osmotic, loop) as prescribed.

      9) Limit fluid intake.

      10) Maintain skin integrity.

      11) Use semi-Fowler's position. Reposition every 2 hr.

      12) Restrict sodium intake.

III. *Electrolyte Imbalances*

A. **Normal Electrolyte Ranges**

   1. Major Intracellular Electrolytes

      a. Potassium

      b. Phosphorus

      c. Magnesium

   2. Major Extracellular Electrolytes

      a. Sodium

      b. Calcium

      c. Chloride

      d. Bicarbonate

B. **Function**

   1. Maintain homeostasis.

   2. Promote neuromuscular excitability.

   3. Maintain fluid volume.

   4. Distribute water between fluid compartments.

   5. Maintain cardiac stability.

   6. Regulate acid–base balance.

MAJOR ELECTROLYTES: IMBALANCE/INTERVENTIONS

Potassium (K⁺): Hypokalemia

RISK FACTORS	Adverse effects of medications > Corticosteroids > Diuretics > Digitalis > Laxatives (abuse of)	Body fluid loss > Vomiting > Diarrhea > Wound drainage > Nasogastric suction	Excessive diaphoresis Kidney disease Dietary deficiency Alkalosis
MANIFESTATIONS	Muscle weakness, cramping Fatigue Nausea, vomiting	Irritability, confusion Decreased bowel motility Paresthesia	Dysrhythmias Flat and/or inverted T waves (ECG)
INTERVENTIONS	Monitor respiratory status. Initiate fall precautions. Initiate and monitor potassium replacement (oral, IV).	Monitor ECG. Monitor I&O. Monitor arterial HCO_3 and pH.	Reinforce client teaching. > Dietary sources > Medications
	NOTE: NEVER give K⁺ IV bolus. MUST dilute. NOTE: "No P = No K." If the client is not urinating, do NOT administer potassium.		

Potassium (K⁺): Hyperkalemia

RISK FACTORS	Renal failure Adrenal insufficiency	Acidosis Excessive potassium intake	Medications > Potassium-sparing diuretics > ACE inhibitors
MANIFESTATIONS	Peaked T-waves (ECG) Ventricular dysrhythmias	Muscle twitching and paresthesia (early) Ascending muscle weakness (late)	Increased bowel motility
INTERVENTIONS	Monitor ECG. Monitor bowel sounds. Initiate dialysis. Dietary restriction and teaching.	Administer medications. > Kayexalate (monitor bowel sounds) > 50% glucose with insulin > Calcium gluconate	> Bicarbonate > Loop diuretics

Sodium (Na⁺): Hyponatremia

RISK FACTORS	GI loss SIADH Adrenal insufficiency NPO status	Restricted-sodium diet Water intoxication Excessive diaphoresis	Medications > Diuretics > Anticonvulsants > SSRIs > Lithium > Demeclocycline
MANIFESTATIONS	Weakness Lethargy Confusion Seizures	Headache Anorexia, nausea, vomiting Muscle cramps, twitching Hypotension	Tachycardia Weight gain, edema
INTERVENTIONS	Sodium replacement (oral, GI tube, IV) Restrict oral fluid intake.	Weigh the client daily. Monitor I&O.	Medication: Conivaptan hydrochloride
	NOTE: Risk with hypertonic solutions: cerebral edema		

Sodium (Na⁺): Hypernatremia

RISK FACTORS	Dehydration GI loss Hyperaldosteronism	Hypertonic tube feedings Diabetes insipidus Kidney failure	Burns Heatstroke Corticosteroids
MANIFESTATIONS	Fever Swollen, dry tongue Sticky mucous membranes Hallucinations	Lethargy, restlessness, irritability Seizures Tachycardia Hypertension	Hyperreflexia, twitching Pulmonary edema
INTERVENTIONS	Daily weight I&O Seizure precautions	IV infusion of hypotonic or isotonic fluid Diuretics	Dietary sodium restriction and education Increased oral fluid intake

Calcium (Ca++): Hypocalcemia

RISK FACTORS	Hypoparathyroidism Hypomagnesemia Kidney failure	Vitamin D deficiency Inadequate intake GI loss (wound drainage, diarrhea)	Disease process > Celiac disease > Lactose intolerance > Crohn's disease > Alcohol use disorder
MANIFESTATIONS	Tetany, cramps Paresthesia Dysrhythmias	Trousseau's sign Chvostek's sign Seizures	Hyperreflexia Impaired clotting time
INTERVENTIONS	Seizure precautions IV calcium replacement	Daily calcium supplements Vitamin D therapy	Monitor for orthostatic hypotension. Dietary increase and education
	NOTE: IV calcium must be administered slowly and the site monitored for extravasation. It is diluted in D_5W, NEVER in NS.		

Calcium has an inverse relationship with phosphorus.

Calcium (Ca++): Hypercalcemia

RISK FACTORS	Hyperparathyroidism Malignant disease Prolonged immobilization Dehydration	Vitamin D excess Thiazide diuretics Lithium Glucocorticoids	Digoxin toxicity Overuse of calcium supplements Hyperthyroidism
MANIFESTATIONS	Muscle weakness Hypercalciuria/kidney stones Dysrhythmias Lethargy/coma	Hyporeflexia Pathologic fractures Flank pain Deep bone pain	Polyuria, polydipsia, dehydration Hypertension Nausea, vomiting
INTERVENTIONS	Increase mobility Isotonic IV fluids Dialysis Cardiac monitoring	Medications > Furosemide > Calcitonin > Glucocorticoids	 > Bisphosphonates > Calcium chelators

Calcium has an inverse relationship with phosphorus.

Magnesium (Mg++): Hypomagnesemia

RISK FACTORS	GI loss Alcohol use disorder Hypocalcemia Hypokalemia Diabetic ketoacidosis (DKA)	Hyperparathyroidism Malabsorption Total parenteral nutrition (TPN) Laxative abuse Acute MI	Medications > Cisplatin > Cyclosporine > Aminoglycoside antibiotics > Diuretics > Amphotericin B
MANIFESTATIONS	Paresthesias Dysrhythmias Trousseau's sign Chvostek's sign	Agitation, confusion Hyperreflexia Hypertension	Insomnia, irritability Anorexia, nausea, vomiting Dysphagia
INTERVENTIONS	Seizure precautions Monitor swallowing. Dietary measures and education	Administer medications. > IV magnesium sulfate > PO magnesium salts	Monitor urine output. Monitor respirations.
	NOTE: Monitor for signs of magnesium toxicity with IV replacement, and treat with calcium gluconate.		

Magnesium (Mg⁺⁺): Hypermagnesemia

RISK FACTORS	Renal failure Excessive Mg⁺⁺ therapy	Adrenal insufficiency Laxative overuse	Lithium toxicity Extensive soft tissue injury or necrosis
MANIFESTATIONS	Hypotension Drowsiness Bradycardia	Bradypnea Coma Cardiac arrest	Hyporeflexia Nausea, vomiting Facial flushing
INTERVENTIONS	Mechanical ventilation IV fluids (lactated Ringer's or NS)	Administer medications. > IV calcium gluconate > Loop diuretics	Monitor respirations and blood pressure. Monitor deep-tendon reflexes.

NOTE: Magnesium should not be administered to clients in renal failure.

Phosphorus: Hypophosphatemia

RISK FACTORS	Vitamin D deficiency Refeeding after starvation Alcohol use disorder DKA Alkalosis	Hypomagnesemia Hypokalemia Excessive loss of body fluids (sweat, diarrhea, vomiting, hyperventilation) Burns	TPN Overuse of antacids
MANIFESTATIONS	Paresthesia Muscle weakness Bone pain and deformities	Chest pain Confusion	Seizures Nystagmus
INTERVENTIONS	Oral phosphate replacement Careful IV administration of phosphorus (for severe cases)	Gradual introduction of solution for clients on TPN Protection from infection	Dietary management and education Seizure precautions

Phosphorus has an inverse relationship with calcium.

Phosphorus: Hyperphosphatemia

RISK FACTORS	Renal failure Chemotherapy Acute pancreatitis	High vitamin D High phosphorus intake Hypoparathyroidism	Excessive enema use Acidosis
MANIFESTATIONS	Tetany, cramps Paresthesias Dysrhythmias	Trousseau's sign Chvostek's sign Hyperreflexia	Anorexia, nausea, vomiting Soft tissue calcifications
INTERVENTIONS	Medications > Vitamin D > Aluminum hydroxide > Diuretics	IV normal saline Dialysis Dietary management and education	

Phosphorus has an inverse relationship with calcium.

IV Acid-Base Balance

A. **Definition:** Acid–base imbalances range from simple to complex. The four basic imbalances include the following.

ACID-BASE IMBALANCES

	PH	PCO₂	HCO₃
Normal value	7.35 to 7.45	35 to 45 mm Hg	21 to 28 mEq/L
Metabolic acidosis	↓	Normal	↓
Metabolic alkalosis	↑	Normal	↑
Respiratory acidosis	↓	↑	Normal
Respiratory alkalosis	↑	↓	Normal

B. **ROME:** "**R**espiratory **O**pposite, **M**etabolic **E**qual"

ROME

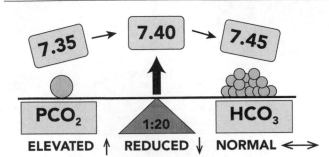

1. Remember the normal	2. Remember the possibilities	3. Use arrows
pH 7.35 to 7.45 PCO₂ 35 to 45 HCO₃ 21 to 28	Normal Abnormal (uncompensated) Partially compensated Fully compensated	Normal Elevated Reduced

Abnormals

Respiratory acidosis	Metabolic acidosis
Respiratory alkalosis	Metabolic alkalosis

Tips

If all three are normal, ABGs are NORMAL.

If two are abnormal, ABGs are fully compensated when pH has returned to normal and uncompensated when two values are abnormal.

If three are abnormal, ABGs are partially compensated or combined disorder.

C. **Regulation of acid–base balance is primarily controlled by**

1. Lungs (regulate carbonic acid through respiration)
2. Kidneys (regulate bicarbonate by retention or excretion)

ACID-BASED IMBALANCE INTERVENTIONS

Metabolic Acidosis

RISK FACTORS	Diarrhea Fever Hypoxia Starvation Seizure	Overdose (salicylates or ethanol) Renal failure DKA Dehydration
MANIFESTATIONS	Vital signs: Bradycardia, weak pulses, hypotension, tachypnea Flaccid paralysis Confusion	Hyporeflexia Lethargy Warm, flushed, dry skin Kussmaul respirations
INTERVENTIONS	Treat underlying cause. Administer fluids, electrolytes.	

Metabolic Alkalosis

RISK FACTORS	Ingestion of antacids GI suction Hypokalemia	TPN Blood transfusion Prolonged vomiting
MANIFESTATIONS	Dizziness Paresthesia	Hypertonic muscles Decreased respirations
INTERVENTIONS	Treat underlying cause. Administer fluids, electrolytes.	

Respiratory Acidosis

RISK FACTORS	Respiratory depression Pneumothorax	Airway obstruction Inadequate ventilation
MANIFESTATIONS	Dizziness Palpitations	Muscle twitching Convulsions
INTERVENTIONS	Maintain patent airway. Administer reversal agents for narcotics.	Provide regulation ventilation therapy. Administer bronchodilators. Administer mucolytics.

Respiratory Alkalosis

RISK FACTORS	Hyperventilation Hypoxemia Altitude sickness	Asphyxiation Asthma Pneumonia
MANIFESTATIONS	Tachypnea Anxiety, tetany Paresthesia	Palpitations Chest pain
INTERVENTIONS	Regulate oxygen therapy. Reduce anxiety. Use rebreathing techniques.	

ACID-BASE WORKSHEET

	PH	PCO₂	HCO₃	ACID-BASE IMBALANCE	COMPENSATION
1.	7.24	83 mm Hg	24 mEq/L		
2.	7.58	48 mm Hg	36 mEq/L		
3.	7.47	29 mm Hg	22 mEq/L		
4.	7.30	59 mm Hg	29 mEq/L		
5.	7.48	39 mm Hg	32 mEq/L		
6.	7.27	37 mm Hg	16 mEq/L		

Answer Key: 1. Respiratory acidosis, uncompensated; 2. Metabolic alkalosis, partially compensated; 3. Respiratory alkalosis, uncompensated; 4. Respiratory acidosis, partially compensated; 5. Metabolic alkalosis, uncompensated; 6. Metabolic acidosis, uncompensated

SECTION 2

Respiratory System Alterations

The respiratory system includes upper airways, lungs, lower airways, and alveolar air sacs (base of lungs). The lungs aid the body in oxygenation and tissue perfusion.

I Diagnostic Tests for Respiratory Disorders

A. **Noninvasive Procedures**

1. Chest x-ray (CXR): Use lead shield for adults of childbearing age.
2. Pulse oximetry
3. Pulmonary function tests
4. Sputum culture
5. Computed tomography (CT)
6. Magnetic resonance imaging (MRI)

B. **Invasive Procedures**

1. **Arterial blood gas** (ABGs via arterial puncture or arterial line): Allows the most accurate method of assessing respiratory function

   a. Perform Allen test if no arterial line.
   b. Sample is drawn into heparinized syringe.
   c. Keep on ice and transport to laboratory immediately.
   d. Document amount and method of oxygen delivered for accurate results.
   e. Apply direct pressure to puncture site at least 5 min (longer for clients at risk for bleeding).
   f. Monitor for hematoma.

2. **Bronchoscopy**: Visualize larynx, trachea, bronchi; obtain tissue biopsy; foreign body removal

   a. Obtain informed consent.
   b. Maintain NPO 8 to 12 hr.
   c. Provide local anesthetic throat spray.
   d. Position the client upright.
   e. Administer medications as prescribed (atropine [to reduce oral secretions], sedation, antianxiety).

   f. Label specimens.
   g. Observe postprocedure.
      1) Gag reflex
      2) Bleeding
      3) Respiratory status, vital signs, and level of consciousness

3. **Mantoux test**: Positive test indicates exposure to tuberculosis. Diagnosis must be confirmed with sputum culture for presence of acid-fast bacillus (AFB).

   a. Administer 0.1 mL purified protein derivative intradermal to upper half inner surface of forearm. (Insert needle bevel up.)
   b. Monitor for reaction in 48 to 72 hr following injection. Induration (hardening) of 10 mm or greater is considered a positive test. 5 mm can be considered significant if immunocompromised.

4. **QuantiFERON–TB Gold test (QFT–GT) and T–SPOT.TB**: Identify the presence of *Mycobacterium tuberculosis* infection by measuring the immune response to the TB bacteria in whole blood

5. **Thoracentesis**: Surgical perforation of the pleural space to obtain specimen, to remove fluid or air, or to instill medication

   a. Obtain informed consent.
   b. Reinforce client education (remaining still, feeling of pressure, positioning).
   c. Position the client upright.
   d. Monitor respiratory status and vital signs.
   e. Label specimens.
   f. Document client response, and amount, color, and viscosity of fluid. (Maximum amount of fluid to be removed at one time is 1 L.)
   g. Chest tube at bedside.
   h. Obtain CXR before and after procedure.

II Disorders of the Respiratory System: Airflow Problems

A. **Asthma:** Chronic inflammatory disorder of the airways resulting in intermittent and reversible airflow obstruction of the bronchioles

1. Contributing Factors

   a. Extrinsic: Antigen–antibody reaction triggered by food, medications, or inhaled substances
   b. Intrinsic: Pathophysiological abnormalities within the respiratory tract
   c. Older adult clients: Beta receptors are less responsive to agonist and trigger bronchospasms

2. Manifestations

   a. Sudden, severe dyspnea with use of accessory muscles
   b. Sitting up, leaning forward
   c. Diaphoresis and anxiety
   d. Wheezing, gasping
   e. Coughing
   f. Cyanosis (late sign)
   g. Barrel chest

3. Diagnostic Procedures
   a. ABGs
   b. Sputum cultures
   c. Pulmonary function tests
4. Collaborative Care
   a. **Nursing Interventions**
      1) Remain with the client during the attack.
      2) Position the client in high-Fowler's.
      3) Monitor lung sounds and pulse oximetry.
      4) Administer oxygen therapy.
      5) Maintain IV access.
   b. Medications
      1) Bronchodilators
         a) Short-acting inhaled: albuterol for rapid relief
         b) Methylxanthines: theophylline (Monitor therapeutic range for toxicity.)
      2) Anti-inflammatory
         a) Corticosteroids: fluticasone and prednisone
         b) Leukotriene antagonists: montelukast
      3) Combination agents
         a) Ipratropium and albuterol
         b) Fluticasone and salmeterol

NOTE: With inhaled agents, administer bronchodilators BEFORE anti-inflammatory medication.

   c. Therapeutic Measures
      1) Respiratory treatments
      2) Oxygen administration
   d. Client Education and Referral
      1) Avoid allergens and triggers.
      2) Properly use inhaler and peak flow monitoring.

B. **Status asthmaticus** is a life-threatening episode of airway obstruction that is often unresponsive to treatment.
   1. Manifestations
      a. Extreme wheezing
      b. Labored breathing
      c. Use of accessory muscles
      d. Distended neck veins
      e. High risk for cardiac or respiratory arrest
   2. **Nursing Interventions**
      a. Place the client in high-Fowler's position.
      b. Prepare for emergency intubation.
      c. Administer oxygen, epinephrine, and systemic steroid as prescribed.
      d. Provide emotional support.

C. **Chronic obstructive pulmonary disease (COPD)** encompasses pulmonary emphysema and chronic bronchitis. COPD is not reversible.
   1. **Pulmonary emphysema**: Destruction of alveoli, narrowing of bronchioles, and trapping of air resulting in loss of lung elasticity
      a. Contributing Factors
         1) Cigarette smoking (main causative factor); passive smoke inhalation
         2) Advanced age
         3) Exposure to air pollution
         4) Alpha-antitrypsin deficiency (inability to break down pollutants)
         5) Occupational dust and chemical exposure
      b. Manifestations
         1) Dyspnea with productive cough
         2) Difficult exhalation, use of pursed-lip breathing
         3) Wheezing, crackles
         4) Barrel chest
         5) Shallow, rapid respirations
         6) Respiratory acidosis with hypoxia
         7) Weight loss
         8) Clubbed fingernails
         9) Fatigue
   2. **Chronic bronchitis**: Inflammation and hypersecretion of mucus in the bronchi and bronchioles caused by chronic exposure to irritants
      a. Contributing Factors
         1) Cigarette smoking (main causative factor)
         2) Exposure to air pollution and other environmental irritants
      b. Manifestations
         1) Productive cough
         2) Thick, tenacious sputum
         3) Hypoxemia
         4) Respiratory acidosis
      c. Diagnostic Procedures for COPD
         1) Chest x-ray
         2) Pulmonary function tests: air remains trapped in lungs
         3) Pulse oximetry: Often less than 90%
         4) ABGs: Chronic respiratory acidosis
         5) Computed tomography (CT)
      d. Collaborative Care
         1) **Nursing Interventions**
            a) Monitor respiratory status.
            b) Monitor cardiac status for signs of right-sided failure.
            c) Position the client upright and leaning forward.
            d) Schedule activities to allow for frequent rest periods.
            e) Administer oxygen therapy as prescribed.
            f) Use incentive spirometry, breathing techniques, and effective coughing.

g) Encourage fluids 2 to 3 L/day unless contraindicated.

h) Encourage a high-calorie diet.

i) Provide emotional support.

j) Reinforce teaching about immunizations for pneumonia and influenza.

2) Medications

a) Bronchodilators

b) Beta-adrenergic agents

c) Cholinergic antagonists

d) Corticosteroids

e) Methylxanthines

f) Anti-inflammatory agents

g) Mucolytic agents

3) Therapeutic Measures

a) Chest physiotherapy/pulmonary drainage

b) Lung reduction surgery

4) Client Education and Referral

a) Breathing techniques

b) Oxygen therapy

c) Medications

d) Nutrition

e) Refraining from smoking

f) Infection prevention measures

g) Pulmonary rehabilitation

h) Activity pacing

3. Complications of COPD

a. **Cor pulmonale:** Right-sided heart failure caused by pulmonary disease

1) Manifestations

a) Hypoxia and hypoxemia

b) Extreme dyspnea

c) Cyanotic lips

d) Jugular venous distention

e) Dependent edema

f) Hepatomegaly

g) Pulmonary hypertension

2) Collaborative Care

a) **Nursing Interventions**

(1) Monitor respiratory status.

(2) Monitor cardiac status and for indications of right-sided heart failure.

(3) Administer oxygen therapy as prescribed.

(4) Ensure adequate rest periods.

(5) Encourage a low-sodium diet.

(6) Maintain fluid balance; possible fluid restriction.

(7) Administer medications as prescribed.

b) Medications

(1) Diuretics

(2) Digoxin

c) Therapeutic Measures

(1) Mechanical ventilation

D. **Carbon Dioxide Toxicity:** Stuporous secondary to increased CO_2 retention

1. Contributing Factors

a. Carbon dioxide retention

b. Excessive oxygen delivery

2. Manifestations

a. Alteration in level of consciousness

b. Tachypnea

c. Increased blood pressure

d. Tachycardia with dysrhythmias

3. Collaborative Care

a. Monitor pulse oximetry and ABGs.

b. Avoid excessive concentrations of oxygen.

c. Provide pulmonary hygiene.

d. Provide ventilatory support with CPAP, BiPAP, or mechanical ventilation.

E. **Pneumonia** is an inflammatory process in the lungs that produces excess fluid and exudate that fill the alveoli; classified as bacterial, viral, fungal, or chemical.

1. Contributing Factors

a. Advanced age

b. No pneumococcal vaccination within the last 5 years

c. No influenza vaccine within the last year

d. Chronic lung disease

e. Immunocompromised

f. Mechanical ventilation

g. Postoperative

h. Sedation and opioid use

i. Prolonged immobility

j. Tobacco use

k. Enteral tube feeding

2. Manifestations

a. Tachypnea and tachycardia

b. Sudden onset of chills, fever, flushing, diaphoresis

c. Productive cough

d. Dyspnea with pleuritic pain

e. Crackles

f. Elevated WBC

g. Decreased O_2 saturation

3. Diagnostic Procedures

a. Chest x-ray

b. Pulse oximetry

c. Sputum culture and sensitivity

4. Collaborative Care

  a. **Nursing Interventions**

    1) Monitor respiratory status.

    2) Administer oxygen.

    3) Monitor sputum.

    4) Monitor vital signs.

    5) Encourage 3 L of fluid per day.

    6) Provide pulmonary hygiene.

    7) Encourage mouth care.

    8) Promote nutrition.

  b. Medications

    1) Anti-infectives

    2) Antipyretics

    3) Bronchodilators

    4) Anti-inflammatories

  c. Client Education

    1) Medication administration

    2) Preventive measures

    3) Pneumonia and influenza vaccine

F. **Tuberculosis** is an infectious disease caused by *Mycobacterium tuberculosis* and transmitted through aerosolization (an airborne route).

  1. Contributing Factors

    a. Older adult clients

    b. People who do not have a permanent dwelling

    c. People who have low socioeconomic status

    d. Foreign immigrants

    e. Those in frequent contact with untreated persons

    f. Overcrowded living conditions

  2. Manifestations

    a. Cough, hemoptysis

    b. Positive sputum culture for acid-fast bacillus (AFB)

    c. Low-grade fever with night sweats

    d. Anorexia, weight loss

    e. Malaise, fatigue

  3. Diagnostic Procedures

    a. Mantoux test

    b. Sputum culture and smear for AFB to confirm diagnosis

    c. Serum analysis, QFT-GT

    d. Chest x-ray

  4. Collaborative Care

    a. **Nursing Interventions**

      1) Initiate airborne isolation precautions.

      2) Obtain sputum sample before administering medications.

      3) Maintain adequate nutritional status.

    4) Remind the client to avoid foods containing tyramine when taking isoniazid (INH).

    5) Inform the client that rifampin can alter the metabolism of certain other medications.

    6) Monitor laboratory findings for liver and kidney function.

  b. Medications: Combination drug therapy

    1) Administer medications on an empty stomach at the same time every day.

    2) Medications should be taken for 6 to 12 months, as directed.

    3) Reinforce teaching to the client to watch for indications of hepatotoxicity, nephrotoxicity, and visual changes, and to notify a provider if any of these are noted.

    4) Medications to treat TB

      a) Isoniazid (INH)

      b) Rifampin

      c) Pyrazinamide

      d) Ethambutol

      e) Fluoroquinolones and aminoglycosides (if TB is resistance to anti-TB drugs)

  c. Client Education and Referral

    1) Follow infection control measures.

    2) Adhere to medication and follow-up care.

  5. Cases of diagnosed TB are reported to local or state health department.

    a. Refer all high-risk clients to the local health department for testing and prophylactic treatment regimen.

G. **Laryngeal Cancer:** Malignant cells occurring in the mucosal tissue of the larynx; more common in men age 55 to 70

  1. Contributing Factors

    a. Smoking

    b. Radiation exposure

    c. Chronic laryngitis and/or straining of vocal cords

  2. Manifestations

    a. Hoarseness longer than 2 weeks

    b. Dysphagia

    c. Dyspnea

    d. Cough

    e. Persistent sore throat

    f. Hard, immobile lymph nodes in neck

    g. Weight loss, anorexia

  3. Diagnostic Procedures

    a. MRI

    b. Direct laryngoscopy with biopsy

    c. X-ray and CT

    d. Bone scan and positron emission tomography (PET) scan

4. Collaborative Care
   a. **Nursing Interventions**
      1) Maintain patent airway.
      2) Follow swallowing precautions.
      3) Provide emotional support.
      4) Provide adequate nutrition.
      5) Provide pain management.
      6) Administer medications as elixir when possible.
   b. Therapeutic Measures
      1) Partial or total laryngectomy
      2) Radiation therapy
   c. Client Education and Referral
      1) Communication method
      2) Stoma care
      3) Swallowing maneuvers
      4) Speech therapy

H. **Lung Cancer:** Leading cause of cancer-related deaths for both men and women in the U.S.; primary or metastatic disease; most commonly occurs from ages 45 to 70 years

1. Contributing Factors
   a. Smoking (first- and second-hand smoke)
   b. Radiation exposure
   c. Chronic exposure to inhaled irritants
   d. Older adult
2. Manifestations
   a. Chronic cough
   b. Chronic dyspnea
   c. Hemoptysis
   d. Hoarseness
   e. Fatigue, weight loss, anorexia
   f. Clubbing of fingers
   g. Chest wall pain
3. Diagnostic Procedures
   a. Chest x-ray and CT scan
   b. CT-guided needle aspiration
   c. Bronchoscopy with biopsy
   d. TNM system for staging
      1) T: Tumor
      2) N: Nodes
      3) M: Metastasis
4. Collaborative Care
   a. **Nursing Interventions**
      1) Maintain patent airway.
      2) Suction as indicated by manifestations.
      3) Monitor vital signs and pulse oximetry.
      4) Monitor nutritional status.
      5) Position the client in high-Fowler's.
      6) Provide emotional support.
      7) Monitor and treat stomatitis.
      8) Ensure protection for immunocompromised clients.

   b. Medications
      1) Chemotherapeutic agents
      2) Opioid narcotics
   c. Therapeutic Measures
      1) Palliative care
         a) Medication
         b) Thoracentesis
      2) Surgical
         a) Tumor excision
         b) Pneumonectomy, lobectomy, wedge resection
         c) Radiation
   d. Client Education and Referral
      1) Medications
      2) Constipation prevention and management
      3) Mouth and skin care
      4) Nutrition
5. Respiratory services
6. Radiology
7. Rehabilitation
8. Nutrition
9. Hospice

III Respiratory Emergencies

A. **Pulmonary Embolism:** A life-threatening hypoxic condition caused by a collection of particulate matter (solid, gas, liquid) that enters venous circulation and lodges in the pulmonary vessels causing pulmonary blood flow obstruction

1. Contributing Factors
   a. Chronic atrial fibrillation
   b. Hypercoagulability
   c. Long bone fracture
   d. Long-term immobility
   e. Oral contraceptive or estrogen therapy
   f. Obesity
   g. Postoperative
   h. Peripheral vascular disease, deep vein thrombosis (DVT)
   i. Sickle cell anemia
   j. Central venous catheters
2. Manifestations
   a. Dyspnea, tachypnea
   b. Sharp, stabbing pain on inspiration
   c. Tachycardia, hypotension
   d. Sense of impending doom
   e. Diaphoresis
   f. Decreased SaO_2
   g. Pleural effusion
   h. Crackles and cough

NOTE: Petechiae over chest and axilla are present with fat emboli.

3. Diagnostic Procedures
   a. ABGs
   b. D-dimer
   c. Chest x-ray
   d. Ventilation–perfusion (VQ) scan
   e. Pulmonary angiography
4. Collaborative Care
   a. **Nursing Interventions**
      1) Monitor respiratory status and vital signs.
      2) Provide respiratory support.
      3) Provide oxygen therapy.
      4) Position the client in high-Fowler's.
      5) Assist with initiating IV access.
      6) Provide emotional support.
   b. Medications
      1) Thrombolytics
      2) Anticoagulants
   c. Therapeutic Measures
      1) Embolectomy
      2) Vena cava filter
   d. Client Education and Referral
      1) Preventive measures
      2) Dietary precautions with vitamin K
      3) Follow-up for PT or INR
      4) Bleeding precautions
      5) Home oxygen therapy
5. Cardiology and pulmonary services
   a. Respiratory care

B. **Pneumothorax:** A collection of air or gas in the chest or pleural space that causes part or all of a lung to collapse due to a loss of negative pressure

C. **Tension Pneumothorax:** Occurs when air enters the pleural space during inspiration through a one-way valve and is not able to exit upon expiration. The trapped air causes pressure on the heart and the lung. As a result, the increase in pressure compresses blood vessels and limits venous return, leading to a decrease in cardiac output. Death can result if not treated immediately.

D. **Hemothorax:** Accumulation of blood in the pleural cavity
1. Contributing Factors
   a. Blunt chest trauma
   b. COPD
   c. Closed/occluded chest tube
   d. Advanced age
   e. Penetrating chest wounds
2. Manifestations
   a. Respiratory distress
   b. Tracheal deviation to unaffected side (tension pneumothorax)
   c. Reduced or absent breath sound (affected side)
   d. Asymmetrical chest wall movement

e. Hyperresonance on percussion due to trapped air (pneumothorax)
   f. Subcutaneous emphysema
   g. Chest pain
3. Diagnostic Procedures
   a. Chest x-ray
   b. Thoracentesis (hemothorax)
4. Collaborative Care
   a. **Nursing Interventions**
      1) Monitor respiratory status.
      2) Administer oxygen.
      3) Position in high-Fowler's.
      4) Monitor chest tube and dressing.
      5) Provide emotional support.
   b. Therapeutic Measures
      1) Chest tube insertion
         a) Chest tube: Inserted to pleural space for draining fluid, blood, or air; re-establishes a negative pressure; facilitates lung expansion
            (1) Position the client supine or semi-Fowler's.
            (2) Verify informed consent is signed.
            (3) Prepare chest drainage system prior to insertion.
            (4) Administer pain and sedation medication as prescribed.
            (5) Assist provider as needed during insertion.
            (6) Apply dressing to insertion site.
            (7) Maintain chest tube system.
            (8) Monitor respiratory status, pulse oximetry, vital signs, and client response.
            (9) Monitor for complications.

CHEST TUBE COMPLICATIONS

COMPLICATION	NURSING INTERVENTIONS
Air leak (continuous rapid bubbling in the water seal chamber)	Start at the chest and move down tubing to locate leak. Tighten connection or replace drainage system. Keep connection taped securely.
No tidaling in water seal chamber	Check for kinks in the tubing. Check breath sounds (lungs re-expanded).
No bubbling in suction control chamber	Verify tubing is attached. Verify water is filled to prescribed level. Check wall suction regulator.
Chest tube disconnected from system	Insert open end of the chest tube into sterile water until system can be replaced.
Chest tube accidentally pulled from client	Cover insertion site with sterile dressing, taped on three sides. Contact provider. Prepare for reinsertion.

IV Airway Management

A. **Oxygen Therapy** is used in many acute and chronic respiratory problems to improve cellular oxygenation and prevent hypoxia or hypoxemia.

1. Manifestations (hypoxia and hypoxemia)

MANIFESTATIONS OF HYPOXIA AND HYPOXEMIA

EARLY	LATE
Tachypnea	Bradypnea
Tachycardia	Bradycardia
Restlessness	Confusion and stupor
Pale skin and mucous membranes	Cyanotic skin and mucous membranes
Elevated blood pressure	Hypotension
Use of accessory muscles, nasal flaring, adventitious lung sounds	Cardiac dysrhythmias

2. Collaborative Care

OXYGEN DELIVERY DEVICES

DEVICE	FIO$_2$/FLOW RATE
Nasal cannula	24% to 44% at 1 to 6 L/min
Simple face mask	40% to 60% at 6 to 8 L/min
Partial rebreather mask	50% to 75% at 8 to 11 L/min
Nonrebreather mask	80% to 100% at 12 L/min
Venturi mask	24% to 40% at 4 to 8 L/min
Aerosol mask, face tent	30% to 100% at 8 to 10 L/min
T-piece	30% to 100% at 8 to 10 L/min

3. Client Education

   a. Identify electrical hazards.
   b. Post "oxygen in use" sign.
   c. Wear cotton gown.
   d. Refrain from smoking.

B. **Suctioning:** Use of a suction machine and catheter to remove secretions from the airway

1. Manifestations (indicating a need for suctioning)

   a. Restlessness
   b. Tachypnea
   c. Tachycardia
   d. Decreased SaO$_2$
   e. Adventitious breath sounds
   f. Visualization of secretions
   g. Absence of spontaneous cough

2. Collaborative Care

   a. Perform hand hygiene.
   b. Explain the procedure.
   c. Don required PPE.
   d. Position client to semi- or high-Fowler's.
   e. Obtain baseline breath sounds, vital signs, and SaO$_2$.
   f. Use medical aseptic technique (oral suction).
   g. Use surgical aseptic technique for all other types.
   h. Hyperoxygenate client.

   i. Suction 10 to 15 seconds (rotating motion). Limit to two to three attempts.
   j. Allow recovery between attempts (20 to 30 seconds).
   k. Document amount, color, and consistency of secretions, as well as client response.

C. **Tracheostomy Care:** Care of a tracheostomy to maintain a patent airway and optimal ventilation

1. Collaborative Care

   a. Explain the procedure.
   b. Position client in semi- or high-Fowler's.
   c. At all times, keep two extra tracheostomy tubes (one the client's size and one a smaller size) at the bedside in the event of accidental decannulation.
   d. Suction client only as clinically indicated (never on routine schedule). Surgical asepsis is used for tracheal suctioning.
   e. Monitor for respiratory distress.
   f. Provide tracheostomy care every 8 hr and as needed.
   g. Change tracheostomy tubes as prescribed.

2. Client Education and Referral

   a. Tracheostomy care
   b. Prevention of respiratory infections
   c. Nutrition
   d. Home health care agency
   e. Community support group

D. **Mechanical ventilation** provides respiratory support through the controlled delivery of ventilation and oxygenation via an endotracheal tube, tracheostomy tube, or noninvasive ventilation via mask through continuous positive airway pressure (CPAP) or bi-level positive airway pressure (BiPAP).

1. Indication

   a. During surgery
   b. Acute respiratory distress
   c. Respiratory failure

2. **Nursing Interventions**

   a. Explain the procedure to the client.
   b. Establish means of communication (asking yes/no questions, providing writing materials, using a dry erase or a picture communication board, lip reading).
   c. Maintain patent airway:

      1) Ensure advanced airway device is secured (endotracheal tube or tracheostomy tube).
      2) Monitor position and placement of tube. Document in centimeters at the client's lips or teeth.
      3) Prevent accidental extubation. Wrist restraints can be required.
      4) Suction oral and tracheal secretions as indicated by assessment data.
      5) Monitor respiratory status every 1 to 2 hr and as needed.

6) Monitor ventilator settings and alarms. Never turn off ventilator alarms. If the cause of an alarm cannot be identified and corrected, and the client's respiratory status begins to decline, ventilate the client using a manual resuscitation bag until the issue is resolved.

   a) Low–pressure alarm: Indicates low volume and is usually associated with tube disconnection, cuff leak, or tube dislodgement

   b) High–pressure alarm: Indicates increased pressure, which can be caused by secretions, kinking of tube, pulmonary edema, or the client coughing or biting the tube

   c) Apnea alarm: Indicates there has been no spontaneous breath within a preset time period

7) Maintain adequate but not excessive cuff pressure. (Less than 20 mm Hg is recommended to reduce risk of tracheal necrosis.)

8) Administer medications as prescribed.

   a) Analgesics

   b) Sedation

   c) Neuromuscular blocking agents

9) Reposition endotracheal tube every 24 hr or by protocol. Monitor skin for breakdown.

d. Prevent complications.

   1) Pneumonia

      a) Hand hygiene

      b) Elevate head of bed

      c) Oral hygiene

   2) Pneumothorax

      a) Caused by high ventilation pressures

      b) Auscultate lung sounds frequently

      c) Consider if sudden respiratory distress

      d) Requires immediate action (chest tube)

RESPIRATORY END-OF-SECTION REVIEW

1. The client who is experiencing respiratory distress should be placed in _____ position unless contraindicated.

2. The first inhaled medication to be given to a client experiencing an acute asthma attack is a _____.

3. The client who has a history of COPD should receive _____ concentrations of oxygen to prevent a decrease in his hypoxic drive to breathe.

4. The nurse teaches the client who has a diagnosis of COPD to use _____ breathing to facilitate the exhalation of trapped air from the lungs.

5. A client is considered to have a positive Mantoux test when induration is _____ or greater in the nonimmunocompromised client. The Mantoux test indicates exposure to TB not _____ disease. The diagnosis of tuberculosis is confirmed with a _____ acid-fast bacillus (AFB) sputum culture.

6. The client who has a suspected diagnosis of TB should be placed on _____ precautions.

7. _____ should be obtained prior to administering antibiotics to a client who has the diagnosis of pneumonia.

8. The most precise noninvasive oxygen delivery system is the _____ mask.

9. The most common cause of a low-pressure ventilator alarm is a _____; the most common cause of a high-pressure ventilator alarm is _____. If the nurse cannot quickly resolve the issue causing the ventilator alarm and the client's respiratory status begins to decline, the nurse should _____ the client.

10. The client who has had a laryngectomy needs to be placed on _____ precautions to prevent aspiration.

WORD BANK

10 mm

Active

Airborne

Blood cultures

High-Fowler's

Leak

Low

Manually ventilate

Occlusion

Positive

Pursed-lip

Short-acting bronchodilator

Swallowing

Venturi

Answer Key: 1. High-Fowler's; 2. Short-acting bronchodilator; 3. Low; 4. Pursed-lip; 5. 10 mm, active, positive; 6. Airborne; 7. Blood cultures; 8. Venturi; 9. Leak, occlusion; manually ventilate 10. Swallowing

Perioperative Care

A. **Preoperative Phase:** Procedures or teaching completed prior to a surgical procedure reduce potential complications and postoperative discomfort, relieve anxiety, and increase participation in care

1. Care of the client before surgery

    a. **Nursing Interventions**

        1) Take client history.

        2) Identify risk factors (infants, older adult clients, chronic illness, malnutrition, respiratory conditions, obesity, emergent procedures).

        3) Check for informed consent. (A nurse can witness only.)

        4) Verify baseline assessment is complete.

        5) Collect data to identify allergies.

        6) Verify NPO status.

    b. Medications

        1) Anesthesia

            a) Inhalation

            b) Intravenous

            c) Regional

            d) Topical

        2) Antibiotics

        3) Anticholinergics

        4) Narcotics

        5) Sedatives

    c. Diagnostic Tests

        1) Laboratory profile

        2) Chest x-ray

        3) ECG

        4) Pregnancy test

    d. Client Education

        1) Fears and anxiety

        2) Medications

            a) Hold anticoagulants for 7 to 10 days prior to surgery (warfarin, aspirin)

        3) Invasive procedures

        4) Incentive spirometry

        5) Turn, position, and perform early ambulation, including leg exercises

        6) Analgesics and pain control methods

        7) Routine and expected postoperative care

        8) Pre-, intra-, and postoperative routines

B. **Intraoperative Phase:** Begins when client enters the surgical suite and ends with transfer to postanesthesia recovery area. Nursing focus is on safety, client advocacy, and health team collaboration.

1. The Universal Protocol (safety initiative from Joint Commission)

    a. Conduct a preprocedure verification process.

    b. Mark the procedure site.

    c. Perform a "time out" before starting the procedure.

2. Collaborative Care

    a. Perioperative Nursing Staff

        1) Holding

        2) Circulator

        3) Scrub

        4) Specialty

    b. **Nursing Interventions**

        1) Implement role according to established standards.

        2) Maintain safe environment.

        3) Ensure strict asepsis.

        4) Apply grounding devices.

        5) Ensure correct sponge, needle, and instrument count.

        6) Position the client.

        7) Remain alert to complications.

        8) Communicate with the surgical team.

    c. Therapeutic Measures

        1) Blood transfusion

        2) Radiology

        3) Biopsy

        4) Laboratory profiles

C. **Postoperative Phase:** Begins when client enters the postanesthesia recovery area and continues until discharge from the health care facility

1. Collaborative Care

    a. **Nursing Interventions**: Immediate recovery period

        1) Ongoing assessment

            a) Pulmonary

                (1) Verify airway and check gag reflex.

                (2) Check for bilateral breath sounds.

                (3) Encourage coughing and deep breathing.

            b) Circulatory

                (1) Compare vital signs to baseline.

                (2) Monitor tissue perfusion.

            c) Neurological

                (1) Evaluate the level of consciousness.

                (2) Monitor reflexes and movement.

            d) Genitourinary

                (1) Monitor I&O.

                (2) Monitor urinary output (color, clarity, amount).

e) Gastrointestinal
  (1) Monitor bowel sounds.
  (2) Monitor for abdominal distention.
f) Integument
  (1) Monitor color.
  (2) Monitor wound.
  (3) Monitor drainage insertion sites.
g) **Nursing Interventions**
  (1) Verify IV fluid type, rate, and site.
  (2) Check dressings for type and amount of drainage.
  (3) Identify drainage including color and amount
  (4) If NG tube, determine type and amount of suction prescribed.
  (5) Position in semi-Fowler's to facilitate maximum oxygenation.
  (6) Monitor O_2 saturation.
  (7) Ensure thermoregulation.
  (8) Provide pain management.
  (9) Maintain NPO until the client is alert and a gag reflex returns.
  (10) Prevent complications (see table).
  (11) Transfer or discharge the client to a unit or home.

COMMON POSTOPERATIVE COMPLICATIONS

Atelectasis

OCCURRENCE	First 48 hr	
MANIFESTATIONS	Tachycardia	Shallow respirations
	Tachypnea	
INTERVENTIONS	Incentive spirometer	Hydration
	Turn, cough, deep breathe (TCDB) every 2 hr.	Monitor respiratory rate and rhythm
	Early ambulation	

Hypostatic pneumonia

OCCURRENCE	After 48 hr	
MANIFESTATIONS	Febrile	Tachypnea
	Tachycardia	Crackles, rhonchi
INTERVENTIONS	Incentive spirometer	Hydration
	TCDB every 2 hr	Mucolytics
	Early ambulation	

Respiratory depression

OCCURRENCE	Immediate to 48 hr	
MANIFESTATIONS	Bradypnea	Decreased LOC
	Shallow respirations	
INTERVENTIONS	Monitor respiratory rate and rhythm.	Oxygen therapy
	Monitor LOC.	Narcotic antagonist: naloxone
	Regulate narcotics.	

Hypoxia

OCCURRENCE	Immediate to 48 hr	
MANIFESTATIONS	Confusion	Tachypnea
	Increased BP, pulse	
INTERVENTIONS	Monitor vital signs.	Resolve underlying problem.
	Oxygen therapy	

Nausea

OCCURRENCE	Immediate to 48 hr	
MANIFESTATIONS	Nausea	
INTERVENTIONS	Comfort measures	Antiemetic
	Relaxation	NG tube to decompress stomach
	Mouth care	

Shock

OCCURRENCE	Immediate to 48 hr	
MANIFESTATIONS	Decreased BP, pulse, urinary output	Lethargy
		Stupor
	Cold, clammy, pale skin	
INTERVENTIONS	Monitor vital signs.	I&O
	Replace fluids.	Monitor LOC.
	Position in modified Trendelenburg.	Administer vasopressors as prescribed.

Urinary retention/hesitancy

OCCURRENCE	Immediate to 3 days	
MANIFESTATIONS	Inability to void	Restlessness
	Bladder distention	Increased BP
INTERVENTIONS	Privacy	Offer bedpan
	Bladder scan	I&O

Decreased peristalsis/Paralytic ileus

OCCURRENCE	2 to 4 days
MANIFESTATIONS	Hypoactive/absent bowel sounds
	No flatus
INTERVENTIONS	NG to decompress stomach
	Limit narcotics.
	Ambulation
	Prokinetic agents: metoclopramide as prescribed

Wound hemorrhage

OCCURRENCE	Immediate to discharge
MANIFESTATIONS	Bleeding from drainage tubes or surgical site
	Signs of shock
INTERVENTIONS	Monitor site.
	Identify early signs.
	Monitor drainage device, keep patent.
	Avoid tension at surgical site.

Thrombophlebitis

OCCURRENCE	7 to 14 days
MANIFESTATIONS	Redness, warmth, calf tenderness/pain, edema at site
INTERVENTIONS	Early ambulation Apply antiembolic stockings or sequential compression devices as prescribed. Avoid actions that decrease venous flow. Anticoagulant prophylaxis

Delayed wound healing

OCCURRENCE	5 to 6 days
MANIFESTATIONS	Edema, redness, pallor, separation at edges, absence of granulation tissue
INTERVENTIONS	Splint incision as needed. Use incision support devices (abdominal binder). Promote high-protein diet.

Wound infection

OCCURRENCE	3 to 5 days
MANIFESTATIONS	Signs of delayed healing with purulent/discolored drainage, pain in incisional area
INTERVENTIONS	Promote healthy diet, adequate fluid intake, adequate rest, and exercise. Provide wound care. Administer antibiotics as prescribed.

Wound dehiscence/evisceration

OCCURRENCE	4 to 15 days
MANIFESTATIONS	Open wound revealing underlying tissue (dehiscence) or organs (evisceration)
INTERVENTIONS	Position client to decrease tension at suture line. Apply sterile saline-soaked gauze. Notify surgeon. Instruct the client not to cough or strain. Provide emotional support.

Urinary tract infection

OCCURRENCE	5 to 8 days
MANIFESTATIONS	Frequency, urgency, dysuria Malodorous, cloudy urine
INTERVENTIONS	Wipe front to back after urination. Limit use of indwelling catheters. Encourage voiding. Increase fluids 3 L/day. Provide cranberry juice. Administer antibiotics as prescribed. Administer analgesics as prescribed.

Gastrointestinal, Hepatic, and Pancreatic Disorders

A. **Impaired function of the GI tract, pancreas, and liver resulting from structural, mechanical, motility, infection, or cancerous conditions**

B. **Contributing Factors**
1. History of autoimmune disorder
2. Alcohol use disorder
3. Dietary patterns
4. NSAID use
5. Age
6. Family history
7. Previous abdominal surgery
8. Allergies
9. Musculoskeletal impairment (CVA, MS)
10. Obesity
11. Smoking
12. Sedentary lifestyle
13. Stress

Diagnostic Procedures

A. **Laboratory Profiles: Gastric Aspirate**
1. Hydrochloric acid and pepsin (evaluate Zollinger–Ellison syndrome)
   a. NPO 12 hr.
   b. Avoid alcohol, tobacco, and medications that change gastric pH for 24 hr.
   c. Insert NG tube.
   d. Aspirate gastric contents.
   e. Obtain pH.

B. **Laboratory Profiles: Hepatic or Pancreatic Disease**
1. Albumin
2. Ammonia: Liver's ability to break down protein by-products
3. Bilirubin: Measured directly in the blood
4. Cholesterol
   a. Total cholesterol
   b. LDL ("bad")
   c. HDL ("good")
   d. Triglycerides
5. Liver enzymes
   a. ALT/SGPT
   b. AST/SGOT
   c. ALP
6. Pancreatic enzymes
   a. Amylase
   b. Lipase
   c. Prothrombin time

C. **Laboratory Profiles: GI Parasites, Bacteria, or Bleeding**

1. Stool sample
   a. Inspect for color, consistency
   b. Tests
      1) Ova and parasites
      2) *Clostridium difficile (C. diff)*
      3) Urobilinogen
      4) Fecal fat (steatorrhea)
      5) Fecal nitrogen
      6) Food residues
      7) Cytotoxic assay (preferred vs. stool culture)

KEY POINT: When obtaining a stool sample, have the client defecate into a bedpan or bedside commode. Use an approved specimen container. It must be uncontaminated by urine or toilet paper and sent promptly to the lab.

2. Fecal screening tests (can be obtained at home and mailed in)
   a. Fecal occult blood test
      1) Recommended annually to detect colon cancer.
      2) Remind the client to avoid red meat, aspirin, turnips, and horseradish at least 72 hr prior to testing to avoid false positive results. Ingestion of vitamin C-rich foods or supplements can result in a false negative.
      3) NSAIDs and anticoagulants should be discontinued 7 days prior to testing.
   b. Fecal immunochemical test
   c. Stool DNA

D. **Breath Tests**

1. Hydrogen breath test
   a. To evaluate carbohydrate absorption
   b. Aids in the detection of bacterial overgrowth in intestine
2. Urea breath test
   a. To detect presence of *H. pylori*
   b. Remind clients to avoid antibiotics and bismuth subsalicylate 1 month before the test; proton pump inhibitors and sucralfate 1 week before testing; and H_2 inhibitors for 24 hr before testing.

E. **Endoscopy:** Allows direct visualization of tissues, cavities, and organs using a flexible fiber-optic tube

1. Colonoscopy: Exam of the entire large intestine
   a. Bowel prep to clear fecal contents (1 to 3 day prep)
   b. Clear liquid diet 12 to 24 hr before procedure
   c. NPO except water 6 to 8 hr before procedure
   d. IV sedation
   e. Monitor postprocedure for excessive bleeding or severe pain

2. Virtual colonoscopy
   a. Bowel prep as for traditional colonoscopy
   b. Performed using MRI or CT
   c. Small tube is placed in the rectum
   d. Images viewed on screen
3. Sigmoidoscopy: Exam of rectum and sigmoid colon
   a. Clear liquid diet 24 hr before procedure.
   b. Laxative the evening before the procedure.
   c. Enema the morning of the procedure.
   d. Sedation is not required.
   e. Tissue biopsy can be performed.
   f. Report excessive bleeding.
4. Small bowel capsule endoscopy: Video exam of small bowel, including distal ileum
   a. Only water is allowed 8 to 10 hr before test.
   b. Maintain NPO status 2 hr before test.
   c. Client's abdomen is marked for location of placement for sensors.
   d. Client wears abdominal belt housing data recorder.
   e. Administer video capsule with full glass of water.
   f. Resume normal diet 4 hr after swallowing pill.
   g. Return to the facility with capsule equipment for download of data.
   h. Procedure takes approximately 8 hr.
   i. Capsule will be excreted via stool (might not be seen). No action is needed.
5. Esophagogastroduodenoscopy (EGD): Exam of esophagus, stomach, and duodenum (to identify bleeding, Crohn's disease, colitis)
   a. NPO 6 to 8 hr before procedure.
   b. Avoid anticoagulants, aspirin, or NSAIDs for several days before test.
   c. Maintain IV sedation.
   d. Administer atropine to dry secretions.
   e. Local anesthetic is sprayed to inactivate gag reflex.
   f. Prevent aspiration.
   g. Monitor for signs of perforation, pain, bleeding, or fever.
   h. Provide comfort measures for hoarseness or sore throat (several days).
6. Endoscopic retrograde cholangiopancreatography (ERCP): Exam of liver, gallbladder, bile ducts, pancreas
   a. Maintain NPO status 6 to 8 hr before procedure.
   b. Avoid anticoagulants, aspirin, or NSAIDs for several days before test.
   c. Verify any allergies to x-ray dye.
   d. Maintain IV sedation.
   e. Clients can have colicky abdominal discomfort.
   f. Monitor for severe pain, fever, nausea, or vomiting (indicates perforation).

F. **Radiographic Studies (with or without contrast)**

1. Barium series: X-ray visualization from the mouth to the duodenojejunal junction; can include a small bowel follow-through

2. Preprocedure

   a. Maintain NPO status 8 hr before procedure.

   b. Avoid opioid analgesics and anticholinergic medications for 24 hr before the test.

   c. Avoid smoking or chewing gum.

   d. Have the client drink 16 oz barium liquid.

   e. Client will assume multiple positions during the x-ray exam.

   f. Postprocedure

      1) Reinforce teaching with the client to include additional fiber and fluids to promote barium elimination.

      2) Visualize stool for barium contents for the next 24 to 72 hr (will be chalky white).

      3) Brown stool should return when barium is evacuated.

      4) Administer mild laxative or stool softener as needed to promote bowel elimination.

G. **Liver Biopsy:** Needle inserted through abdominal wall to obtain sample for biopsy or tissue examination; performed under fluoroscopy

1. Preparation

   a. Obtain informed consent.

   b. Monitor coagulation studies (PT, aPTT, INR, platelet count).

   c. NPO 8 to 10 hr before procedure.

   d. Position on affected side to promote hemostasis.

   e. Monitor for bleeding complications.

H. **Paracentesis:** Needle inserted through abdominal wall into peritoneal cavity, withdrawing fluid accumulated due to ascites

1. Have the client void.

2. Obtain baseline vital signs.

3. Position the client upright.

4. Administer mild sedation.

5. Administer prescribed IV fluids or albumin to restore fluid balance (as much as 4 to 6 L of fluid is slowly drained from the abdomen).

6. Monitor vital signs.

7. Record weight before and after procedure.

8. Measure abdominal girth before and after procedure.

9. Monitor laboratory profile before and after procedure (albumin, amylase, protein, BUN, creatinine).

Gastrointestinal Therapeutic Procedures

GASTROINTESTINAL TUBES

TUBE	PURPOSE	NURSING INTERVENTIONS
Nasogastric > **Levin**: single lumen > **Salem sump**: double lumen » Suction, aspiration » Vent	Decompress stomach (ileus, gastric atony, intestinal obstruction) Obtain specimens for analysis (pH of gastric fluid and the presence of blood)	Elevate head of bed. Verify placement. Provide frequent mouth care. Maintain NPO.
Miller-Abbott: double lumen > Aspiration > Inflate balloon at tip	Small bowel suction	Reposition every 1 hr. Do NOT tape tube to nose. Monitor advancement of tube. Monitor color of gastric contents.
Sengstaken-Blakemore: triple lumen > Esophageal balloon > Gastric balloon > Suction, irrigation	For treatment of esophageal varices Can cause potential trauma and complications for the client, such as rebleeding, pneumonia, and respiratory obstruction	Monitor for respiratory distress. (Most clients have endotracheal tube.) Keep scissors at bedside. Monitor for signs of shock.

A. **Enteral Feeding Tubes:** Delivery of a nutritionally complete feeding directly into the stomach, duodenum, or jejunum

KEY POINT: The auscultatory method of checking placement is NOT considered reliable. Initial placement of the nasogastric or nasointestinal tube should be checked by x-ray. Subsequent placement should be checked by aspirating stomach or intestinal contents and measuring pH. Gastric pH should be 1.5 to 4. Intestinal aspirate pH is around 6. Respiratory aspirate pH is 7 or higher.

1. Small-bore nasogastric feeding tubes

   a. Obtain x-ray to determine placement.

   b. Verify gastric pH before each feeding (every 4 hr for continuous feeding).

   c. Maintain a semi-Fowler's position while feeding is infusing.

   d. Verify residual in the stomach and refeed the residual, unless it exceeds the maximum.

   e. Provide nose and mouth care.

   f. Replace tube every 4 weeks.

KEY POINT: If residual exceeds 100 mL for intermittent feedings (or 2 hr worth of a continuous feeding), hold or stop the feeding. Do NOT refeed aspirate. Notify the provider.

2. Small-bore nasointestinal/jejunostomy tubes: Inserted through the skin and occasionally sutured in place for long-term feeding

   a. Obtain x-ray to determine placement (prior to initial feeding).

   b. Monitor length of exposed tubing (tube migration).

   c. Monitor placement prior to feeding using intestinal pH.

   d. Maintain a semi-Fowler's position.

   e. Monitor residual. (Greater volume indicates upward migration.)

3. Monitor for complications.

   a. Refeeding syndrome can be life-threatening.

   b. Bleeding.

   c. Infection.

   d. Tube misplacement/dislodgement, aspiration: Immediately remove any tube suspected of being dislodged or misplaced.

   e. Abdominal distention, nausea, vomiting, diarrhea, constipation.

   f. Fluid imbalance: Hyperosmolar preparations can lead to dehydration.

   g. Electrolyte imbalance: The most common are hyponatremia and hyperkalemia.

4. Percutaneous endoscopic gastrostomy (PEG)

   a. Monitor skin integrity.

   b. Monitor residual volume.

   c. Allow feeding to infuse slowly (raise/lower syringe).

   d. Flush with 30 mL warm water before and after feeding.

   e. Maintain semi-Fowler's position 1 to 2 hr after feeding.

B. **Parenteral Nutrition:** IV administration of a hypertonic IV solution made of glucose, insulin, minerals, lipids, electrolytes, and other essential nutrients. Used when the client cannot effectively use the GI tract for nutrition.

   1. Partial or peripheral parenteral nutrition (PPN)

      a. Used when client can eat, but cannot take in enough nutrients to meet needs

      b. Administered through a large distal arm vein or PICC line

   2. Total parenteral nutrition (TPN)

      a. Used when the client requires intensive nutritional support for an extended time period

      b. Delivered through a central vein

   3. Contributing Factors

      a. Gastrointestinal mobility disorders

      b. Inability to achieve or maintain adequate nutrition for body requirements

      c. Short bowel syndrome

      d. Chronic pancreatitis

      e. Severe burns

      f. Malabsorption disorders

   4. Collaborative Care

      a. **Nursing Interventions**

         1) Confirm placement by chest x-ray.

         2) Monitor central line insertion site for local infection.

         3) Maintain strict surgical asepsis for dressing change (every 72 hr).

         4) Change tubing and remaining TPN every 24 hr.

         5) Monitor for signs of systemic infection.

         6) Monitor glucose, electrolytes, and fluid balance.

         7) Prevent air embolism.

         8) Use infusion pump.

         9) Keep 10% dextrose in water available.

         10) For clients receiving fat emulsions, monitor for fat overload syndrome (Fever, increased triglycerides, clotting problems, multi-system organ failure). Discontinue infusion and notify the provider immediately.

III Oral and Esophageal Disorders

A. **Dental caries**

   1. An erosive process of the tooth that occurs when acid is formed by the action of bacteria on fermentable carbohydrates

   2. Contributing Factors

      a. Dental plaque

      b. Poor oral hygiene

      c. Lack of fluoridated water

      d. High intake of refined carbohydrates

      e. Decrease in saliva

   3. Manifestations

      a. Halitosis

      b. Tooth pain

      c. Tooth erosion, discoloring

   4. Collaborative Care

      a. **Nursing Interventions**

         1) Remind clients to regularly use preventive measures.

            a) Brush teeth after eating.

            b) Floss.

            c) Increase intake of fresh fruits and vegetables, nuts, cheese, plain yogurt.

            d) If water is not fluoridated, obtain fluoride from another source.

            e) Dental sealants.

            f) Twice-yearly dental cleaning and screening.

B. **Salivary Gland, Oral Mucosa, and Pharyngeal Disorders**
1. Salivary glands consist of the parotid, submandibular, sublingual, and buccal glands. Disorders can affect lubrication, protection from harmful bacteria, and digestion. Disorders include candidiasis (thrush), parotitis, sialadenitis, salivary calculus, stomatitis, and cancer.
2. Contributing factors
   a. Tobacco use
   b. Alcohol use disorder
   c. Aging
   d. Dehydration
   e. Radiation
   f. Stress
   g. Malnutrition
   h. Poor oral hygiene
   i. Immunosuppression
3. Manifestations
   a. Pain
   b. Cheesy white plaque (candidiasis)
   c. Inflammation and redness
   d. Persistent, painless oral lesion that does not heal (cancer)
   e. Xerostomia
4. Collaborative Care
   a. **Nursing Interventions**
      1) Monitor nutritional status. Refer to a dietitian PRN.
      2) Monitor swallowing ability.
      3) Implement alternatives to oral communication PRN.
      4) Ensure adequate food and fluid intake.
      5) Perform and reinforce teaching about regular and thorough oral hygiene.
      6) Minimize pain.
      7) Monitor for indications of infection.
      8) Promote a positive self-image.

C. **Gastroesophageal Reflux Disease**
1. A condition in which the lower esophageal sphincter (LES) does not close properly, allowing stomach contents to back up into the esophagus.
2. Contributing Factors
   a. Older Adults
   b. Obesity
   c. Smoking
   d. Heavy alcohol use
   e. Ingestion of very large meals
   f. Obstructive sleep apnea
3. Manifestations
   a. Dyspepsia
   b. Regurgitation
   c. Eructation
   d. Flatulence
   e. Coughing, hoarseness, wheezing
   f. Water brash
   g. Dysphagia
   h. Odynophagia

4. Collaborative Care
   a. **Nursing Interventions**
      1) Reinforce teaching with the client about dietary management.
         a) Limit or eliminate foods that decrease LES pressure (chocolate, caffeine, fried or fatty foods, alcohol, carbonated beverages, spicy and acidic foods.)
         b) Eat four to six small meals per day.
         c) Eat slowly, and chew thoroughly.
         d) Eating nothing for at least 3 hr before going to bed.
      2) Reinforce teaching to elevate the head of bed 6 to 12 inches.
      3) Reinforce teaching to sleep on the right side.
      4) Refer to smoking and alcohol cessation programs PRN.
      5) Encourage maintenance of proper weight.
      6) Reinforce teaching to wear loose clothing.
      7) Medications
         a) Histamine blockers: cimetidine, famotidine
         b) Antacids
         c) Proton pump inhibitors: omeprazole, esomeprazole, or pantoprazole (can be administered IV short-term)
      8) Endoscopic procedures

D. **Hiatal Hernia**
1. A portion of the stomach protrudes through the esophageal hiatus of the diaphragm into the chest

HIATAL HERNIA

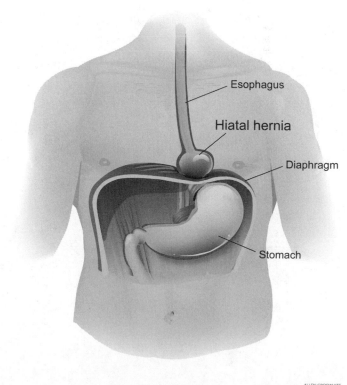

Esophagus

Hiatal hernia

Diaphragm

Stomach

2. Contributing Factors
   a. High-fat diet
   b. Caffeinated beverages
   c. Tobacco products
   d. Medications: Ca⁺⁺ channel blockers, anticholinergics, nitrates
   e. Obesity
3. Manifestations
   a. Regurgitation
   b. Persistent heartburn and dysphagia
   c. Belching
   d. Epigastric pain
   e. Dysphagia
   f. Breathlessness or feeling of suffocation after eating
   g. Chest pain that mimics angina
   h. Symptoms worsen after a meal or when supine
4. Collaborative Care
   a. **Nursing Interventions**
      1) Prepare for barium swallow with fluoroscopy.
      2) Monitor dietary history.
      3) Encourage small, frequent meals.
      4) Avoid eating 3 hr prior to bedtime.
      5) Sit upright for 1 to 2 hr after meals.
      6) Elevate the head of the bed.
      7) Encourage weight reduction for clients who have BMI greater than 25.
      8) Avoid straining or vigorous exercise.
      9) Wear loose clothing around the abdomen.
      10) Monitor for complications.
          a) Bleeding or esophageal ulcers
          b) Barrett's esophagus
          c) Aggravation of asthma, chronic cough, and pulmonary fibrosis
   b. Medications
      1) Antacids
      2) Histamine₂ receptor antagonists
      3) Prokinetic agents
      4) Proton pump inhibitors
   c. Client Education
      1) Dietary medication regimen
      2) Precautions to prevent aspiration
   d. Therapeutic Measures
      1) Hiatal hernia: fundoplication if other measures ineffective

IV **Gastrointestinal Disorders**

A. **Peptic Ulcer Disease (PUD)**
   1. Ulcerations in the stomach or duodenum as a result of mucosal tissue destruction. High risk of perforation and bleeding. Can be referred to as gastric, duodenal or esophageal ulcer, depending on location.
   2. Contributing Factors
      a. NSAIDs
      b. Corticosteroids
      c. *H. pylori* infection
      d. Uncontrolled stress
      e. Smoking
      f. Caffeine
      g. Alcohol use
      h. Type O blood
      i. Age 40 to 60 years
   3. Manifestations
      a. Dyspepsia
      b. Dull, gnawing, burning, midepigastric, or back pain with localized tenderness
      c. Symptoms worsen with empty stomach
      d. Relief noted with antacids
      e. Belching
      f. Bloating
      g. Vomiting of undigested food that can be proceeded by nausea
      h. Melena
      i. Decreased hematocrit and hemoglobin
   4. Collaborative Care
      a. **Nursing Interventions**
         1) Refer to smoking or alcohol cessation programs PRN.
         2) Encourage stress-relieving techniques (biofeedback, meditation, relaxation exercises).
         3) Reinforce teaching of dietary modifications.
            a) Avoid very cold and very hot foods.
            b) Eat three regular meals per day. (Small, frequent feedings are not necessary if an antacid or histamine blocker is taken.)
            c) Avoid caffeine, alcohol, decaffeinated coffee, milk, and cream. (Diet is very individual. Some can tolerate these foods better than others.)
         4) If other methods are not effective, prepare the client for surgery (pyloroplasty, antrectomy).
      b. Medications
         1) Triple therapy for 10 to 14 days: Two antibiotics—metronidazole or amoxicillin and clarithromycin—plus a proton pump inhibitor (preferred treatment)
         2) Quadruple therapy that adds bismuth salts to the previous
         3) Mucosal healing agents
         4) Stool softeners
         5) Antacids

6) Histamine$_2$ receptor antagonists
7) Prokinetic agents
8) Proton pump inhibitors

c. Diagnostic Tests
1) EGD
2) Chest and abdominal x-ray
3) Hematocrit and hemoglobin
4) Stool specimen

d. Client Education
1) Symptom management
2) Medication therapy
3) Nutrition therapy
4) Stress reduction

B. **Irritable Bowel Syndrome (IBS)**

1. Chronic disorder with recurrent diarrhea, constipation, and/or abdominal pain and bloating (most common digestive disorder seen in clinical practice)
2. Contributing Factors
a. Smoking
b. Caffeine
c. NSAIDs
d. Stress
e. Mental or behavioral illness
f. High-fat diet
g. Female sex
h. Family history
i. Dairy products
j. Alcohol use
3. Manifestations
a. Weight loss
b. Fatigue and malaise
c. Erratic bowel patterns
d. Abdominal pain relieved by defecation
e. Abdominal distention
f. Mucus with passage of stool
g. Colicky abdomen with diffuse tenderness
4. Collaborative Care
a. **Nursing Interventions**
1) Encourage a diet high in fiber.
2) Encourage regular exercise (walking, yoga).
3) Reinforce stress-reduction techniques.
4) Reinforce teaching to eat at regular times.
5) Reinforce teaching to eat slowly and chew thoroughly.
6) Reinforce importance of adequate fluid intake, but discourage fluids with meals.
7) Encourage a food diary to identify triggers.

b. Medications
1) Bulk agents (such as psyllium)
2) Antidiarrheals
3) Antidepressants
4) Anticholinergics
5) Antispasmodics
6) Probiotics
7) Complementary agents
a) Peppermint oil
b) Artichoke leaf extract
c) Caraway oil

c. Diagnostic Tests
1) Endoscopy
2) Chest and abdominal x-ray
3) Test for *H. pylori*

d. Client Education
1) Keep a diary to identify triggers.
2) Avoid causative agents.
3) Symptom management
4) Medication therapy
5) Nutrition therapy
6) Stress reduction

C. **Inflammatory Bowel Disease**

KEY POINT: Do not confuse inflammatory bowel disease with irritable bowel syndrome, which is much less severe. Inflammatory bowel disease is an autoimmune disorder that includes Crohn's disease and ulcerative colitis.

1. **Crohn's Disease**
a. Inflammation of the GI tract that extends through all layers. It can occur anywhere in the intestinal tract, but most commonly occurs in the distal (terminal) ileum. It is characterized by the cobblestone appearance of ulcers that are separated by normal tissue.

CROHN'S DISEASE

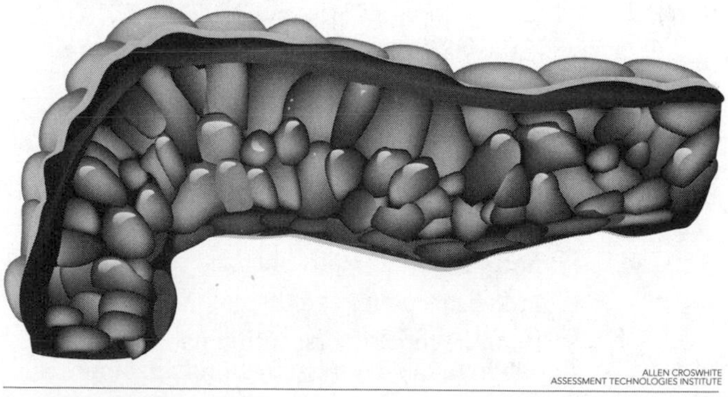
ALLEN CROSWHITE
ASSESSMENT TECHNOLOGIES INSTITUTE

b. Contributing Factors
1) Family history
2) Jewish ancestry
3) Bacterial infection
4) Smoking
5) Adolescents or young adults (age 15 to 40 year)
6) Living in an urban area

c. Manifestations

1) Abdominal pain (right lower quadrant)

   a) Does not resolve with defecation

   b) Pain is aggravated by eating

2) Low-grade fever

3) Diarrhea, steatorrhea

4) Weight loss (can become emaciated)

5) Formation of fistulas (abnormal tracts between bowel and skin/bladder or vagina)

6) Usually there is no bleeding (which helps differentiate from ulcerative colitis)

7) Low-grade fever, leukocytosis

8) Can be accompanied by arthritis, skin lesions, conjunctivitis, or oral ulcers

9) "String sign" on x-ray indicates constriction in a segment of the terminal ileum

10) Decreased hematocrit and hemoglobin, elevated ESR

d. Collaborative Care

1) **Nursing Interventions**

   a) Promote adequate rest periods.

   b) Record color, volume, frequency, and consistency of stools.

   c) Monitor and prevent fluid deficit.

   d) Nutrition therapy includes high-calorie, protein, low-fiber, no dairy.

   e) Provide supportive care.

   f) Monitor for complications.

     (1) Intestinal obstruction

     (2) Perianal disease

     (3) Fluid electrolyte imbalances

     (4) Malnutrition

     (5) Fistula, abscess

   g) If the above measures are not effective, prepare for surgery (bowel resection with possible ileostomy or stricturoplasty).

   h) Refer the client to a support group.

2) Medications

   a) Steroids

   b) Anti-infective: Metronidazole

   c) Aminosalicylates (5-ASAs)

   d) Immune modulators: Infliximab, adalimumab, certolizumab, natalizumab

   e) TPN

3) Therapeutic Measures

   a) Bowel resection (possible ileostomy)

   b) Stricturoplasty

   c) Laboratory profiles: Hct, hemoglobin, C-reactive protein, WBC, ESR

   d) Abdominal x-ray

4) Client Education

   a) Referral to support group

   b) Dietary guidelines

   c) Health promotion and relaxation

2. **Ulcerative Colitis**

a. Recurrent ulcerative and inflammatory disease of the superficial mucosa of the colon. It usually begins in the rectum and spreads proximally through the entire colon. It is characterized by contiguous ulcers.

b. Contributing Factors

1) Family history

2) Jewish ancestry

3) Isotretinoin use

4) Young and middle adults (females 15 to 25 years; males 55 to 65 years)

5) Caucasian ethnicity

6) Low-fiber diet

c. Manifestations

1) Liquid, bloody stool (10 to 20 per day)

2) Low-grade fever

3) Abdominal distention along the colon

4) High-pitched bowel sounds

5) Rebound tenderness (indicates perforation/peritonitis)

6) Passage of mucous and pus from the bowel

7) Left lower quadrant abdominal pain

8) Anorexia and weight loss

9) Vomiting and dehydration

10) Sensation of an urgent need to defecate

11) Hypocalcemia, anemia

12) Associated arthritis, conjunctivitis, skin lesions or liver problems

KEY POINT: Bleeding is common with ulcerative colitis. This helps differentiate it from Crohn's disease, in which bleeding is rare.

d. Collaborative Care

1) **Nursing Interventions**

   a) Promote adequate rest periods.

   b) Record color, volume, frequency, and consistency of stools.

   c) Maintain NPO status during acute phase.

   d) Monitor for dehydration. Maintain fluid balance.

   e) Monitor electrolytes. IV fluids can be indicated for imbalances.

   f) Provide dietary management and reinforce client education.

     (1) Increase oral fluids.

     (2) Eat a low-residue, high-calorie, high-protein diet.

   g) Administer multivitamin and supplemental iron.

   h) Refer the client to a support group.

   i) If the above measures are not successful, prepare for surgery (proctocolectomy with ileostomy).

2) Medications

   a) Antidiarrheals (monitor for megacolon)

   b) Aminosalicylates (5-ASAs)

   c) Immune modulators: infliximab, adalimumab, certolizumab, and natalizumab

   d) TPN

   e) Corticosteroids (oral, parenteral, topical)

3) Therapeutic Measures

   a) Surgical management is indicated for bowel perforation, toxic megacolon, hemorrhage, and colon cancer.

      (1) Colectomy and ileostomy

      (2) Total proctocolectomy with permanent ileostomy

      (3) Laboratory profiles: Hct, hemoglobin, C–reactive protein, WBC, ESR

      (4) Abdominal x–ray

4) Client Education

   a) Referral to support group

   b) Dietary guidelines

   c) Health promotion and relaxation

D. **Diverticular Disease**

1. Includes three conditions that involve numerous small sacs or pockets in the wall of the colon

   a. Diverticulosis: The presence of pouch-like herniations (diverticula) along the wall of the intestines; most common in the sigmoid colon

   b. Diverticular bleeding: Results from injury of small vessels near the diverticula

   c. Diverticulitis: Inflammation of one or more diverticula

2. Contributing Factors

   a. Aging

   b. Constipation

   c. Diet risk: Low-fiber, high-fat, red meat

   d. Connective tissue disorders causing weakness in the colon wall

3. Manifestations (Diverticulitis)

   a. Alternating diarrhea with constipation

   b. Painful cramps or tenderness in the lower abdomen (lower left quadrant)

   c. Chills or fever

   d. Tachycardia, nausea, vomiting

4. Collaborative Care

   a. **Nursing Interventions**

      1) Dietary management

         a) Diverticulitis: Begin with clear liquids; advance to a low-fiber diet.

         b) Diverticulosis: Provide a high-fiber diet.

         c) Reinforce education about fiber sources.

         d) Reinforce teaching to avoid foods with nuts, seeds, or kernels (such as popcorn).

         e) Increase fluid intake to 3 L/day.

         f) Refer for nutritional counseling.

2) Manage pain.

3) Avoid laxatives.

4) Monitor bowel elimination patterns.

5) Monitor for complications (obstruction, hemorrhage, infection).

6) In event of complications, prepare for surgery (colon resection).

b. Medications

   1) Bulk laxatives (preventive)

   2) Metronidazole

   3) Trimethoprim/sulfamethoxazole

   4) Ciprofloxacin

   5) Antispasmodics (oxyphencyclimine)

   6) Analgesics (meperidine)

> **KEY POINT:** Morphine is contraindicated because it can increase pressure in the colon, exacerbating symptoms.

c. Therapeutic Measures

   1) Emergency colon resection for peritonitis, bowel obstruction, or abscess

d. Client Education

   1) High-fiber vs. low-fiber diet

   2) Collaboration with nutritionist

   3) Preventive measures

E. **Abdominal Hernia**

1. Protrusion of bowel through the muscle wall of abdominal cavity (umbilical, ventral, inguinal/femoral). Classified as reducible, irreducible, or strangulated.

> **KEY POINT:** Absent bowel sounds can indicate strangulation, which cuts off the blood supply to the bowel. This is a medical emergency that can result in ischemia and obstruction, leading to necrosis and perforation. Manifestations are abdominal distention, nausea, vomiting, pain, fever, and tachycardia.

FEMORAL HERNIA

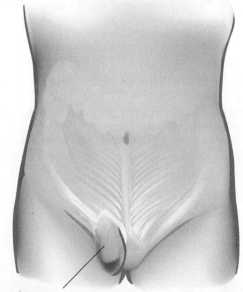

femoral hernia

2. Contributing Factors
   a. Aging
   b. Male sex
   c. Obesity
   d. Heavy lifting or straining
   e. Abdominal surgery
   f. Pregnancy
   g. Congenital or acquired muscle weakness
   h. Ascites, distension
3. Manifestations
   a. Client reports "lump" felt at the involved site
   b. Pain in groin when bending, coughing, or lifting
   c. Absent bowel sounds (strangulated)
   d. Palpation of mass
4. Collaborative Care
   a. **Nursing Interventions**
      1) Encourage wearing an abdominal binder for support of herniated tissue.
      2) Encourage increased fluid intake.
      3) Monitor for complications (strangulation, perforation).
      4) Prepare for surgery: Minimally invasive inguinal hernia repair (MIIHR, herniorrhaphy) or laparoscopic repair; bowel resection for strangulation.
      5) Postsurgical care
         a) Allow male clients to stand to void.
         b) For inguinal repair: Elevate scrotum and apply ice.
         c) Reinforce teaching to avoid coughing during recovery period.
         d) Reinforce teaching to avoid lifting or straining for 4 to 6 weeks.
      6) Medications
         a) Analgesics
         b) Stool softeners
   b. Therapeutic Procedures
      1) Herniorrhaphy laparoscopic repair

F. **Peritonitis**
1. Inflammation of peritoneum and lining of abdominal cavity
   a. Results from infection of the peritoneum due to puncture (surgery or trauma), septicemia, or rupture of part of the gastrointestinal tract
   b. Can be life-threatening
2. Manifestations
   a. Rigid, board-like abdomen (hallmark sign)
   b. Nausea, vomiting
   c. Tachycardic, febrile
   d. Rebound abdominal tenderness

3. **Nursing Interventions**
   a. Positioning: Fowler's or semi-Fowler's
   b. Nasogastric tube to low intermittent suction
   c. Oxygen
   d. Monitor fluid and electrolytes
   e. Antibiotics as prescribed
4. Therapeutic Procedures
   a. Exploratory surgery as needed based on client condition

G. **Intestinal Obstruction**
1. Partial or complete blockage of intestinal contents; can be the result of mechanical obstruction (adhesions, tumors, volvulus), neurogenic (such as paralytic ileus), or vascular (such as mesenteric artery occlusion)
2. Etiology: Any disorder that causes a mechanical or functional intestinal obstruction
3. Contributing Factors
   a. Crohn's disease
   b. Radiation therapy
   c. Fecal impaction
   d. Carcinomas
   e. Surgical procedures
   f. Narcotics
   g. Hypokalemia
   h. Diverticulitis
4. Manifestations
   a. Inability to pass flatus or stool for more than 8 hr
   b. Abdominal distention
   c. Hyperactive bowel sounds above site of obstruction
   d. Hypoactive or active bowel sounds below site of obstruction

COMPARISON OF INTESTINAL OBSTRUCTION MANIFESTATIONS

Small Bowel	Large Intestine
Sporadic, colicky pain	Diffuse and constant pain
Visible peristaltic waves	Significant abdominal distention
Profuse, projectile vomitus with fecal odor (vomiting relieves pain)	Infrequent vomiting, leakage of fecal fluid around impaction

5. Collaborative Care
   a. **Nursing Interventions**
      1) Maintain NPO.
      2) Monitor bowel sounds.
      3) Provide IV fluids.
      4) Provide preoperative care.
      5) Maintain NG tube for decompression.
      6) Prevent fluid and electrolyte deficit.

b. Therapeutic Measures

   1) Abdominal x-rays

   2) Endoscopy

   3) CT scan

   4) Surgical intervention (remove obstruction, resection)

c. Client Education

   1) Preventive measures based on etiology

   2) Diet

V Gastric Surgical Procedures

A. **Bariatric Surgery for Morbid Obesity**

1. Morbid obesity is more than two times ideal body weight, which places clients at high risk for multiple health problems. Bariatric surgery is performed when nonsurgical attempts at weight reduction fail. Methods include restrictive (gastric banding reduces volume of the stomach) and malabsorptive (Roux-en-Y gastric bypass interferes with food and nutrient absorption).

2. Indications for surgery

  a. BMI greater than 40

  b. BMI greater than 35 with other diseases

  c. Repeated failure of nonsurgical weight reduction

3. Collaborative Care

  a. **Nursing Interventions**

    1) Preoperative care

      a) Ensure thorough psychological preparation.

      b) Reinforce teaching about postoperative changes: Diet of liquids and pureed foods for first 6 weeks.

      c) Reinforce healthy lifestyle changes.

      d) Ensure support systems are available.

    2) Postoperative care

      a) Immediate priority is airway.

      b) Ensure abdominal binder is in place.

      c) Place the client in semi-Fowler's position.

      d) Assist the client to ambulate as soon as able the day of surgery.

      e) Measure and compare abdominal girth. Listen for bowel sounds.

      f) Collaborate with a dietitian to introduce six small feedings per day. Begin with 1 oz cups of clear liquids. Increase amount as tolerated.

      g) Monitor for manifestations of dumping syndrome (tachycardia, nausea, diarrhea, abdominal cramping, diaphoresis, anastomotic leak).

> **KEY POINT:** Anastomotic leaks are the most common complication and can be life-threatening. Monitor for increasing back, shoulder, and abdominal pain; restlessness; tachycardia; and oliguria. Report to provider immediately.

    3) Medications

      a) Analgesics

      b) Antispasmodics

      c) Multivitamin

    4) Long-term management

      a) To prevent dumping syndrome

        (1) Eat small meals throughout the day.

        (2) Consume high-fat and -protein; low-carbohydrate and -roughage; and no milk, sweets, or sugars.

        (3) Drink liquids only between meals.

        (4) Lie flat with head slightly elevated for 30 to 60 min after eating.

      b) Encourage increase in physical activity.

      c) Provide ongoing psychological support.

B. **Colostomy:** A surgical procedure that brings the end of the colon through the abdominal wall, creating an opening for the evacuation of fecal material. Can be temporary or permanent.

1. Indications

  a. Cancer or tumors

  b. Obstructive bowel disease

  c. Colectomy

  d. Severe diverticulitis or Crohn's disease

  e. Trauma

2. Collaborative Care

  a. **Nursing Interventions**

    1) Monitor ostomy site.

    2) Monitor output from stoma. (The higher an ostomy is placed in the small intestine, the more liquid and acidic the output will be.)

    3) Empty ostomy bag when ¼ to ½ full.

    4) Fit appliance to prevent leakage.

    5) Monitor for complications (fluid and electrolyte imbalances, ischemia of ostomy, bleeding, infection, peristomal skin irritation).

    6) Offer emotional support.

    7) Refer to support group.

  b. Client Education

    1) How to fit, care for, and change appliance.

    2) Refer to ostomy nurse for additional teaching.

    3) A breath mint can be placed in bag to reduce odor.

    4) Dietary management

      a) Avoid hard-to-digest foods (nuts, popcorn, celery, seeds, coconut).

      b) Maintain adequate fluid intake.

      c) Reintroduce foods one at a time.

      d) Foods that can contribute to odor and gas (cruciferous vegetables, asparagus, fish, eggs, garlic, beans).

VI Hepatic Disorders

A. **Cirrhosis:** A chronic disease characterized by extensive, irreversible scarring of the liver that disrupts structure and function.

1. Contributing Factors
   a. Alcohol consumption (Laennec's)
   b. Postnecrotic (hepatitis, chemicals)
   c. Biliary disease
   d. Severe right-sided heart failure

2. Manifestations
   a. Early stage
      1) Enlarged liver
      2) Jaundice
      3) Gastrointestinal disturbances
      4) Weight loss
   b. Late stage
      1) Liver becomes smaller and nodular
      2) Splenomegaly
      3) Ascites, distended abdominal veins; increased pressure in the portal system
      4) Bleeding tendencies; decreased vitamin K and prothrombin; anemia
      5) Esophageal varices, internal hemorrhoids; increased pressure in the portal area
      6) Dyspnea from ascites and anemia
      7) Pruritus from dry skin
      8) Clay-colored stools; no bile in stool
      9) Tea-colored urine; bile in urine
   c. End Stage—Portal Systemic Encephalopathy
      1) Prodromal: Slurred speech, vacant stare, restlessness, neurological deterioration
      2) Impending: Asterixis (flapping tremors), apraxia, lethargy, confusion
      3) Stuporous: Marked mental confusion, somnolence
      4) Coma: Unarousable, fetor hepaticus, seizures, high mortality rate

3. Collaborative Care
   a. **Nursing Interventions**
      1) Encourage rest.
      2) Weigh the client daily and measure abdominal girth.
      3) Monitor skin integrity frequently.
      4) Monitor I&O.
      5) Monitor for bleeding and hemorrhoids.
      6) Avoid hepatotoxic medications.
      7) Maintain a high-calorie, low-protein (20 to 40 g/day), low-fat, low-sodium diet.
      8) Limit sodium and fluid intake as prescribed.
      9) Monitor liver enzymes, bilirubin, and hematologic testing (CBC, WBC, platelets, PT/INR, ammonia levels).
   b. Medications
      1) Diuretics: spironolactone, furosemide
      2) Neomycin and metronidazole: Reduces intestinal bacteria
      3) Lactulose: Decreases ammonia levels.
      4) Supplemental vitamins (B_1 and B complex, A, C, and K; folic acid; thiamine) as prescribed
      5) Fat-soluble vitamin supplements and folic acid can need to be given IV
      6) Proton pump inhibitors and H_2 receptor antagonist
      7) Albumin IV to decrease ascites
   c. Therapeutic Measures
      1) Liver biopsy
      2) EGD
      3) Paracentesis
      4) Transjugular intrahepatic portosystemic shunt (TIPS)
   d. Client Education
      1) Abstain from alcohol.
      2) Follow dietary guidelines.
      3) Bleeding risk and precautions

4. Referral and Follow-up
   a. Alcohol recovery program
   b. Nutrition
   c. Social services

B. **Hepatitis**

1. Inflammation of the liver caused by infectious organisms, chemicals, or toxins. Cases must be reported to the local health department.

CHARACTERISTICS OF HEPATITIS

Mode of transmission

TYPE A (HAV)	Fecal-oral route Person-to-person	Food/water contamination
TYPE B (HBV)	Unprotected sex Sharing needles Needlesticks	Blood products; organ transplant before 1992
TYPE C (HCV)	Blood-to-blood Illicit IV drug sharing Unprotected sex	Blood products; organ transplant before 1992

Manifestations

TYPE A (HAV)	Mild course Flu-like Advanced age and chronic disease increase severity	
TYPE B (HBV)	Can be asymptomatic Right upper quadrant pain Anorexia, nausea, vomiting Fatigue	Febrile Dark urine Light-colored stool Jaundice
TYPE C (HCV)	Most are asymptomatic Diagnosis with blood testing Chronic inflammation progresses to cirrhosis	

CHARACTERISTICS OF HEPATITIS (CONTINUED)

Prevention

TYPE A (HAV)	Hand washing Vaccine for age 2 years and older Two doses 6 to 18 months apart
TYPE B (HBV)	Vaccine infants and high-risk populations Three doses over 6-month period
TYPE C (HCV)	Avoid high-risk behaviors.

Treatment

TYPE A (HAV)	Symptom-specific Can have change in medication regimen to "rest liver"
TYPE B (HBV)	Administer antiviral drugs.
TYPE C (HCV)	Administer peginterferon-alpha 2B. Monitor kidney function.

C. **Nonviral Hepatitis**

1. Definition: Liver injury and inflammation caused by ingestion of drugs and chemicals (industrial toxins, alcohol, drugs)

2. Contributing Factors
   a. Inhalation of hepatotoxic agents
   b. Drug toxicity
   c. Alcohol
   d. Secondary infection can occur with Epstein-Barr, herpes simplex, varicella-zoster, and cytomegalovirus

3. Manifestations
   a. Jaundice
   b. Liver enlargement
   c. Liver necrosis

4. Collaborative Care
   a. Monitor for signs of liver impairment.
   b. Monitor for right upper quadrant pain.
   c. Monitor the client's weight.
   d. Treatment is specific to symptoms and causative factors.

D. **Gallbladder Disease**

1. Types
   a. Cholecystitis: Inflammation of the gallbladder
   b. Cholelithiasis: Presence of stones in the gallbladder

2. Contributing Factors
   a. More common in females
   b. Obesity
   c. High-fat diet
   d. Older adult clients
   e. Type 2 diabetes mellitus

3. Manifestations
   a. Sharp right upper quadrant, epigastric, or shoulder pain
   b. Nausea and vomiting after ingestion of high-fat food
   c. Murphy's sign
   d. Flatulence
   e. Dyspepsia
   f. Dark urine, clay-colored stool

4. Diagnostic Procedures
   a. Ultrasound
   b. Hepatobiliary (HIDA) scan
   c. Endoscopic retrograde cholangiopancreatography (ERCP)
   d. Cholangiography

5. Collaborative Care
   a. **Nursing Interventions**
      1) Administer analgesics as prescribed.
      2) Prevent F&E imbalances.
      3) Maintain low-fat diet.
      4) Provide postoperative care.
      5) Cholecystectomy client can have T-tube 1 to 2 weeks postoperative.
         a) Monitor drainage. Keep below level of gallbladder.
         b) Empty collection bag every 8 hr.
         c) Report drainage amounts greater than 1,000 mL/day.
         d) Never irrigate without physician order.
      6) Observe color of stool.
      7) Monitor for indications of postcholecystectomy syndrome (manifestations of cholecystitis after surgery) and report to the provider.
   b. Medications
      1) Analgesics: morphine or hydromorphone (acute biliary pain); ketorolac (mild to moderate pain)
      2) Antiemetics
      3) Anticholinergics
      4) Ursodeoxycholic acid and chenodiol can be used to nonsurgically dissolve stones
      5) Antibiotics
   c. Therapeutic Measures
      1) Sphincterotomy with stone removal can be done with ERCP
      2) Extracorporeal shock wave lithotripsy (ESWL) to break up stones (only for small cholesterol stones)
      3) Cholecystectomy
   d. Client Education
      1) Resume regular low-fat diet.
      2) Prevent dumping syndrome.
      3) Care for T-tube (following discharge).

VII Pancreatic Disorders

A. **Acute Pancreatitis**

1. Inflammation of the pancreas caused by autodigestion by exocrine enzymes. It is life-threatening.

B. **Chronic Pancreatitis:** Progressive disease of the pancreas characterized by remissions and exacerbations resulting in diminished function

1. Contributing Factors
   a. Alcohol use disorder
   b. Gallstones
   c. Illegal drug use
   d. Infection
   e. Blunt abdominal trauma
   f. Operative manipulation and trauma

2. Manifestations
   a. Severe midepigastric or left upper quadrant pain
   b. Pain intensifies after meals and when lying down
   c. Nausea and vomiting
   d. Weight loss
   e. Abdominal tenderness; ascites
   f. Elevated amylase and lipase
   g. Steatorrhea
   h. Turner's sign
   i. Cullen's sign

3. Diagnostic Procedures
   a. Laboratory profiles: Liver enzymes, bilirubin, pancreatic enzymes
   b. CT scan with contrast

4. Collaborative Care
   a. **Nursing Interventions**
      1) Provide dietary management.
         a) NPO initially.
         b) After 24 to 48 hr, begin jejunal feedings.
         c) When food is tolerated, advance to small, frequent, moderate- to high-carbohydrate, high-protein, low-fat meals.
      2) Nasogastric tube for the severely ill, with intractable vomiting or biliary obstruction
      3) Provide pain management.
      4) Position for comfort (fetal position, sitting up, leaning forward).
      5) Monitor bowel sounds.
      6) Monitor I&O.
      7) Monitor for indications of hypocalcemia and hypomagnesemia.
      8) Monitor respirations.
      9) Reassure clients, and carefully explain procedures to reduce anxiety.

   b. Medications
      1) Antibiotics
      2) Opioid analgesics: morphine or hydromorphone; **meperidine is contraindicated**
      3) Anticholinergics
      4) Pancreatic enzymes
      5) H_2 blockers or proton pump inhibitors

   c. Therapeutic Measures
      1) TPN
      2) ERCP to create an opening in sphincter of Oddi if cause is gallstones
      3) Cholecystectomy
      4) Pancreaticojejunostomy (Roux-en-Y) to "reroute" pancreatic secretions to the jejunum

   d. Client Education for Chronic Pancreatitis
      1) Take enzymes before meals and snacks.
      2) Follow up with all scheduled laboratory testing.
      3) Nutrition: High caloric needs.
      4) Abstain from alcohol.
      5) Limit fat intake.

5. Referral and Follow-up
   a. Alcohol recovery program
   b. Home health for clients requiring long-term TPN
   c. Referral to a dietitian

C. **Pancreatic Cancer**

1. Carcinoma has vague symptoms and is usually diagnosed in late stages after liver or gallbladder involvement. It has a high mortality rate.

2. Contributing Factors
   a. Older adult clients
   b. Tobacco use
   c. Chronic pancreatitis
   d. Diabetes mellitus
   e. Cirrhosis
   f. High intake of red meat, processed meat
   g. Obesity
   h. Small number have an inherited risk

3. Manifestations
   a. Fatigue, anorexia, flatulence
   b. Pruritus
   c. Weight loss, palpable abdominal mass, abdominal pain that can radiate to the back
   d. Hepatomegaly, jaundice (late sign when cancer blocks the bile duct)
   e. Ascites
   f. Clay-colored stools; dark urine
   g. Glucose intolerance

4. Diagnostic Procedures
   a. Carcinoembryonic antigen (CEA) levels
      1) Expected findings: less than 2.5 ng/mL nonsmoker; less than 5 ng/mL smoker
      2) Critical findings: greater than 6 ng/mL
   b. Elevated serum amylase and lipase
   c. Elevated alkaline phosphatase and bilirubin
   d. ERCP
   e. Ultrasound, CT scan
5. Collaborative Care
   a. **Nursing Interventions**
      1) Provide palliative care measures.
      2) Provide pain management.
      3) Monitor blood glucose levels.
      4) Provide nutritional support (enteral supplements, TPN).
   b. Medications
      1) Opioid analgesics: morphine or hydromorphone
   c. Therapeutic Measures
      1) Chemotherapy can be used to shrink the tumor size. Monitor for myelosuppression and pancytopenia.
      2) Radiation therapy
      3) Partial pancreatectomy for small tumors
      4) **Whipple procedure:** Pancreatoduodenectomy is the most common operation to remove (resect) pancreatic cancers. Procedure is done when cancer is located in the head of the pancreas. It involves removing the head of the pancreas, duodenum, parts of the jejunum and stomach, gallbladder, and possibly spleen. The pancreatic duct is reconnected to the common bile duct, and the stomach is connected to the jejunum. This can be done laparoscopically.
         a) **Nursing Interventions**
            (1) Provide routine postoperative care.
            (2) Monitor NG output. Observe for bloody or bile-tinged drainage, which can indicate anastomotic disruption.
            (3) Maintain a semi-Fowler's position to prevent stress on suture line.
            (4) Facilitate coughing and deep breathing and use of incentive spirometer.
            (5) Monitor blood glucose and administer insulin as needed.
            (6) Provide analgesia.
   d. Client Education
      1) Seek palliative care at home, cancer support group, and available community resources.
      2) Use support measures for pain, anorexia, and weight loss.

Disorders of the Musculoskeletal System

Diagnostic Tests for Musculoskeletal Disorders

A. **Arthroscopy:** Visualizes internal structures of shoulder or knee joints. Cannot be done if infection present. Client must be able to bend joint at least 40°.
   1. Apply ice and elevate 24 hr postprocedure.
   2. Collaborate with physical therapist for exercises.

B. **Bone Scan:** Radioactive medium is injected for viewing the entire skeleton, primarily to detect tumors, arthritis, osteomyelitis, osteoporosis, vertebral compression fractures, and unexplained bone pain.
   1. Technician or physician administers the isotope 4 to 6 hr prior to testing.
   2. The client must lie still for 30 to 60 min as imaging is performed.
   3. Increase fluids postprocedure.

C. **Dual-Energy X-ray Absorptiometry (DEXA) Scan:** Most common screening tool for measuring bone mineral density for diagnosis of osteopenia and osteoporosis
   1. Baseline for female clients in their 40s.
   2. Clients should wear loose clothing without zippers or metal.
   3. Clients must remove jewelry.
   4. Instruct clients to stop vitamin D and calcium supplementation 48 hr prior to scan.

D. **Electromyography (EMG) and Nerve Conduction Studies:** Used to evaluate muscle weakness by emission of low-frequency electrical stimulation (ALS, carpal tunnel, myasthenia gravis, Guillain-Barré)
   1. Client performs activities for measurement of muscle activity.
   2. Observe needle insertion sites for hematoma.
   3. Support client who has anxiety related to testing.

E. **Magnetic Resonance Imaging (MRI):** Imaging produced through interaction of magnetic fields, radio waves, and atomic nuclei to diagnose muscle, tissue, and bone disorders
   1. Client must remove all metal objects. (Inquire about surgical implanted devices, nonvisible piercings.) Canes, crutches, and walkers generally must be left outside of the MRI room. Assist clients as necessary to the stretcher.
   2. MRI is contraindicated for clients who have pacemakers, stents, and surgical clips.
   3. Clients who have titanium joint replacements can have an MRI.
   4. Monitor clients for claustrophobia if closed scanner is used.
   5. Monitor clients for ability to lie still in supine position for 45 to 60 min.

F. **Laboratory**
   1. Serum calcium
   2. Serum phosphorus
   3. Alkaline phosphatase
   4. Creatine kinase
   5. Lactic dehydrogenase
   6. Aspartate aminotransferase
   7. Aldolase

‖ Arthritis

Inflammation of one or more joints, which results in pain, swelling, stiffness, and limited movement

A. **Osteoarthritis:** Progressive degenerative deterioration and loss of cartilage in one or more joints

1. Contributing Factors
   a. Aging
   b. Female sex
   c. Metabolic disease
   d. Obesity
   e. Repetitive use or abuse of joints
   f. Smoking

2. Manifestations
   a. Chronic joint pain and stiffness
   b. Pain diminished after rest and worse after activity
   c. Crepitus
   d. Limited movement
   e. Heberden's nodes (closest to the end of the fingers and toes)
   f. Bouchard's nodes (middle joints of fingers or toes)
   g. Excess joint fluid (especially with knee involvement)
   h. Skeletal muscle atrophy from disuse

ARTHRITIS MANIFESTATIONS

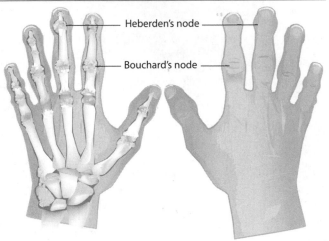

Heberden's node

Bouchard's node

ALLEN CROSWHITE
ASSESSMENT TECHNOLOGIES INSTITUTE

3. Diagnostic Procedures
   a. X-rays
   b. MRI
   c. Erythrocyte sedimentation rate (ESR) and serum C-reactive protein (CRP) show slight elevation

4. Collaborative Care
   a. **Nursing Interventions**
      1) Monitor and manage pain.
      2) Remind clients to use ice or heat for comfort.
      3) Encourage clients to perform range of motion and isometric exercises.
      4) Encourage adequate rest and sleep as needed to relieve pain.
      5) Involve physical therapy as appropriate.
      6) Use assistive devices to help increase independence and complete activities of daily living.

   b. Medications
      1) NSAIDs
      2) Corticosteroids
      3) Topical analgesics
      4) Supplements
         a) Glucosamine
         b) Chondroitin sulfate
   c. Therapeutic Measures
      1) Total joint arthroplasty
      2) Total joint replacement
   d. Client Education
      1) Use of mobility devices and safety
      2) Prevention of complications
      3) Performing exercises per treatment plan

5. Referral and Follow-up
   a. Physical therapy
   b. Rehabilitation therapy

B. **Rheumatoid Arthritis:** Chronic, progressive autoimmune connective tissue disorder primarily affecting synovial joints

1. Contributing Factors
   a. Physical and emotional stress
   b. Female sex
   c. Young to middle adult
   d. Family history

2. Manifestations
   a. Morning stiffness; pain at rest or after immobility
   b. Bilateral joint inflammation with decreased range of motion
   c. Joint deformity in late stages
   d. Warmth, redness, and edema of affected areas
   e. Dry eyes and mouth (Sjögren's syndrome)
   f. Numbness, tingling, or burning in hands and feet

3. Diagnostic Procedures
   a. X-ray
   b. MRI
   c. Positive rheumatoid factor
   d. Synovial fluid analysis
   e. Antinuclear antibody test
   f. ESR
   g. CRP

4. Collaborative Care
   a. **Nursing Interventions**
      1) Reinforce teaching with the client to use ice or heat for comfort.
      2) Encourage physical activity to maintain joint mobility (within client's capacity).
      3) Monitor for indications of fatigue.
      4) Monitor for complications related to therapy (secondary osteoporosis, vasculitis).

5) Complementary therapies
   a) Hypnosis
   b) Imagery
   c) Acupuncture
   d) Music therapy
   e) Omega-3
   f) Tai chi
b. Medications
   1) NSAIDs
   2) Corticosteroids
   3) Disease-modifying antirheumatic drugs (DMARDs)
      a) Methotrexate
      b) Leflunomide
      c) Hydroxychloroquine
   4) Biologic-response modifiers (administered parenterally)
      a) Etanercept
      b) Adalimumab
c. Therapeutic Measures
   1) Plasmapheresis for severe, life-threatening exacerbation
   2) Synovectomy
   3) Total joint arthroplasty if unresponsive to medication
d. Client Education
   1) Use of mobility devices and safety
   2) Prevention of complications
   3) Performing exercises per treatment plan
5. Referral and Follow-up
   a. Occupational/physical therapy
   b. Rehabilitation therapy
   c. Arthritis support group
C. **Gouty Arthritis:** Systemic inflammatory disease caused by problems with purine metabolism (primary gout) or hyperuricemia (secondary gout)
   1. Contributing Factors
      a. Family history
      b. Excessive alcohol intake
      c. High intake of foods with purines (organ meats, yeast, sardines, spinach)
      d. Obesity
      e. Comorbid conditions of diabetes mellitus or kidney disease
   2. Manifestations
      a. Excruciating pain and inflammation in one or more small joints (great toe is most common joint; appears warm and red)
      b. Appearance of tophi (deposits of sodium urate crystals; generally appear after years of gouty arthritis)
      c. Progressive joint damage and deformity
      d. Increased incidence of uric acid renal stone
   3. Diagnostic Procedures
      a. Serum uric acid greater than 7 mg/dL
      b. ESR
      c. Synovial fluid analysis (will show uric acid crystals)

4. Collaborative Care
   a. **Nursing Interventions**
      1) Maintain bed rest during acute attacks.
      2) Use bed cradle to keep linen elevated above affected joint.
      3) Promote fluid intake 3 L/day.
      4) Limit foods high in purine.
   b. Medications
      1) Acute phase: colchicine
      2) Chronic treatment: allopurinol
      3) NSAIDs
      4) Corticosteroids
      5) Injection of corticosteroid into affected joint by provider
   c. Client Education
      1) Foods to avoid include those high in purine.
      2) Keep a diary of triggering factors.
      3) Avoid alcohol.
      4) Lose weight slowly. (Rapid weight loss can precipitate a flare-up or increase the incidence of uric acid renal stones.)

III Fractures
A break or disruption in the continuity of bone tissue
A. **Types of Fractures**
   1. Closed
   2. Comminuted (fragmented)
   3. Compression
   4. Displaced
   5. Greenstick
   6. Impacted
   7. Oblique
   8. Open (compound)
   9. Pathologic (caused by tumors, infection, bone disease)
   10. Spiral
   11. Stress (small crack in bone)

TYPES OF BONE FRACTURES

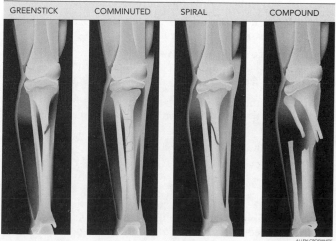

| GREENSTICK | COMMINUTED | SPIRAL | COMPOUND |

ALLEN CROSWHITE
ASSESSMENT TECHNOLOGIES INSTITUTE

B. **Collaborative Care**

1. Monitor neurovascular status (6 P's), noting bilateral comparisons.

   a. Pain

   b. Pressure

   c. Paralysis

   d. Pallor

   e. Pulselessness

   f. Paresthesia

2. Monitor for changes in skin temperature.

3. Monitor for complications of fat embolism (most common with long bone fractures):

   a. Confusion, anxiety

   b. Tachycardia

   c. Chest pain

   d. Tachypnea

   e. Hemoptysis

   f. Petechiae over neck, upper arms, chest, abdomen (late sign)

4. Monitor for complications of compartment syndrome (irreversible if compromise persists beyond 4 to 6 hr).

   a. Pain unrelieved by positioning or medication

   b. Cyanosis

   c. Tingling

   d. Paralysis

5. Maintain correct body alignment.

6. Provide nursing care specific to therapeutic measures of fracture reduction.

C. **Therapeutic Measures**

1. Cast: Application of plaster or fiberglass to immobilize and maintain alignment of the bone

   a. Collaborative Care

      1) Monitor neurovascular status.

      2) Allow plaster cast to air-dry. Handle cast with palms while drying.

      3) Elevate affected extremity.

      4) Monitor for complications.

      5) Client can "petal" plaster cast if irritation around edges develops.

      6) To help reduce risk of infection, remind the client to not place objects down the cast.

2. Traction

   a. Skin traction: Provides a mechanical pulling force to overcome muscle spasms, immobilize, or relieve pain

      1) Buck's

      2) Bryant's

      3) Cervical halter

      4) Pelvic

   b. Skeletal traction: Applied directly to a bone to reduce a fracture or maintain surgically manipulated bone alignment

      1) Pins or wires inserted through skin and soft tissue into the bone

      2) Balanced suspension using splints, slings, weights

D. **External Fixation Device:** Rigid metal frames with attached percutaneous pins or wires used to align and immobilize

1. Collaborative Care

   a. Monitor pulses and vascular status.

   b. Maintain proper body alignment.

   c. Verify weights are free hanging.

   d. Monitor skin for pressure points or breakdown.

   e. Promote strengthening exercises for uninjured areas.

   f. Consult with physical therapy.

   g. Pin site care per agency protocol.

   h. Administer medications (opioids, NSAIDs, muscle relaxants).

IV Osteoporosis

Chronic disease in which bone loss causes decreased density and possible fracture. Osteopenia is the precursor of osteoporosis.

A. **Contributing Factors**

1. Primary Osteoporosis

   a. Females age 65 and older

   b. Males age 75 and older

   c. Asian and Caucasian ethnicity

   d. Family history

   e. Estrogen or androgen deficiency

   f. Protein deficiency

   g. Sedentary lifestyle

   h. Smoking and alcohol intake

2. Secondary Osteoporosis

   a. Bone cancer

   b. Cushing's syndrome

   c. Diabetes mellitus

   d. Medications: corticosteroids, phenytoin, cytotoxic agents, immunosuppressants, loop diuretics

   e. Paget's disease

   f. Prolonged immobilization

   g. Rheumatoid arthritis

B. **Manifestations**

1. Shortened height

2. History of fractures

3. Thoracic kyphosis

4. Decreased bone mass

C. **Collaborative Care**

1. **Nursing Interventions**

   a. Encourage safe weight-bearing exercises.

   b. Reinforce teaching about strengthening exercises. Encourage walking.

   c. Remind clients to increase foods rich in calcium and vitamin D.

   d. Refer clients to smoking cessation program.

   e. Implement fall precautions.

EXTERNAL FIXATION DEVICES

Cervical Traction

Buck's Traction

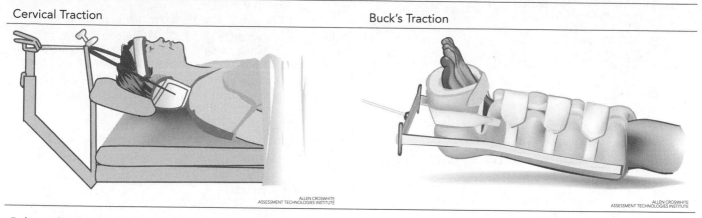

Balanced Suspension Skeletal Traction

Halo Traction

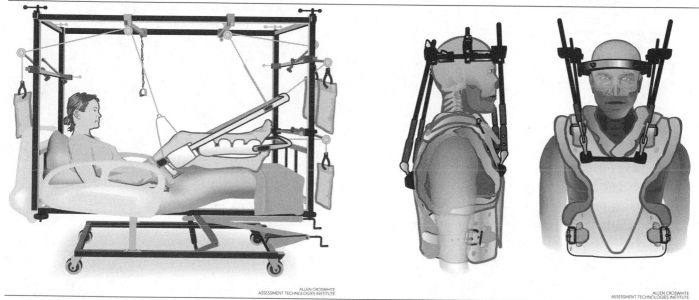

2. Medications
   a. Biophosphonates
   b. Calcium supplements
   c. Vitamin D supplements
   d. Estrogen agonists/antagonists
   e. Calcitonin
   f. Parathyroid hormone (prepared as teriparatide): Reinforce teaching to administer subcutaneously each day.
3. Client Education
   a. Continue health screenings and diagnostic evaluations.
   b. Avoid activities with increased risk of falls (ice, slippery surfaces).
   c. Take medications as prescribed.

ⅴ Osteomyelitis

An acute or chronic bone infection

A. **Contributing Factors**
   1. Diabetes
   2. Hemodialysis
   3. Injection drug use
   4. Poor blood supply
   5. Recent trauma

B. **Manifestations**
   1. Bone pain
   2. Fever
   3. General discomfort, uneasiness, or ill feeling (malaise)
   4. Local swelling, redness, and warmth
   5. Other possible manifestations
      a. Chills
      b. Excessive sweating
      c. Low-back pain
      d. Swelling of the ankles, feet, and legs

C. **Diagnostic Procedures**

1. Bone biopsy (which is then cultured)
2. Bone scan
3. Bone x-ray
4. Complete blood count (CBC)
5. CRP
6. ESR
7. MRI of the bone
8. Needle aspiration of the area around affected bones

D. **Collaborative Care**

1. **Nursing Interventions**

   a. Initiate IV antibiotic therapy as soon as possible.
   b. In the presence of wound drainage, implement contact precautions.
   c. Reinforce that the full course of antibiotics must be completed, even if manifestations disappear.
   d. Implement wound irrigation.
   e. Refer to wound care nurse as needed.

2. Medications

   a. Antibiotics
   b. Analgesics

3. Therapeutic Measures

   a. Surgical excision of dead and infected bone can be needed.
   b. Bone grafting can be performed in large impacted areas.

VI Total Joint Arthroplasty (Replacement)

Surgical procedure performed to replace a joint with a prosthetic system. Arthroplasty can be performed for ankle, finger, elbow, shoulder, toe, and wrist. The hip and knee arthroplasties are the most commonly performed procedures.

KNEE REPLACEMENT

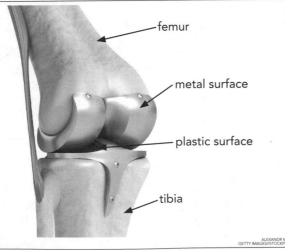

femur

metal surface

plastic surface

tibia

ALEXANDR MITIUC
GETTY IMAGES/ISTOCKPHOTO

A. **Contributing Factors**

1. Impaired mobility and uncontrolled pain related to osteoarthritis
2. Congenital anomalies
3. Trauma
4. Osteonecrosis

B. **Collaborative Care**

1. **Nursing Interventions**

   a. Position clients correctly, maintaining alignment.
      1) Hip arthroplasty: Keep abductor pillow in place while in bed. Do not flex hip more than 90°. (Do not position the client on the operative site.)
      2) Knee arthroplasty: Maintain continue passive motion (CPM) machine to promote joint mobility.
   b. Monitor for pain, rotation, and extremity shortening.
   c. Monitor neurovascular status.
   d. Use aseptic technique for wound care and emptying of drains.
   e. Monitor for indications of infection.
   f. Ambulate the day of surgery, after stabilization and discharge from PACU.
   g. Use a toilet seat extender.
   h. Reinforce teaching of exercises to reduce risk of DVT (ankle dorsiflexion, circles with the feet, pushing feet into bed while tightening quads, straight-leg raises).

2. Medications

   a. Anticoagulants
   b. NSAIDs
   c. Opioid narcotics; extended-release epidural morphine or PCA
   d. Antibiotics

3. Client Education

   a. Participate in exercise regimen.
   b. Use of ambulatory devices.

C. **Referral and Follow-up**

1. Physical therapy for ambulation, transfer, and joint movement
2. Occupational therapy to meet goals of independence and self-care

VII Amputations

Removal of a part of the body; can be elective or traumatic

A. **Types of Amputations**

1. Above-the-knee
2. Below-the-knee
3. Mid-foot
4. Toe

B. **Contributing Factors**

1. Peripheral vascular disease
2. Severe crushing of tissues or significant vessels
3. Malignant tumors
4. Osteomyelitis
5. Thermal injuries

C. **Collaborative Care**

1. **Nursing Interventions**
   a. Monitor neurovascular status.
   b. Monitor psychosocial status.
   c. Monitor client's willingness and motivation to withstand prolonged rehabilitation.
   d. Manage phantom limb and residual limb pain.
   e. Monitor for signs of wound healing.
   f. Monitor for complications
      1) Hemorrhage
      2) Infection
      3) Phantom limb pain
      4) Flexion contractures
   g. Promote mobility and range of motion.
   h. Promote independence.
   i. Maintain aseptic technique with dressing changes.
   j. Wrap residual limb with figure-8 elastic bandage after surgical dressing is removed.

FIGURE-8 BANDAGE

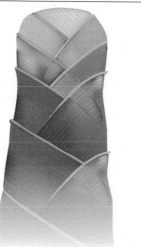

ALLEN CROSWHITE
ASSESSMENT TECHNOLOGIES INSTITUTE

2. Medications
   a. Opioids for residual limb pain
   b. Calcitonin to reduce phantom pain
   c. Antispasmodics for muscle spasms
   d. Beta blockers for constant, dull, burning pain
   e. Antiepileptic drugs for knifelike or sharp burning pain
3. Client Education
   a. Types of pain and management regimen
   b. Measures to prevent contractures
   c. Use of ambulatory devices or prosthetics
D. **Referral and Follow-Up**
1. Rehabilitation therapy
2. Support group

Endocrine System Functions and Disorders

Overview of the endocrine system: The endocrine system is made up of glands, organs, and hormones. The endocrine system works with the nervous system to regulate body function and maintain homeostasis through feedback loops. Endocrine glands include the hypothalamus, pituitary gland, adrenal glands, thyroid gland, parathyroid glands, islet cells of the pancreas, and gonads.

I Pituitary Gland

A. **Anterior pituitary gland:** Secretion of these hormones is controlled by the hypothalamus.
   1. Adrenocorticotropic hormone (ACTH)
   2. Follicle-stimulating hormone (FSH)
   3. Luteinizing hormone (LH)
   4. Gonadotropic hormones
   5. Prolactin
   6. Growth hormone (GH)
   7. Thyroid-stimulating hormone (TSH)
B. **Posterior pituitary gland**
   1. Vasopressin (antidiuretic hormone [ADH])
   2. Oxytocin

II Disorders of the Anterior Pituitary Gland

A. **Acromegaly:** Hypersecretion of GH that occurs after puberty
   1. Manifestations
      a. Enlargement of skeletal extremities; increase in adult height; change in ring or shoe size
      b. Protrusion of the jaw and orbital ridges
      c. Headache, visual problems, blindness
      d. Muscle weakness
      e. Organ enlargement
      f. Decalcification of the skeleton
      g. Endocrine disturbances similar hyperthyroidism
   2. Diagnostic Procedures
      a. Serum studies show elevated GH levels.
      b. CT and MRI of pituitary can show pituitary tumor.
      c. X-rays show abnormal bone growth.
   3. Collaborative Care
      a. **Nursing Interventions**
         1) Provide emotional support.
         2) Provide symptomatic care.
         3) Prepare the client for surgery or radiation if indicated for tumor treatment.
      b. Medications
         1) Octreotide: synthetic GH analogue
         2) Bromocriptine mesylate or pergolide: dopamine agonists

c. Therapeutic Measures

  1) Surgical removal of pituitary gland (transsphenoidal hypophysectomy); surgery is generally the first treatment option.

  2) Replacement therapy will be needed following surgical removal of the pituitary gland and can be needed following radiation therapy.

    a) Corticosteroids

    b) Thyroid hormones

  3) Radiation therapy

4. Client Education and Referral

  a. Adhere to medications.

  b. Continue adherence to follow-up appointments with all providers.

B. **Gigantism:** Hypersecretion of GH that occurs in childhood prior to closure of the growth plates

1. Manifestations

  a. Proportional overgrowth in all body tissue

2. Diagnostic Procedures/Collaborative Care: Same as acromegaly

C. **Dwarfism:** Hyposecretion of GH during fetal development or childhood that results in limited growth congenital or result from damage to the pituitary gland.

1. Manifestations

  a. Head and extremities disproportionate to torso

    1) Face can appear younger than peers'

  b. Short stature; slow or flat growth rate

  c. Progressive bowed legs and lordosis

  d. Delayed adolescence or puberty

2. Diagnostic Procedures

  a. Comparison of height/weight against growth charts: slowed growth rate will be noted.

  b. Serum growth hormone level; most providers also evaluate other hormonal levels to ensure that no secondary deficiencies exist.

  c. MRI of the head (to assess pituitary gland).

3. Collaborative Care

  a. **Nursing Interventions**

    1) Reinforce teaching with the child and family about adaptive measures available for ADLs.

    2) Reinforce with the child and family how to administer supplemental GH.

     a) The earlier the therapy is initiated, the better the prognosis.

     b) GH therapy does not work in all children.

    3) Provide positive feedback to child to promote positive self-esteem.

  b. Medications

    1) Human growth hormone injections

III *Disorders of the Posterior Pituitary Gland*

A. **Diabetes Insipidus (DI):** A deficiency of antidiuretic hormone (ADH or vasopressin) due to a disorder of the posterior pituitary gland that results in the inability of the kidneys to conserve water appropriately. DI is caused by head trauma, tumor, surgery, radiation, CNS infections, malignant tumors, or failure of renal tubules. The underlying cause of DI should be identified and treated.

1. Manifestations

  a. Urine chemistry (dilute)

    1) Decreased urine specific gravity

    2) Decreased urine osmolality

  b. Serum chemistry (concentrated)

    1) Hypernatremia

    2) Increased serum osmolality

  c. Polyuria and polydipsia

    1) Increased urinary output

    2) Craving ice water in excessive amounts

  d. Dehydration, weight loss, muscle weakness, and dry skin

  e. Hemoconcentration

2. Diagnostic Procedures

  a. Water (fluid) deprivation test

    1) Monitor body weight, vital signs, and hourly urine output.

    2) Monitor serum and urine osmolality.

  b. Vasopressin test

    1) Performed only if fluid deprivation test is inconclusive.

    2) IV vasopressin is administered.

    3) Client urine and serum chemistries will improve.

  c. MRI of hypothalamus and pituitary

  d. 24-hr urine

3. Collaborative Care

  a. **Nursing Interventions**

    1) Weigh the client daily.

    2) Monitor urine output and urine specific gravity.

    3) Monitor blood pressure and heart rate.

    4) Maintain fluid and electrolyte balance.

  b. Medications

    1) Desmopressin acetate

    2) Vasopressin

    3) If DI is nephrogenic in origin, thiazide diuretics will be prescribed.

  c. Client Education and Referral

    1) Lifetime vasopressin replacement therapy.

    2) Report weight gain or loss, polyuria, or polydipsia to the provider.

    3) Monitor fluid intake and urine output.

    4) Avoid foods with diuretic action.

B. **Syndrome of Inappropriate Secretion of Antidiuretic Hormone (SIADH):** The excessive release of ADH resulting in the inability to excrete an appropriate amount of urine thus developing fluid retention and dilutional hyponatremia. Caused by neoplastic tumors, head injury, meningitis, respiratory disorders, and some medications (vincristine, phenothiazines, tricyclic antidepressants, thiazide diuretics), and nicotine.

1. Manifestations
    a. Urine chemistry (concentrated)
        1) Increased urine specific gravity and osmolality
    b. Serum chemistry (dilute)
        1) Hyponatremia
        2) Decreased serum osmolality
    c. Mental confusion, irritability, lethargy, and seizures (due to hyponatremia)
    d. Weakness, anorexia, nausea, and vomiting (due to hyponatremia)
    e. Increased ADH (vasopressin) levels
    f. Weight gain
2. Collaborative Care
    a. **Nursing Interventions**
        1) Restrict oral fluids to 500 to 1,000 mL/day.
        2) Monitor I&O.
        3) Weigh the client daily.
        4) Monitor for increased blood pressure, tachycardia, and hypothermia.
        5) Monitor mental status frequently. Initiate seizure precautions.
    b. Medications
        1) Hypertonic saline infusion (3% to 5% sodium chloride)
        2) Loop diuretics; used to treat hypervolemic hyponatremia
        3) Declomycin
        4) Vasopressin receptor antagonists
            a) Conivaptan
    c. Therapeutic Measures
        1) Treat the underlying cause with surgery, chemotherapy, and/or radiation.

IV Adrenal Gland

The adrenal cortex produces glucocorticoids (cortisol), mineralocorticoids (aldosterone), and sex hormones. The adrenal medulla produces the catecholamines epinephrine and norepinephrine.

V Disorders of the Adrenal Cortex

A. **Addison's disease (adrenal insufficiency):** The hyposecretion of adrenal cortex hormones caused by autoimmune disease, TB, histoplasmosis, adrenalectomy, tumors, HIV; can be induced by abrupt cessation of steroid medications

MEMORY HINT: With Addison's you need to **add** cortisol.

1. Manifestations
    a. Weakness and fatigue
    b. Nausea and vomiting
    c. Hyperpigmentation
    d. Hypotension; increased heart rate
    e. Hypoglycemia, hyponatremia, hyperkalemia, hypercalcemia
    f. Craving salty foods
    g. Emotional lability and depression
    h. Diminished libido
2. Diagnostic Procedures
    a. Serum adrenocortical hormone levels
    b. ACTH stimulation test
    c. Electrolyte panels
    d. Abdominal/renal CT scan
3. Collaborative Care
    a. **Nursing Interventions**
        1) Monitor blood pressure and heart rhythm.
        2) Monitor fluid and electrolyte balance.
        3) Monitor and treat hypoglycemia.
        4) Monitor for Addisonian crisis (also known as adrenal crisis), characterized by signs of shock (hypotension, tachycardia, tachypnea, pallor). It occurs secondary to stressors (infection, trauma, surgery, pregnancy, emotional stress). The client requires IV fluid replacement and IV steroids and can require respiratory support.
        5) Monitor for adverse effects of hormone replacement therapy, which are the same manifestations as hypersecretion of the adrenal cortex.
    b. Medications—adrenocorticoid replacement
        1) Hydrocortisone
        2) Prednisone
        3) Cortisone

c. Client Education and Referral

1) Provide emotional support and reinforce teaching about lifelong disease management (medications, prompt treatment of infection and illness, stress management).

2) Reinforce teaching about lifelong medication replacement, including the a potential need for increased steroid therapy during times of stress or illness.

   a) Manifestations of excessive or insufficient hormone replacement

   b) Promptly notify the provider in cases of infection, injury, and stress. Doses of hormones need to be individually adjusted during these times.

3) Indications of Addisonian crisis.

4) Avoid using caffeine and alcohol.

5) Have appropriate medical identification at all times in case of emergency.

6) Eat a high-protein, high-carbohydrate diet.

B. **Cushing's Disease and Cushing's Syndrome:** The hypersecretion of the glucocorticoids caused by hyperplasia of the adrenal cortex or pituitary gland tumor. Cushing's syndrome is caused by exogenous use of steroid medications.

1. Manifestations

   a. Upper body obesity and thin extremities; moon face, buffalo hump, and neck fat

   b. Skin fragility with purple striae

   c. Osteoporosis

   d. Hyperglycemia, hypernatremia, hypokalemia, and hypocalcemia

   e. Hirsutism

   f. Amenorrhea

   g. Elevated triglycerides and hypertension

   h. Sexual dysfunction; decreased libido, erectile dysfunction in men

   i. Immunosuppression

   j. Peptic ulcer disease

   k. Slowed growth rate in children

   l. Backache, bone pain, or tenderness

   m. Increased thirst and urination

2. Diagnostic Procedures

   a. Dexamethasone suppression test (dexamethasone administered at 2300; plasma cortisol levels obtained at 0800). Suppression of cortisol indicates the hypothalamic–pituitary–adrenal axis is functioning properly.

   b. Nighttime salivary cortisol levels

3. Collaborative Care

   a. **Nursing Interventions**

   1) Monitor for infection.

   2) Protect the client from accidents and falls.

   3) Monitor and treat hyperglycemia.

   4) Monitor blood pressure and heart rhythm.

b. Medications

1) Adrenal enzyme inhibitors (metyrapone, aminoglutethimide, mitotane, ketoconazole)

c. Therapeutic Measures

1) For a pituitary adenoma, the client can need a transsphenoidal adenomectomy.

2) For an adrenal carcinoma, the client can need a unilateral or bilateral adrenalectomy.

3) Monitor for adrenal insufficiency following postsurgery.

4) Slowly taper corticosteroid therapy.

d. Client Education and Referral

1) Explain the risks associated with long-term hormone suppression therapy with Cushing's disease. Steroid doses must be tapered in Cushing's syndrome.

2) Eat foods high in protein and calcium, low in carbohydrates and sodium, with potassium supplementation.

3) Practice infection prevention, fall precautions, and skin care.

4 S's OF CUSHING'S AND ADDISON'S DISEASE

	CUSHINGS DISEASE (Big S's) ↑	ADDISONS DISEASE (Small S's) ↓
Steroid	↑	↓ (need to "add")
Sugar	↑	↓
Sodium	↑	↓
Skin	Thin, fragile, striae	Hyperpigmented

C. **Hyperaldosteronism (Conn's syndrome):** The hypersecretion of aldosterone from the adrenal cortex (usually due to a tumor), manifestations of Cushing's syndrome.

1. Manifestations

   a. Hypokalemia and hypernatremia

   b. Hypertension

   c. Muscle weakness, numbness, and cardiac problems

   d. Fatigue

   e. Headache

   f. Polyuria and polydipsia

   g. Alkalosis

2. Diagnostic Procedures

   a. Abdominal CT, MRI

   b. ECG

   c. Serum aldosterone/renin and potassium

   d. Urine aldosterone

3. Collaborative Care

   a. **Nursing Interventions**

   1) Provide a quiet environment.

   2) Monitor blood pressure and cardiac activity.

   3) Monitor potassium level and be prepared to replace potassium.

   4) Closely monitor I&O.

b. Medications

   1) Antihypertensive medications: spironolactone

   2) Eplerenone: Blocks action of aldosterone

c. Therapeutic Measures

   1) Surgical removal of tumor/adrenal gland if primary cause

VI Disorders of the Adrenal Medulla

A. **Pheochromocytoma:** A usually benign tumor of the adrenal medulla that causes hypersecretion of epinephrine and norepinephrine

1. Manifestations

   a. Most common signs are the 5 H's

     1) Hypertension

     2) Headache

     3) Hyperhidrosis (excessive sweating)

     4) Hypermetabolism

     5) Hyperglycemia

2. Diagnostic Procedures

   a. Plasma levels of catecholamines and metanephrine (catecholamine metabolite)

   b. 24-hr urine level of catecholamines and their metabolites

   c. CT, MRI, or PET scan

   d. Adrenal biopsy

   e. Clonidine suppression test (in clients who have pheochromocytoma, catecholamines are not suppressed)

3. Collaborative Care

   a. **Nursing Interventions**

     1) Monitor vital signs.

     2) Provide a high-calorie, nutritious diet. Avoid caffeine.

     3) Encourage frequent rest periods.

     4) Provide a quiet environment.

     5) Prevent stroke secondary to hypertensive crisis.

     6) Do not palpate or assess for CVA tenderness, as this can cause rupture of the tumor.

   b. Medications

     1) Alpha (phentolamine) and beta blocker (propranolol) to diminish the effect of norepinephrine prior to surgery

     2) Sodium nitroprusside

     3) Calcium channel blockers (nifedipine)

   c. Therapeutic Measures

     1) Surgical removal of tumor

VII Thyroid Gland

The thyroid gland has a rich blood supply and produces thyroxine (T_4), triiodothyronine (T_3), and calcitonin. T_4 and T_3 regulate metabolism, and calcitonin inhibits mobilization of calcium from bone and reduces blood calcium levels.

VIII Disorders of the Thyroid Gland

A. **Hypothyroidism:** Suboptimal levels of thyroid hormone resulting in decreased metabolism. Occurs most frequently in females age 30 to 60.

1. Manifestations

   a. Fatigue and weakness

   b. Increased sensitivity to cold

   c. Constipation

   d. Dry skin, brittle hair and nails

   e. Weight gain

   f. Deepened, hoarse voice

   g. Joint pain

   h. Hyperlipidemia and anemia

   i. Depression

   j. Menstrual disturbances

2. Diagnostic Procedures/Findings

   a. Low serum T_4 and T_3

   b. Elevated TSH (seen in primary hypothyroidism)

3. Myxedema coma is a rare, life-threatening condition seen in untreated or uncontrolled hypothyroidism. The client is hypothermic with changes in mental functioning ranging from depression to unconsciousness. The severely decreased metabolism causes respiratory depression and cardiovascular collapse. Management is to provide intensive supportive measures along with hemodynamic therapy. High mortality rate.

4. Collaborative Care

   a. **Nursing Interventions**

     1) Provide a warm environment.

     2) Provide a low-calorie, low-cholesterol, low-fat diet.

     3) Increase roughage and fluids.

     4) Avoid sedatives.

     5) Plan rest periods for the client.

     6) Weigh the client daily.

     7) Observe for manifestations of overdose of thyroid preparations (palpitations, insomnia, increased appetite, tremors).

   b. Medications

     1) Levothyroxine

   c. Client Education and Referral

     1) Reinforce education regarding lifelong medication therapy.

     2) Follow up with the provider.

     3) Take medication on an empty stomach each morning.

     4) Know manifestations of medication toxicity.

     5) Eat a diet high in fiber.

     6) Monitor the need for sleep.

B. **Hyperthyroidism:** The excessive secretion of thyroid hormones. Graves' disease is the most common type of hyperthyroid disease and causes overstimulation of the thyroid by circulating immunoglobulins.

1. Manifestations
   a. Anxiety and irritability
   b. Insomnia and fatigue
   c. Tachycardia
   d. Tremors
   e. Diaphoresis
   f. Intolerance of heat
   g. Weight loss (despite food intake)
   h. Exophthalmos
   i. Diarrhea
   j. Light or absent menstrual cycle

2. Diagnostic Procedures/Findings
   a. Elevated T_4 and T_3
   b. Decreased TSH

3. Thyroid storm is a life-threatening condition seen in untreated or uncontrolled hyperthyroidism. Manifestations include hyperpyrexia, tachycardia, hypertension, and other exaggerated symptoms of hyperthyroidism.

4. Collaborative Care
   a. **Nursing Interventions**
      1) Monitor vital signs. Report temperature increase of 1° or greater to provider immediately
      2) Promote comfort.
      3) Encourage the client to get adequate rest in a cool, quiet environment.
      4) Provide a high-calorie diet without extra stimulants.
      5) Weigh the client daily.
      6) Provide emotional support.
      7) Provide eye protection for the client who has exophthalmos by giving ophthalmic medicine, taping the client's eyes at night, and decreasing sodium and water.
      8) Elevate the head of the bed.
   b. Medications
      1) Beta blockers to manage tachycardia, anxiety, and tremors.
      2) Propylthiouracil (PTU): Blocks thyroid hormone production.
      3) Methimazole: Short-term use to block production of thyroxine; usually used no more than 8 weeks. Monitor CBC frequently for occurrence of agranulocytosis.
      4) Iodides decrease vascularity and inhibit the release of thyroid hormones. Administer through a straw to prevent staining of teeth.
         a) Lugol's solution
         b) Saturated solution of potassium iodide (SSKI): used prior to thyroidectomy
      5) A radioactive iodine treatment shrinks the thyroid gland. It can be used alone or prior to surgery. Reinforce teaching about appropriate radiation precautions.

   c. Therapeutic Measures
      1) Thyroidectomy: The removal of all or part of the thyroid gland. Requires a lifelong intake of levothyroxine and possible calcium supplementation.
         a) Preoperative goal: Decrease thyroid function toward normal range (euthyroid) using saturated solution of potassium iodide (SSKI) and antithyroid medication.
         b) Postoperative interventions
            (1) Place the client in the semi-Fowler's position.
            (2) Monitor the client's dressing, especially the back of the neck.
            (3) Observe for respiratory distress. Keep a tracheostomy tray, oxygen, and suction apparatus at the bedside.
            (4) Monitor for signs of hemorrhage.
            (5) Note any hoarseness, which indicates laryngeal nerve injury. Limit talking.
            (6) Observe for signs of tetany (Chvostek's and Trousseau's sign), which can indicate damage or accidental removal of parathyroid glands and subsequent hypocalcemia.
            (7) Keep calcium gluconate IV at the bedside.
            (8) Observe for thyroid storm caused by an increased release of the thyroid hormone due to manipulation of the thyroid gland.
            (9) Gradually increase the range of motion to the neck and support the client when sitting up.

IX Parathyroid Gland

Parathormone (parathyroid hormone) maintains calcium and phosphate balance.

X Disorders of the Parathyroid Gland

A. **Hypoparathyroidism:** The hyposecretion of parathyroid hormone (PTH), resulting in hypocalcemia and hyperphosphatemia usually caused by surgical removal of parathyroid gland tissue during parathyroidectomy, thyroidectomy, or radical neck dissection.

1. Manifestations—from hypocalcemia
   a. Paresthesia
   b. Muscle cramps and tetany
   c. Chvostek's sign: Tapping the side of the cheek causes muscle spasms and twitching around the mouth, throat, and cheeks.
   d. Trousseau's sign: Pressure from the blood pressure cuff induces muscle spasms in the distal extremity.
   e. Circumoral paresthesia with numbness and tingling of the fingers
   f. Severe tetany can lead to bronchospasm, laryngeal spasm, carpopedal spasm, dysphagia, cardiac dysrhythmias, and seizures.

2. Collaborative Care
   a. **Nursing Interventions**
      1) Monitor ECG.
      2) Monitor for signs of neuromuscular irritability.
      3) Provide a high-calcium, low-phosphorous diet.
      4) Institute seizure precautions.
   b. Medications
      1) Acute: IV calcium gluconate
      2) Chronic
         a) Oral calcium salts (generally calcium carbonate) and phosphate binders
         b) Vitamin D

B. **Hyperparathyroidism:** A hypersecretion of PTH (caused by tumor or renal disease) that leads to the loss of calcium from the bones into the serum, resulting in hypercalcemia and hypophosphatemia

   1. Manifestations—might not have symptoms
      a. Kidney stones (containing calcium)
      b. Osteoporosis
      c. Hypercalcemia and hypophosphatemia
      d. Abdominal pain, constipation, nausea, vomiting
      e. Muscle weakness and fatigue; skeletal and joint pain
      f. Polyuria and polydipsia
      g. Hypertension
      h. Cardiac dysrhythmias
   2. Collaborative Care
      a. **Nursing Interventions**
         1) Encourage a minimum of 2,000 mL of fluids daily.
         2) Provide a low-calcium, low-vitamin D diet.
         3) Prevent constipation and fecal impaction.
         4) Strain all of the client's urine.
         5) Reinforce teaching about safety measures to prevent fractures.
         6) Encourage cranberry juice to lower urinary pH.
         7) Monitor for hypercalcemic crisis, which is life-threatening. It usually occurs with serum calcium levels greater than 15 mg/dL.
            a) IV rehydration
            b) Phosphate therapy
            c) Calcitonin
            d) Dialysis
      b. Medications
         1) Calcimimetics (such as cinacalcet) mimic calcium in the blood and can cause the parathyroid to decrease the release of parathormone.
         2) Calcitonin decreases the release of skeletal calcium and increases the kidney excretion of calcium (enhanced if given along with glucocorticoids).
         3) Hydration and diuretics: Furosemide promotes excretion of excess calcium. (Avoid thiazide diuretics.)
         4) Biphosphates
      c. Therapeutic Measures
         1) Surgical removal of the parathyroid gland

XI **Pancreas**

The pancreas has exocrine (secretion of the pancreatic enzymes amylase, trypsin, and lipase, which aid in digestion) and endocrine (secretion of insulin, glucagon, and somatostatin) functions. Insulin lowers blood glucose by facilitating glucose entry into the cell. Somatostatin also lowers blood glucose levels. Glucagon raises blood glucose by converting glycogen to glucose in the liver.

XII *Disorders of the Pancreas*

A. **Diabetes mellitus:** A group of metabolic disorders characterized by hyperglycemia caused by altered insulin production, action, or a combination of both.

   1. **Type 1:** Usually characterized by an acute onset before 30 years old. In type 1 diabetes, the pancreatic beta cells are destroyed by either genetic predisposition (not inherited), immunologic, environmental, or a combination of these factors.
   2. **Type 2:** Usually occurs after 30 years old and is comprised of inadequate insulin production and insulin resistance.
      a. Contributing Factors
         1) Family history of diabetes
         2) Obesity
         3) More prevalent in African American, Native American, and Hispanic populations
         4) Hypertension
         5) History of gestational diabetes
         6) Sedentary lifestyle
   3. **Metabolic Syndrome**
      a. Insulin resistance leads to increase insulin production in attempt to maintain glucose at a normal level.
      b. Characterized by hypertension, hypercholesterolemia, and abdominal obesity.
      c. If the beta cells cannot produce enough insulin to meet the demands, type 2 diabetes will develop.
   4. Diagnostic Criteria
      a. Symptoms of diabetes plus casual plasma glucose of 200 mg/dL or greater, or
      b. Fasting plasma glucose of 126 mg/dL or greater, or
      c. 2-hr postload glucose of 200 mg/dL or greater during an oral glucose tolerance test
   5. Glycemic Control
      a. Glucose control is monitored on a day-to-day basis by capillary blood glucose levels.
         1) Normal preprandial (fasting) blood glucose is 70 to 105 mg/dL.
         2) Normal postprandial blood glucose is less than 180 mg/dL.
      b. Glucose control is monitored on a long-term basis by HbA1c (glycosylated hemoglobin).

6. Manifestations
   a. "3 Polys"
      1) Polyuria
      2) Polydipsia
      3) Polyphagia
   b. Fatigue and weakness
   c. Sudden vision changes
   d. Recurrent infections
   e. Slow wound healing
   f. Type 1 diabetes
      1) Sudden weight loss
      2) Nausea, vomiting, or abdominal pain
7. Long-Term Complications
   a. Neuropathy
   b. Nephropathy
   c. Retinopathy
   d. Cardiovascular disease
   e. Infection and slow wound healing
8. Collaborative Care
   a. **Nursing Interventions**
      1) Monitor blood glucose.
      2) Administer medication as prescribed.
      3) Reinforce client education.
      4) Monitor vital signs and I&O.
      5) Refer clients to a diabetic educator.
      6) Monitor for complications.
   b. Possible Complications
      1) Hypoglycemia occurs when the blood glucose level falls below 60 mg/dL.
         a) Causes: Decreased dietary intake, excess insulin, increased exercise
         b) Manifestations
            (1) Tachycardia
            (2) Diaphoresis
            (3) Weakness, fatigue
            (4) Irritability, anxiety
            (5) Confusion
            (6) Headache, blurred vision
         c) **Nursing Interventions**
            (1) Administer 15 g fast-acting simple carbohydrates.
               (a) Three or four glucose tablets for the equivalent to 15 g carbohydrates
               (b) 4 oz fruit juice or regular soda
               (c) Six to 10 hard candies
               (d) 2 to 3 teaspoons sugar or honey
            (2) If the client is unconscious or unable to swallow, administer glucagon IM or subcutaneous. Repeat in 10 min if client is still unconscious and notify provider.

            (3) Follow the 15/15/15 rule.
               (a) Administer 15 g fast-acting carbohydrates.
               (b) Wait 15 min and recheck blood glucose.
               (c) Administer another 15 g carbohydrates if blood glucose remains less than 70 mg/dL.
               (d) Give 7 g protein when blood glucose is within normal limits.
                  i) 2 tablespoons peanut butter
                  ii) 1 oz cheese
                  iii) 8 oz milk
      2) **Transient Hyperglycemia:** An elevated blood glucose; generally treated with sliding scale insulin to return serum blood glucose to normal range
         a) Prompt treatment is necessary to avoid hyperglycemic emergencies.
            (1) Treat with regular insulin.
            (2) Do not hold insulin when blood glucose is in the normal range.
            (3) Reinforce education on importance and strategies to maintain blood glucose in the normal range.
   c. Medications (see Unit Four: Pharmacology in Nursing)
      1) Insulin pump: An external device that provides a basal dose of rapid-acting or regular insulin with a bolus dose for meals, which is calculated by the client using a predetermined insulin-to-carbohydrate ratio; does not read blood glucose.
         a) Needles are inserted into subcutaneous abdominal tissue. (Change site at least every 3 days.)
         b) Complications are secondary to continuous administration of insulin or from disruption of insulin infusion.
         c) Allows for flexibility of diet.
   d. Client Education
      1) Nutritional therapy as prescribed (exchange, carbohydrate counting, calories, healthy food choices)
      2) Importance of consistent exercise
      3) Self-glucose monitoring and interpretation of results
      4) Medication administration
         a) Medication importance and schedule
         b) Medication route (PO, subcutaneous, insulin pump)
         c) Rotation of injection within an anatomic area

5) Manifestations and management of hypo and hyperglycemia

6) Wear medical alert bracelet.

7) Foot care

   a) Cleanse feet daily in warm, soapy water. Rinse and dry carefully.

   b) Trim nails straight across.

   c) Wear supportive, protective shoes.

   d) Do not go barefoot. Inspect feet daily, including between the toes.

8) Guidelines during illness ("sick day rules")

   a) Take usual doses of insulin or antidiabetic agents.

   b) Test blood glucose and urine for ketones every 3 to 4 hr.

   c) Report elevated blood glucose or urine ketones to the provider.

   d) Consume 4 oz sugar-free, noncaffeinated fluids every 30 min to prevent dehydration.

   e) Eat small, frequent meals of soft foods or liquids to meet carbohydrate needs.

B. **Diabetic Ketoacidosis:** An acute, life-threatening complication of diabetes mellitus due to insufficient insulin. Main manifestations are hyperglycemia (blood glucose levels vary between 300 to 800 mg/dL), acidosis, dehydration, and fluid loss; most common in type 1 diabetes mellitus.

1. Contributing Factors

   a. Decreased or missed dose of insulin

   b. Illness or infection

   c. Undiagnosed or untreated diabetes

2. Manifestations

   a. Exacerbated polyuria, polydipsia, polyphagia

   b. Anorexia, nausea, vomiting, abdominal pain

   c. Metabolic acidosis with ketonuria

   d. Kussmaul respirations

   e. Acetone breath (fruity odor)

   f. Altered mental status, blurred vision, headache

   g. Weak, rapid pulse

   h. Orthostatic hypotension

3. Collaborative Care

   a. **Nursing Interventions**

      1) Monitor blood glucose, LOC, vital signs, and strict I&O.

      2) Administer prescribed IV fluids to promote perfusion.

         a) Normal saline infusion to maintain perfusion.

         b) Follow with 45% saline infusion to replace total body fluid losses.

         c) Add fluids containing dextrose when blood glucose is approximately 250 mg/dL.

      3) Administer insulin.

         a) Insulin infusion usually at 0.1 mg/kg/hr. Regular insulin is the only insulin that can be given IV.

         b) Usually blood glucose checks hourly while on an insulin infusion.

         c) Resume subcutaneous when possible.

      4) Monitor potassium levels and replace as prescribed.

      5) Monitor acid–base balance.

      6) Reinforce strategies to prevent DKA and hyperglycemic hyperosmolar state (HHS).

C. **Hyperglycemic Hyperosmolar State:** An acute, life-threatening complication of diabetes (more commonly in type 2). It is characterized by elevated blood glucose levels greater than 600 mg/dL, a hyperosmolar state, which leads to fluid and electrolyte losses.

1. Contributing Factors

   a. Acute illness (surgery, infection, CVA)

   b. Medications that exacerbate hyperglycemia (such as thiazides)

   c. Treatments (such as dialysis)

2. Manifestations

   a. Clinical signs of dehydration

      1) Hypotension and tachycardia

      2) Elevated BUN

   b. Generally not seen with ketosis

   c. Altered mental status

3. Collaborative Care

   a. **Nursing Interventions**

      1) Replace fluids as prescribed. (Monitor for fluid overload.)

      2) Administer insulin and electrolytes as prescribed.

      3) Monitor blood glucose, LOC, vital signs, electrolyte levels, and acid–base balance.

      4) Reinforce strategies to prevent HHS.

ENDOCRINE END-OF-SECTION REVIEW

1. The client who has syndrome of inappropriate antidiuretic hormone (SIADH) would have _____ serum and concentrated _____. The opposite would be true for diabetes insipidus (DI).

2. A medication that is beneficial in the treatment of diabetes insipidus (DI) is _____.

3. The client who is receiving long-term _____ therapy can have symptoms similar to those of the client who has Cushing's disease. This client is at risk to develop Addisonian crisis, which can cause dehydration and cardiovascular collapse, if this medication therapy is _____ stopped.

4. The client who has pheochromocytoma is at risk for cerebral vascular accident (CVA) secondary to _____ crisis.

5. The client who has _____ would be expected to have the following laboratory findings: thyroid stimulating hormone (TSH) level increased and thyroxine (T_4) and triiodothyronine (T_3) decreased. The medication usually given for this disorder is _____. A potentially life-threatening condition that can be caused when this disorder is untreated can lead to decreased cardiac output and organ failure due to severely decreased metabolism is called _____.

6. The client can develop hypoparathyroidism following surgical removal of the thyroid gland. The client can experience manifestations related to alteration in _____ levels. Potentially life-threatening manifestations that the nurse needs to monitor for in clients who have alteration in this electrolyte are _____, _____, and _____.

7. It is important to reinforce teaching about appropriate foot care to the client who has diabetes mellitus. This includes reminding the client to always wear socks and protective _____ and inspect, wash, and thoroughly _____ the feet daily.

8. The client needs to be taught to _____ injection sites within the same anatomical location when giving insulin injections.

9. A client who has diabetes has a blood glucose level less than 70 mg/dL. The appropriate intervention would be to give the client 15 g carbohydrates, which can include _____. The blood glucose is rechecked in 15 min and is now 90 mg/dL. The appropriate interventions would be to give the client 7 g protein, which can include _____.

10. The priority interventions during the management of diabetic ketoacidosis (DKA) and hyperglycemic hyperosmolar state (HHS) focus on restoration of _____, _____ (particularly potassium), and acid-base balance, and reduction of _____ levels.

WORD BANK

4 oz fruit juice

1 oz cheese

Addison's disease

blood glucose

calcium

corticosteroid

desmopressin acetate (DDAVP)

dilute

dry

dysrhythmias

electrolyte

fluid

hypertensive

hypothyroidism

laryngospasms

myxedema coma

rotate

seizures

shoes

suddenly

levothyroxine

urine

Answer Key: 1. Dilute, urine; 2. Desmopressin acetate (DDAVP); 3. Corticosteroid, suddenly; 4. Hypertensive; 5. Hypothyroidism, levothyroxine, myxedema coma; 6. Calcium, dysrhythmia, laryngospasms, seizures; 7. Shoes, dry; 8. Rotate; 9. 4 oz fruit juice, 1 oz cheese; 10. Fluid, electrolyte, blood glucose

Hematologic Disorders

A. **Anemia:** A deficiency of RBCs characterized by a decreased functional RBC count, Hgb/Hct, or both. Anemia is a clinical condition that results in decreased oxygen delivery to the cells.

1. Contributing Factors
   a. Acute or chronic blood loss (gastrointestinal bleeding)
   b. Greater than normal destruction of RBCs (spleen diseases)
   c. Abnormal bone marrow function (chemotherapy)
   d. Decreased erythropoietin (renal failure)
   e. Inadequate maturation of RBCs (cancer)
   f. Nutritional deficiencies (iron, B_{12}, folic acid, intrinsic factor)

2. Manifestations
   a. Fatigue and weakness
   b. Dizziness and headaches
   c. Pallor: First seen in conjunctiva (light-skinned clients) and mucosal membranes (dark-skinned clients), as well as nail beds, palmar creases, and around the mouth
   d. Tachycardia, murmurs, gallops, and orthostatic hypotension
   e. Decreased activity tolerance
   f. Decreased Hgb, Hct, and RBC levels
   g. Shortness of breath and dyspnea; decreased oxygen saturation levels

3. Collaborative Care
   a. **Nursing Interventions**
      1) Monitor labs (RBC, Hgb, Hct).
      2) Encourage activity as tolerated with frequent rest periods.
      3) Monitor skin integrity and implement measures to prevent breakdown.
      4) Provide oxygen therapy to the client as needed.
      5) Administer blood products and medications as prescribed. (See individual anemias.)
      6) Encourage foods high in iron (meats, poultry, fish).

B. **Types of Anemia**

1. **Anemia secondary to renal disease:** Anemia due to lack of erythropoietin
   a. Medications
      1) Erythropoietin

2. **Iron deficiency anemia:** Anemia resulting from low iron levels. The iron stores are depleted first, followed by hemoglobin stores.
   a. Contributing Factors
      1) Chronic blood loss (bleeding ulcer)
      2) Nutritional deficiency
      3) Common in infants, older adults, and young adult females (due to pregnancy or menses)

   b. Manifestations
      1) Microcytic red blood cells
      2) Weakness and pallor
      3) Low serum ferritin levels
   c. Collaborative Care
      1) **Nursing Interventions**
         a) Monitor for symptoms of bleeding.
         b) Monitor labs.
      2) Medications
         a) Administer iron preparations.
      3) Therapeutic Measures
         a) Follow prescriptions for ulcer treatment.

3. **Aplastic anemia:** Bone marrow suppression of new stem cell production resulting in a deficiency of circulating WBCs, platelets, and/or RBCs. Can be due to medications, viruses, toxins, or radiation exposure.
   a. Manifestations
      1) Hypoxia, fatigue, and pallor (related to anemia)
      2) Increased susceptibility to infection (related to leukopenia)
      3) Hemorrhage, ecchymosis/petechiae (related to thrombocytopenia)
      4) Pancytopenia (decrease in RBCs, WBCs, and platelets)
   b. Collaborative Care
      1) **Nursing Interventions**
         a) Monitor labs.
         b) Provide protective isolation.
         c) Monitor for manifestations of infection.
         d) Provide emotional and psychological support.
         e) Implement protective barrier precautions.
         f) Prepare the client for bone marrow aspiration/biopsy.
      2) Medications
         a) Immunosuppressive therapy (prednisone, cyclosporine)
         b) Chemotherapy medications
      3) Therapeutic Measures
         a) Hematopoietic stem cell transplantation
         b) Splenectomy
         c) Cautious use of blood transfusions

4. **B_{12} deficiency anemias (macrocytic):** Anemia due to a lack of dietary intake or absorption of vitamin B_{12}
   a. Contributing Factors
      1) Atrophy of the gastric mucosa/hypochlorhydria (underproduction of hydrochloric acid by the stomach)
      2) Total gastrectomy (lack of intrinsic factor decreases intestinal vitamin B_{12} absorption)
      3) Malnutrition
   b. Manifestations
      1) Numbness and tingling of extremities (paresthesia)
      2) Hypoxemia
      3) Pallor

4) Jaundice

5) Glossitis

6) Poor balance

c. Diagnostic Procedures

1) Shilling test is used to differentiate malabsorption versus pernicious anemia by measuring absorption of B_{12} with and without intrinsic factor after the client receives an oral dose of radioactive vitamin B_{12}.

2) CBC: Megaloblastic RBCs (macrocytic)

d. Collaborative Care

1) **Nursing Interventions**

a) Monitor labs.

b) Promote rest and encourage a balanced dietary intake.

2) Medications

a) Cyanocobalamin (vitamin B_{12}): Standard dose is 1,000 mcg IM daily for 2 weeks, then weekly until Hct level is therapeutic, then monthly for life. Cyanocobalamin intranasally maintains vitamin B_{12} levels.

5. **Folic acid deficiency anemia:** Anemia due to folic acid deficiency. Symptoms similar to vitamin B_{12} deficiency, but nervous system functions remain normal.

a. Contributing Factors

1) Poor nutrition

2) Malabsorption (secondary to Crohn's disease)

3) Drugs (alcohol use disorder, anticonvulsants, oral contraceptives)

b. Collaborative Care

1) **Nursing Interventions**

a) Identify high-risk clients (clients who have alcohol use disorder, older adult clients, clients who are debilitated).

2) Medications

a) Folic acid replacement

6. **Hemolytic and Aplastic anemia:** A group of anemias that occur when bone marrow is unable to increase production to make up for premature destruction of red blood cells. Sickle cell and thalassemia are hemolytic anemias. Aplastic anemia often occurs with leukopenia, thrombocytopenia, and pancytopenia.

a. Contributing Factors

1) Trauma, crushing injuries

2) Lead poisoning

3) Tuberculosis

4) Infections

5) Transfusion reactions

6) Toxic agents

7) Radiation exposure

b. Manifestations

1) Chills

2) Dark urine

3) Enlarged spleen

4) Pallor

5) Rapid heart rate

6) Shortness of breath

7) Jaundice

c. Collaborative Care

1) **Nursing Interventions**

a) Treat the underlying cause.

b) Hydrate the client.

c) Blood transfusion when kidney function is normal.

2) Medications

a) In severe immune-related hemolytic anemia, steroid therapy is sometimes necessary.

b) Hematopoietic stem cell transplantation for aplastic anemia if other treatments fail.

7. **Sickle cell anemia:** A genetic defect found in clients of African American or Mediterranean origin, in which the Hgb molecule assumes a sickle shape and delivers less oxygen to tissues. The sickle cells become lodged in the blood vessels, especially the brain and the kidneys.

a. Contributing Factors (precipitate crisis by enhancing sickling)

1) Stress

2) Dehydration

3) Hypoxia

4) High altitudes

5) Infections

b. Manifestations

1) Severe pain and swelling

2) Fever

3) Jaundice

4) Susceptibility to infection

5) Hypoxic damage to organs (spleen, liver, heart, kidney, brain)

c. Diagnostic Procedures

1) Percentage of hemoglobin S (Hgb S) seen on electrophoresis. Sickle cell trait has less than 40% Hgb S, and sickle cell disease can have 80% to 100% Hgb S.

d. Collaborative Care

1) **Nursing Interventions**

a) Maintain adequate hydration.

b) Provide oxygen therapy.

c) Encourage the client to rest and avoid high altitudes, alcohol, and temperature extremes.

d) Reinforce teaching with the client to identify triggers and get immunizations in a timely manner. Refer for genetic counseling.

2) Medications

a) Morphine sulfate or hydromorphone to manage pain

b) Hydroxyurea to reduce the amount of sickling and number of painful episodes

8. **Thalassemia:** Inherited blood disorder in which the body makes an abnormal form of hemoglobin, resulting in excessive destruction of red blood cells, which leads to anemia

a. Contributing Factors

1) Must inherit the defective gene from both parents to develop thalassemia major

2) Asian, Mediterranean, or African ethnicity

3) Family history of the disorder

b. Manifestations
   1) Develops during the first year of life
   2) Bone deformities in the face
   3) Fatigue
   4) Growth failure
   5) Shortness of breath
   6) Yellow skin (jaundice)
c. Diagnostic Procedures
   1) Red blood cells appear small and abnormally shaped.
   2) Complete blood count (CBC) reveals anemia.
   3) Hemoglobin electrophoresis shows the presence of an abnormal form of hemoglobin.
   4) Mutational analysis detects alpha thalassemia that cannot be seen with hemoglobin electrophoresis.
d. Collaborative Care
   1) **Nursing Interventions**
      a) Encourage increase of folate in the diet by including dark green, leafy vegetables; dried beans and peas (legumes); and citrus fruits and juices.
      b) Administer blood transfusions.
      c) Encourage rest.
      d) Provide genetic counseling.
   2) Therapeutic Measures
      a) Treatment often involves regular blood transfusions.
      b) Clients receiving blood transfusions should not take iron supplements, as this can cause high iron levels in the blood.
      c) Chelation therapy can be necessary to remove excess iron from the body.
      d) Bone marrow transplant can help treat the disease in some clients, especially children.
   3) Medications
      a) Folic acid

SECTION 8

Cardiovascular System Disorders

I Cardiovascular Overview

A. Efficiently pumps blood to all parts of the body, indicating healthy working cardiac muscles and system.
B. Circulates adequate blood volume to meet the body's needs.
C. Adequate blood pressure is maintained by peripheral vasculature.
D. Normal heart rate is 60 to 100/min.

II Diagnostic Procedures

A. **Laboratory tests**
   1. Serum electrolytes
   2. Erythrocyte sedimentation rate (ESR)
   3. C-reactive protein
   4. Blood coagulation tests
      a. PTT: Most significant if the client is on heparin therapy
      b. PT: Most significant if the client is on warfarin therapy
      c. INR
   5. BUN and creatinine: Reflect renal function and perfusion; levels can increase in MI, CHF, and cardiomyopathy
   6. Total serum cholesterol desirable
      a. Low-density lipids (LDL)
      b. High-density lipids (HDL)
      c. Triglycerides
   7. B-type natriuretic peptide (BNP): Indicator for diagnosing heart failure
      a. Critical value greater than 100 pg/mL
   8. Enzymes: Test indicates death of myocardial muscles, heart attack
      a. Creatinine phosphokinase MB (CK–MB) isoenzyme increases within 4 to 6 hr following a MI and remains elevated from 24 to 72 hr.
      b. Troponin is a protein that is considered the gold standard in diagnosing MI. It remains elevated for 2 to 3 weeks following an event. Normal level is less than 0.2 ng/dL.
      c. Myoglobin rises early in response to tissue injury within the first 2 hr, but also declines quickly after 7 hr from injury. It is less useful than CK–MB and troponin because myoglobin is present in skeletal as well as cardiac muscle.

DIAGNOSTIC TESTING: CARDIAC ENZYMES

Important Lab Findings

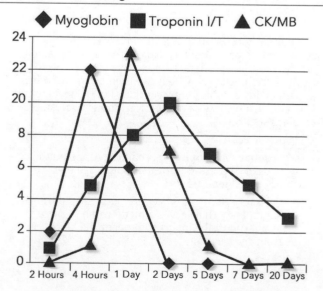

B. **Electrocardiogram (ECG):** A recording of the electrical activity occurring in the heart. A 12-lead ECG should be obtained within 10 min of onset of chest pain to identify any areas of myocardial damage.

1. T-wave inversion: ischemia
2. ST-segment elevation: injury
3. Q-wave enlargement: infarction

ECG WAVE ELEMENTS

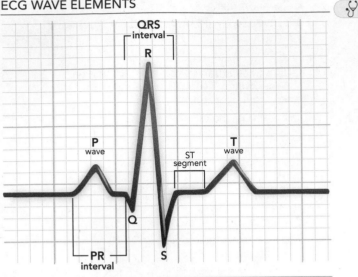

P wave represents atrial depolarization (contraction).

QRS complex (interval) represents ventricular depolarization (contraction) and should be less than 0.12 seconds.

T wave represents ventricular repolarization (relaxation). T wave depression (inversion) indicates myocardial ischemia.

PR interval represents time between SA node and AV node. Should be between 0.12 and 0.20 seconds.

ST segments represents elevation. Indicates myocardial injury.

C. **Cardiac catheterization:** A procedure involving the advancement of a catheter, usually through the femoral artery, into the coronary arteries. Dye can be injected to visualize blockages, which can then be treated with percutaneous coronary intervention (PCI). The femoral vein can also be accessed to perform other assessments of cardiac function.

1. Types of PCI

   a. **Coronary Angioplasty:** A balloon-tipped catheter is used to press the coronary blockage open to improve blood flow.

   b. **Coronary Stent:** A procedure performed during angioplasty that leaves a metal mesh in place as a structural support to prevent the blockage from reoccurring.

2. Purpose

   a. Perform angiography.
   b. Perform PCI.
   c. Obtain information about cardiac structure and blood flow.
   d. Obtain blood samples.
   e. Determine cardiac output.

3. **Nursing Interventions**

   a. Prior to catheterization

      1) Verify that procedural consent has been obtained.
      2) Know approach for shave prep: right (venous) side, or left (arterial) side.
      3) NPO for 6 hr prior to the procedure.
      4) Mark distal (baseline) pulses.
      5) Explain to the client that the procedure can leave a metallic taste, and the client can feel flushed when the dye is injected.
      6) Verify that the client does not have any history of allergy to dye or shellfish.

D. **After catheterization**

1. Monitor blood pressure and apical pulse every 15 min for 2 to 4 hr.
2. Monitor neurovascular status every 15 min for the first 2 hr, then every 30 min until the client can sit up.
3. Monitor for bleeding or hematoma at catheter insertion site.
4. Apply pressure for a minimum of 15 min to prevent bleeding or hematoma formation.
5. Monitor for vasospasm, dysrhythmia, or rupture of the coronary vessel.
6. Monitor for chest pain.
7. Keep the extremity extended for 4 to 6 hr.
8. Maintain bed rest; no hip flexion and no sitting up in bed.
9. Increase fluid intake to enhance flushing of dye.

E. **Transesophageal echocardiogram (TEE):** Diagnostic tool to visualize structures (including valves) and function of the heart. Used for diagnosis of heart failure and murmurs.

1. Preprocedure

   a. NPO 6 to 8 hr prior to the procedure.
   b. Clarify medications to be administered with the provider.

2. Postprocedure

   a. Monitor for adequate gag reflex.
   b. Monitor respiratory effort as client recovers from sedation.
   c. Observe oral secretions (blood-tinged oral secretions common in early recovery).

III Cardiovascular Disorders

A. **Angina:** A manifestation of myocardial ischemia caused by arterial stenosis or blockage, uncontrolled blood pressure, or cardiomyopathy.

1. **Chronic Stable Angina (CSA)** is characterized by the chest discomfort described by the client as typical and usually is relieved with rest or a single nitroglycerin. CSA is attributable most often to fixed or stable atherosclerotic plaque.

2. **Acute Coronary Syndrome (ACS)** describes clients experiencing unstable angina or an acute myocardial infarction (AMI). Unstable angina is characterized by the chest discomfort described by the client as occurring at rest or with activity and can last longer than 15 min unrelieved by nitroglycerin.

3. Types of angina

   a. **Stable (exertional) angina.** Occurs with exercise or emotional stress and is relieved by rest or nitroglycerin.

   b. **Unstable (preinfarction) angina.** Occurs with exercise or at rest, but increases in occurrence, severity, and duration over time.

   c. **Variant (Prinzmetal's) angina.** Due to a coronary artery spasm, often occurring during periods of rest.

B. **Contributing Factors**

1. Coronary artery disease (CAD)

   a. Family history

   b. Advanced age

   c. Hyperlipidemia

   d. Tobacco use

   e. Hypertension

   f. Diabetes mellitus

   g. Obesity

   h. Physical inactivity

C. **Manifestations**

1. Chest pain or discomfort

2. Pain in arms, neck, jaw, shoulder, or back

3. Nausea

4. Fatigue

5. Shortness of breath

6. Anxiety

7. Diaphoresis

8. Dizziness

D. **Diagnostic Procedures**

1. 12-lead ECG

2. Stress test

3. Cardiac catheterization

4. Echocardiogram

5. Cardiac enzymes and biomarkers

E. **Collaborative Care**

1. **Nursing Interventions**

   a. Monitor pain.

      1) Location: Jaw, arm, chest

      2) Character

      3) Duration: Relieved with rest and/or nitroglycerin

      4) Precipitating factors (once identified, eliminate or minimize to avoid attacks)

   b. Administer oxygen as needed.

   c. Provide environment conducive to rest. Avoid activities.

   d. Administer medications.

      1) Aspirin

      2) Nitrates

      3) Beta blockers

      4) Statins

      5) Calcium channel blockers

      6) Angiotensin-converting enzyme (ACE)

   e. Client Education

      1) Lifestyle changes

         a) Avoid constipation.

         b) Avoid excessive activity in cold weather.

         c) Decrease stress.

         d) Exercise.

         e) Consume a low-sodium, low-fat diet.

         f) Maintain a healthy weight.

         g) Rest after meals.

         h) Cease tobacco use.

      2) Practice correct use of nitroglycerin.

         a) Take as needed at onset of chest pain or tightness or in preparation of exertional activity.

         b) Take nitroglycerin as prescribed, at onset of attack, and every 5 min up to three doses. If pain is not relieved after first sublingual tablet, call 911.

         c) Store nitroglycerin in a dark, dry spot, and replace every 6 months.

         d) Side effects of taking nitroglycerin include headache and hypotension.

         e) Types of nitroglycerin are tablets, ointment, patch, and spray.

         f) If the client is given nitroglycerin for prevention, the client must be nitroglycerin-free daily for 12 hr to prevent developing a tolerance.

         g) If the client uses a nitroglycerin patch, apply it in the morning and remove it at bedtime.

         h) Take nitroglycerin while sitting down and stopping all activity.

         i) Erectile dysfunction medication is contraindicated with the use of nitrates.

F. **Myocardial infarction (MI):** The process by which myocardial tissue is destroyed due to reduced coronary blood flow and lack of oxygen. Actual necrosis of the heart muscle (myocardium) occurs.

1. Contributing Factors
   a. Atherosclerotic heart disease
   b. Coronary artery embolism

2. Manifestations
   a. Severe chest pain unrelieved by nitroglycerin or rest
   b. Crushing quality that radiates to jawline, left arm, neck, or back
   c. Females, older adults, and clients who have diabetes mellitus often report no pain.
   d. Diaphoresis, nausea, vomiting, anxiety, fear
   e. Vital sign changes: Tachycardia, hypotension, dyspnea, dysrhythmias

3. Diagnostic Procedures
   a. Laboratory results: Elevated troponin and CK-MB enzymes, elevated myoglobin
   b. 12-lead ECG: Should be obtained ASAP to identify ST changes. Can be an ST elevation MI (STEMI) or non–ST elevation MI (NSTEMI).

4. Collaborative Care
   a. **Nursing Interventions** (aimed at resting the myocardium and preserving the heart muscle)
      1) Early
         a) Administer oxygen.
         b) Administer medications.
            (1) Aspirin
            (2) Antidysrhythmics: amiodarone, lidocaine
            (3) Analgesics: morphine sulfate
            (4) Anticoagulants: heparin IV
            (5) Thrombolytics within 6 hr of a cardiac event: streptokinase, alteplase recombinant
            (6) Vasodilators: nitroglycerin
            (7) Beta blockers: metoprolol
            (8) Calcium channel blockers: verapamil, nifedipine
         c) Frequently monitor vital signs, O_2 saturation, and ECG.
         d) Provide emotional support.
      2) Later
         a) Administer stool softeners to prevent straining with bowel movements or Valsalva maneuver.
         b) Provide a soft, low-fat, low-cholesterol, low-sodium diet.
         c) Use a bedside commode, which requires less energy than using a bedpan.
         d) Promote self-care, but remind the client to stop at the onset of pain.
         e) Plan for cardiac rehabilitation.
         f) Initiate an exercise program, but stop if fatigue or chest pain occurs.
         g) Reinforce teaching and encourage the use of stress management techniques.
      h) Reinforce teaching with the client to modify risk factors.
         (1) Obesity
         (2) Stress
         (3) Diet
         (4) Hypertension
         (5) Tobacco use
         (6) Physical inactivity
      i) Recognize risk factors that cannot be modified.
         (1) Heredity
         (2) Race
         (3) Age
         (4) Sex
      j) Ensure bleeding precautions with anticoagulant and antiplatelet therapy.
      k) Initiate long-term medication therapy.
         (1) Anticoagulants/antiplatelets: heparin, aspirin, warfarin, enoxaparin, clopidogrel
         (2) Antihypertensives
            (a) Beta blockers: metoprolol
            (b) Calcium channel blockers: diltiazem
         (3) Vasodilators: nitroglycerin
         (4) Antilipidemics: simvastatin, atorvastatin

G. **Heart failure:** The inability of the heart to meet the tissue requirements for oxygen. Characterized by manifestations of fluid overload or inadequate tissue perfusion. Has been called congestive heart failure due to the frequent occurrence of pulmonary and peripheral congestion. Most often a chronic condition with a goal of preventing acute exacerbations.

1. Left-sided heart failure: Manifestation primarily related to pulmonary congestion
   a. Dyspnea
   b. Cough
   c. Crackles
   d. Orthopnea
   e. Paroxysmal nocturnal dyspnea
   f. Low oxygen saturation levels
   g. Elevated PAWP

2. Right-sided heart failure: Manifestations primarily related to systemic congestion
   a. Dependent edema
   b. Hepatomegaly
   c. Ascites
   d. Anorexia and vomiting
   e. Weakness
   f. Weight gain
   g. Jugular vein distention
   h. Elevated CVP

HEMODYNAMIC MONITORING

	EXPECTED REFERENCE RANGE	CAUSES OF ABNORMAL RANGE
Central venous pressure (CVP)	1 to 8 mm Hg	Increased: Hypervolemia, right-sided heart failure
		Decreased: Hypovolemia
Pulmonary artery wedge pressure (PAWP)	4 to 12 mm Hg	Increased: Hypervolemia, left-sided heart failure
		Decreased: Hypovolemia

3. Collaborative Care

a. **Nursing Interventions**

1) Respiratory status

a) Auscultate lung sounds to detect crackles and wheezes.

b) Administer oxygen therapy as needed.

c) Fowler's position to help work of breathing

2) Fluid volume

a) Fluid restriction depending on severity

b) Low-sodium diet (2,000 to 3,000 mg/day)

c) Report 2- to 3-lb weight increase in 1 day

3) Pharmacological therapy

a) ACE inhibitors

b) ARBs

c) Hydralazine and nitrates

d) Beta blockers

e) Calcium channel blockers

f) Diuretics

g) Digitalis

h) IV nesiritide

i) IV milrinone

j) IV dobutamine

H. **Valvular disorders:** Result in narrowing of valve that prevents or impedes blood flow (stenosis) or impaired closure that allows backward leakage of blood (regurgitation); can affect mitral, aortic, or tricuspid valve.

1. Contributing Factors

a. History of endocarditis and rheumatic fever is frequently the cause.

2. Manifestations

a. Right-sided heart failure (mitral stenosis, mitral regurgitation, tricuspid stenosis)

b. Left-sided heart failure (aortic stenosis, aortic regurgitation)

c. Murmurs

d. Decreased cardiac output

3. Collaborative Care

a. **Nursing Interventions**

1) Management: Similar as for heart failure.

2) Valvuloplasty: Postprocedure care is similar to that of PCI. Watch for signs of systemic emboli, which can have dislodged from the valve.

3) Valve replacement

a) Mechanical: Will require lifelong anticoagulants using warfarin. Maintain INR 2.0 to 3.0.

b) Biologic: Will require prophylactic anticoagulants for 3 months.

c) All clients who have undergone valve surgery require prophylactic antibiotics prior to any future invasive procedures or tests (including dental procedures) to prevent infective endocarditis.

I. **Aortic aneurysm:** Local distention of the aortic artery wall, usually thoracic or abdominal. Monitored until above 5 cm, when the rate of rupture increases and surgery is usually required.

1. Contributing factors

a. Atherosclerosis (most common cause)

b. Infections/inflammatory disorders

c. Connective tissue disorders

2. Manifestations (frequently asymptomatic)

a. Thoracic: Pain, dyspnea, hoarseness, cough, dysphagia

b. Abdominal: Abdominal pain; persistent or intermittent low-back or flank pain; pulsating abdominal mass

3. Diagnostic Procedures

a. CT scan, MRI

b. X-ray, ultrasound

4. Collaborative Care

a. **Nursing Interventions**

1) Treatment often includes surgery.

a) Preoperative: Maintain systolic pressure at 100 to 120 mm Hg with beta blockers and/or antihypertensives such as hydralazine. Continuous IV nipride can be required. Monitor closely for manifestations of rupture (intense pain, decreasing blood pressure).

b) Postoperative: Careful monitoring of peripheral circulation below the level of the aneurysm. Continue close monitoring of BP. Low BP can indicate hemorrhage. High BP places stress on the arterial suture line.

c) Postoperative complications

(1) Arterial occlusion

(2) Hemorrhage

(3) Infection

(4) Renal failure

J. **Hypertension:** Persistent blood pressure above 140/90 mm Hg; often called the "silent killer."

1. Primary hypertension

a. Most common type (90% of cases)

b. Hereditary disease; cause unknown

c. More common among African American clients

d. Late manifestations: Headaches, fatigue, dyspnea, edema, nocturia, blackouts

e. Usually no manifestations until end-organ involvement occurs

2. Secondary hypertension

a. Due to identifiable cause

b. Pheochromocytoma

c. Renal pathology

3. Collaborative Care

a. **Nursing Interventions**

1) Reinforce weight control methods.

2) Encourage tobacco cessation.

3) Decrease alcohol and caffeine intake.

4) Promote a program of regular physical exercise.

5) Promote a lifestyle with reduced stress.

6) Encourage a sodium-restricted diet.

7) Encourage the DASH Diet—increased fruits, vegetables, low-fat dairy, limited saturated fats.

b. Medications: Initial medications include diuretics and beta blockers.

1) Loop diuretics: Furosemide, bumetanide

2) Thiazide-hydrochlorothiazide (HCTZ), chlorothiazide

a) Interventions for loop and HCTZ diuretics

(1) Administer potassium supplements as prescribed.

(2) Reinforce teaching of dietary sources of potassium.

(3) Hypokalemia increases the risk of digitalis toxicity.

3) Potassium-sparing diuretics

a) Spironolactone

b) Triamterene

c) Monitor for increased potassium level.

4) Beta blockers

a) Propranolol

b) Atenolol

c) Metoprolol

d) **Nursing Interventions** for beta blockers

(1) Monitor for major side effects of bradycardia.

(2) Monitor pulse daily.

(3) Monitor for manifestations of heart failure.

(4) Noncardioselective beta blockers can be contraindicated in clients who have asthma.

(5) Monitor for hypoglycemia in clients who have diabetes mellitus; can mask manifestations.

5) Central-acting alpha-blockers (sympatholytics)

a) Clonidine HCl

b) Guanfacine HCl

c) Methyldopa

6) Angiotensin-converting enzyme (ACE) inhibitors

a) Captopril

b) Enalapril

c) Lisinopril

7) Calcium-channel blockers

a) Nifedipine

b) Verapamil, diltiazem

GERONTOLOGICAL CONSIDERATIONS

1. Medications start at half the dose used in younger clients.

2. Monotherapy desirable due to simplicity and decreased expense.

3. At increased risk for postural hypotension secondary to medications.

K. **Peripheral Vascular Disease:** Includes peripheral arterial disease and peripheral venous disorders

1. **Peripheral Arterial Disease:** Impairs blood flow in the arteries that carry blood away from the heart. Most common in arteries of the legs.

a. Manifestations

1) Intermittent claudication: Pain/cramping when walking; resolves with rest

2) Calf muscle atrophy

3) Skin that appears shiny with hair loss and thickened toenails

4) Poor neurovascular integrity

5) Necrotic ulcers (looks punched-out; no edema present)

6) Tingling and numbness of the toes

7) Cool extremities with poor pulses

b. Collaborative Care

1) **Nursing Interventions**

a) Exercise therapy: Walk to the point of pain three times per week.

b) Encourage tobacco cessation.

c) Promote weight reduction.

d) Dependent position relieves pain.

2) Administer Medications

a) Administer pentoxifylline and cilostazol.

3) Therapeutic Measures

a) Surgical treatment

(1) Femoral popliteal bypass surgery

(2) Angioplasty or stenting

2. **Peripheral Venous Disease:** Disorder that interferes with adequate return of blood flow from legs. Includes venous insufficiency, venous thromboembolism (VTE), and varicose veins.

a. Contributing Factors

1) Prolonged sitting or standing

2) Obesity

3) Pregnancy

4) Thrombophlebitis

b. Manifestations

1) Stasis dermatitis (brown discoloration)

2) Edema

3) Stasis ulcers (typically found around ankles)

c. Collaborative Care

1) **Nursing Interventions**

a) Elevate legs four to five times throughout the day.

b) Avoid the following: crossing legs, constrictive clothing, tight socks.

c) Apply compression stockings.

L. **Venous Thromboembolism:** The collective condition of DVT and pulmonary embolism (PE).

1. Contributing Factors
   a. Immobility
   b. Surgery
   c. Trauma
   d. Obesity
   e. Age older than 65
   f. Spinal cord injury
   g. Disorders of coagulation
   h. Pregnancy
   i. Oral contraceptives

2. Manifestations of DVT
   a. Edema of affected limb
   b. Local swelling, bumpy, knotty
   c. Red, tender, local induration
   d. Venous ulcers usually around the ankle; reddened and bluish; edema often present

3. Diagnostic Procedures
   a. MRI, CT scan, ultrasound

4. Collaborative Care
   a. **Nursing Interventions**
      1) Heparin: Monitor PTT.
      2) Warfarin: Monitor INR.
      3) Thrombolytic therapy: alteplase
      4) Monitor for bleeding and thrombocytopenia.
      5) Elevate affected extremity and apply warm, moist compresses.
      6) Monitor for manifestations of PE: dyspnea, chest pain, tachycardia, anxiety.

KEY NURSING INTERVENTIONS: Prevention of VTE includes early mobilization, leg exercises, compression stockings or intermittent pneumatic compression devices, and prophylactic subcutaneous heparin.

M. **Varicose veins:** Enlarged, twisted and superficial veins, most common in the lower extremities and the esophagus

1. Contributing Factors
   a. Prolonged standing
   b. Pregnancy
   c. Obesity
   d. Heredity

2. Manifestations
   a. Enlarged, tortuous veins in lower extremities, visible just below skin
   b. Muscle cramping, pain after sitting
   c. Edema (after standing)

3. Collaborative Care
   a. **Nursing Interventions**
      1) Avoid prolonged sitting or standing.
      2) Reinforce teaching to wear supportive antiembolism stockings, especially during air flights and pregnancy.
      3) Avoid crossing legs. Engage in daily exercise. Maintain an ideal body weight.
      4) Elevate lower extremities to reduce edema and promote venous return.
      5) Promote circulation with thigh-high antiembolism stockings, ambulation, and elevation.

4. Medical Management
   a. **Sclerotherapy:** Chemical injection
   b. **Ligation and stripping:** Surgery
   c. **Thermal ablation:** Nonsurgical use of energy or lasers

N. **Buerger's disease (thromboangiitis obliterans):** Recurring inflammation of the arteries and veins of the lower and upper extremities, resulting in thrombus with occlusion (cause unknown)

1. Contributing Factors
   a. Thought to have a genetic predisposition
   b. Cigarette smoking and chewing tobacco use
   c. Occurs most often in males age 20 to 35

2. Manifestations
   a. Intermittent pain in the legs, feet, arms, and hands. Pain eases when activity is stopped (claudication).
   b. Inflammation along a vein below the skin's surface (due to a blood clot in the vein).
   c. Cold sensitivity of the Raynaud type frequently occurs in the hands.
   d. Painful open sores on fingers and toes.
   e. Ulcerations and gangrene with amputation are common.

3. Collaborative Care
   a. Interventions
      1) Promote smoking cessation.
      2) Avoid cold or constrictive clothing.

O. **Raynaud's syndrome:** Vasospastic or obstructive condition of the arteries/arterioles of upper and lower extremities resulting from exposure to cold/stress; more common in female clients.

1. Contributing Factors
   a. Factors that cause Raynaud's attacks are not clearly understood.
   b. Blood vessels in hands and feet appear to overreact to cold or stress.

2. Manifestations
   a. Coldness, pallor, and pain in extremities secondary to vasospasm
   b. Occasional ulceration of the fingertips
   c. Color changes from white to blue to red (can be bilateral or symmetrical)

3. Diagnostic Procedures

  a. Cold-stimulation test: Placing the hands in cool water or exposing to cold air to trigger an episode of Raynaud's

4. Collaborative Care

  a. **Nursing Interventions**

    1) Reinforce teaching with the client to avoid the cold and keep extremities warm. Wear warm, nonconstrictive gloves.

    2) Encourage the client to stop smoking and to limit caffeine intake.

  b. Medications

    1) Administer nifedipine.

IV Cardiac Surgery

A. **Coronary artery bypass graft (CABG):** A surgical procedure to bypass occluded coronary arteries and reestablish perfusion to the heart muscle.

1. Most procedures require an open chest/heart approach with a bypass machine. However, newer techniques may not use bypass, resulting in fewer complications and a shorter recovery period for some clients.

2. Collaborative Care

  a. Preoperative/general care

    1) Obtain baseline vital signs, physical assessment, and history.

    2) Provide psychological support. Administer anxiolytic agents as needed (diazepam, lorazepam).

    3) Inform the client and family what to anticipate postoperatively (intubation, IV lines, urinary catheter, arterial line, chest tubes).

    4) Shower with an antiseptic solution.

  b. Postoperative care

    1) Monitor hourly for first 8 hr.

      a) Neurologic: Responsiveness, pupils, reflexes

      b) Cardiac: BP, CVP, PAWP, heart rate and rhythm, cardiac sounds

      c) Respiratory: Chest movement, breath sounds, ventilator settings, chest tube drainage, ABGs

      d) Peripheral vascular status: Pulses, edema, skin color and temperature

      e) Renal: Urinary output, urine specific gravity

      f) F&E: I&O, electrolytes

      g) Pain: Type, location, intensity

    2) Monitor for complications

      a) Decreased cardiac output

      b) Fluid volume and electrolyte imbalance

      c) Impaired gas exchange

      d) Impaired cerebral circulation

V Shock

Inadequate delivery of oxygen and nutrients to support vital organs and cellular function. Results in impaired tissue perfusion.

A. **Types**

1. Cardiogenic: Failure of the heart to pump adequately

2. Hypovolemic: Decreased circulating blood volume

3. Distributive (circulatory): Vasodilation that causes blood to pool in the peripheral vessels.

  a. Neurogenic: Caused by spinal cord injury, some medications, or hypoglycemia. Characterized by warm, dry skin and bradycardia.

  b. Anaphylactic: Hypersensitivity reaction that causes a sudden onset of hypotension and is life-threatening. Can also experience respiratory distress and cardiac arrest.

  c. Septic: Most common type of circulatory shock. It results from a systemic infection and is characterized by warm, dry skin, bounding pulses, and tachypnea.

B. **Manifestations (related to decreased tissue perfusion)**

1. Tachycardia with hypotension

2. Tachypnea

3. Oliguria

4. Cold, moist skin (except neurogenic and septic)

5. Color ashen, pallor

6. Metabolic acidosis

7. Decreased level of consciousness

C. **Collaborative Care**

1. **Nursing Interventions**

  a. Position the client in modified Trendelenburg.

  b. Secure a large-bore IV line (16– or 18–gauge).

  c. Administer oxygen.

  d. Record vital signs every 5 min.

  e. Promote rest and decrease movement.

  f. Monitor urine output.

2. Treatment

  a. Hypovolemic: Volume replacement

  b. Cardiogenic: Increase contractility and reduce afterload (BP).

  c. Septic: IV fluids, vasopressors and antibiotics.

  d. Anaphylactic: Epinephrine and diphenhydramine.

  e. Neurogenic: Treat cause (e.g., stabilize spinal cord).

VI Cardiopulmonary Resuscitation (CPR)

A. **Indications**
1. Absence of palpable carotid pulse
2. Absence of breath sounds

B. **Purpose**
1. Establish effective circulation and respiration.
2. Prevent irreversible cerebral anoxic damage.

C. **Procedure**
1. Follow the American Heart Association 2010 recommendations.
   a. Call 911.
   b. Send someone for the automated external defibrillator (AED).
   c. Immediately begin CPR if an adult victim is unresponsive and not breathing normally.
   d. Early, uninterrupted chest compressions are important. Follow the acronym CAB (Compressions, Airway, Breathing).
   e. Untrained rescuers should perform hands-only compressions. Push hard and fast on the center of the victim's chest, or follow the directions of EMS dispatchers.
   f. Trained rescuers should provide 30 compressions and two rescue breaths to improve outcomes.
   g. Depth: Compress the chest at least 2 inches (5 cm) in adults and ⅓ the depth of chest in children and infants.
   h. Rate: Provide compressions 100/min, to the beat of the Bee Gees song "Stayin' Alive."
   i. Recoil: Allow the chest to recoil fully between compressions.
   j. Minimize interruptions: Do not delay or interrupt chest compressions to check pulse or rhythm.
   k. When necessary to check for a pulse, do not exceed 10 seconds.
2. Complications
   a. Fractured ribs
   b. Punctured lungs
   c. Lacerated liver
   d. Abdominal distension
3. Stop CPR when
   a. A provider pronounces the client dead.
   b. The rescuer is exhausted.
   c. Help arrives.
   d. The client's heartbeat returns.
4. Automated external defibrillator: A computerized defibrillator that analyzes cardiac rhythm once pads are placed on the client's chest
   a. Do not stop compressions while defibrillator is being applied and set up.
   b. Stop compressions and rescue breaths while rhythm is being analyzed.
   c. A mechanical voice tells the rescuer if/when to deliver shock to the client.
   d. AED is frequently found in public locations because it is easy for nontrained individuals to use.

5. Obstructed airway
   a. Conscious
      1) Establish that the client is choking.
      2) Perform the Heimlich maneuver until it is successful or the client becomes unconscious.
   b. Unconscious
      1) If a conscious choking adult becomes unresponsive, look for the foreign object in the pharynx. If object is seen, perform a finger sweep.
      2) If not breathing, begin CPR. Every time you open the airway to give breaths, look for the object.
      3) Continue CPR.

HEART

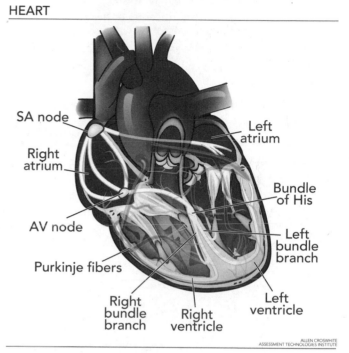

SA node
Right atrium
AV node
Purkinje fibers
Right bundle branch
Right ventricle
Left atrium
Bundle of His
Left bundle branch
Left ventricle

ALLEN CROSWHITE
ASSESSMENT TECHNOLOGIES INSTITUTE

VII Adjunctive Management

If medications are ineffective in eliminating dysrhythmias, electrical cardioversion and defibrillation can be used for tachydysrhythmias and pacemaker therapy for bradycardia.

A. **Cardioversion:** Treats tachydysrhythmias by delivering an electrical current to the heart in an effort to convert the client to a normal rhythm
1. Synchronized (timed to coincide with the client's own electrical cardiac cycle).
2. Used when the client has a pulse.
3. Can be scheduled.
4. TEE can be performed to rule out right atrial or ventricular clot formation prior to cardioversion.
5. Sedation is commonly used.

B. **Defibrillation:** Also delivers an electrical current to the heart, but used only for life-threatening dysrhythmias in an effort to convert the client to a more stable rhythm
1. Used for VF or pulseless VT.
2. Unsynchronized (not timed as with cardioversion).
3. Delivery is required immediately (not scheduled).
4. Used ONLY when client is pulseless.
5. Not effective for treatment of asystole.

C. **Pacemaker Therapy:** An electronic device that provides repetitive electrical stimuli to the heart muscle to control the heart rate

1. Types

   a. Permanent pacemakers

      1) Surgically placed in the subcutaneous tissue of the chest.

      2) Instruct the client to avoid raising arms above the head until the wound heals.

      3) Observe for hiccups (sign of accidental dislodgement).

      4) Client Education

         a) Avoid large magnets (MRIs).

         b) Carry wallet notification or health ID especially for airport travel.

         c) Know set rate and check pulse daily.

         d) Recognize and report signs of battery failure.

         e) Wear loose-fitting clothing.

         f) Avoid contact sports.

   b. Temporary pacemakers (transvenous)

      1) Monitor ECG.

      2) Check heart rate.

      3) Monitor site for hematoma and infection.

      4) Administer analgesics as needed.

      5) Maintain electrically safe environment.

   c. Transcutaneous (skin)

      1) Externally placed for use in emergency situations only.

      2) Causes significant discomfort.

      3) Prepare for alternate interventions (temporary pacemaker).

      4) Remove transdermal patches from chest area. Arching can cause burns.

      5) Clip chest hair as needed to improve pad adherence and reduce burns.

2. Settings

   a. Ventricular demand: Fires at a preset rate when heart rate drops below a predetermined/preprogrammed rate.

   b. Ventricular fixed: Fires constantly at a preset/preprogrammed rate, regardless of heart rate.

   c. Dual chamber: Stimulates both the atria and the ventricles.

   d. Atrial demand: Fires as needed when the atria do not originate a rhythm.

   e. Variable rate: Senses oxygen demands and increases the firing rate to meet the client's needs.

IDENTIFY THE FOLLOWING ECG RHYTHMS

Calculating Heart Rate: To estimate heart rate, count the number of R waves in 6 seconds and multiply by 10. For example, if there are seven R waves in a 6-second strip, the estimated heart rate is 70/min (7 × 10 = 70).

1. Name the rhythm.

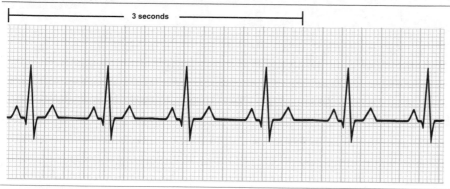

3 seconds

Characteristics

> Rate: Atrial (P wave) and ventricular (QRS complex) rates are 60 to 100/min.

> Rhythm: Atrial (P wave) and ventricular (QRS complex) rhythms are regular.

> P waves: Consistent and one before each QRS complex.

> PR interval: 0.12 to 0.20 seconds and consistent.

> QRS complex: Less than 0.12 seconds and consistent.

2. Name the rhythm.

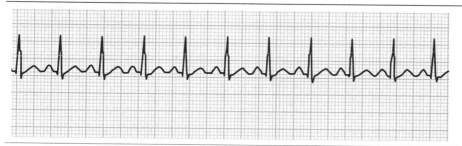

Characteristics

> Rate: Atrial (P wave) and ventricular (QRS complex) rates greater than 100/min.

> Rhythm: Atrial (P wave) and ventricular (QRS complex) rhythms are regular.

> P waves: Consistent and one before each QRS complex.

> PR interval: 0.12 to 0.20 seconds and consistent.

> QRS complex: Less than 0.12 seconds and consistent.

Causes: Shock, fever, stress, exercise, anxiety, pain, stimulants

Treatment: Usually none other than treating the cause.

3. Name the rhythm.

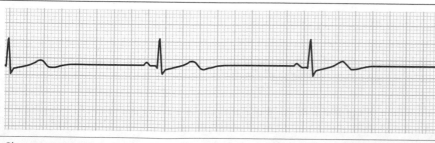

Characteristics

> Rate: Atrial (P wave) and ventricular (QRS complex) rates less than 60/min.

> Rhythm: Atrial (P wave) and ventricular (QRS complex) rhythms are regular.

> P waves: Consistent and one before each QRS complex.

> PR interval: 0.12 to 0.20 seconds and consistent.

> QRS complex: Less than 0.12 seconds and consistent.

Causes: Lower metabolic needs (sleep, hypothyroidism, athletic individuals), vagal stimulation (vomiting, straining during a bowel movement), medications (beta blockers, calcium channel blockers)

Treatment: Directed at the cause if possible (discontinuing medication, preventing vagal stimulation) or signs of hemodynamic instability (hypotensive, dyspneic, altered mental status, angina). If the client is unstable, IV atropine 0.5 mg is the medication of choice, given 3 to 5 min apart to a maximum total of 3 mg.

4. Name the rhythm.

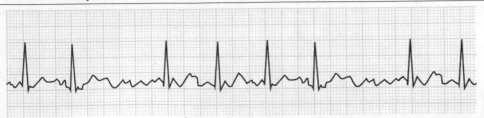

Characteristics

> Rate (atrial): Multiple rapid impulses from many areas of the atria result in a fibrillatory line.

> Ventricular: Usually responds at a rate of 120 to 200/min.

> Rhythm: Ventricular rhythm is irregular.

> P waves: No clear P wave.

> PR interval: No clear P wave so unable to determine.

> QRS complex: Less than 0.12 seconds and consistent.

Causes: Usually occurs in people of advanced age who have heart disease.

Treatment: Depends on the cause and the duration of the dysrhythmia. Many clients convert to a NSR spontaneously within 24 hr. If a client is unstable (hypotensive, dyspneic, altered mental status, angina), electrical cardioversion can be indicated. If a client has been in this rhythm for more than 48 hr, treatment with anticoagulants should occur first with warfarin for 3 to 4 weeks to avoid the formation of emboli, which can cause a cerebrovascular accident (CVA). Heart failure can occur due to loss of atrial kick. Medications can also be effective in converting the client back to a NSR. If atrial fibrillation is chronic, treatment with daily anticoagulant is common to prevent CVA.

5. Name the rhythm.

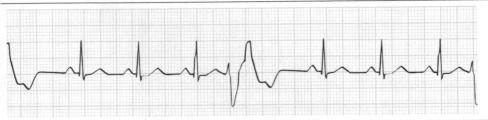

Characteristics: Not a rhythm, but isolated abnormal beats that arise from an irritable area within a ventricle that causes the ventricle to contract prematurely. Might cause palpitations.

Causes: Can occur in healthy individuals. Often associated with nicotine, caffeine, and alcohol intake. Can be caused by myocardial ischemia or infarction, heart failure, acidosis, hypoxia, and electrolyte imbalances, especially hypokalemia.

Treatment: If they occur in the absence of heart disease and are not causing a problem for the client, there might not be any treatment indicated. Treating the cause, if possible, and administering amiodarone or sotalol can be indicated depending on the severity and symptoms of the client. Manifestations can include slowing of the heart rate, decreased blood pressure, and signs of impaired tissue perfusion.

6. Name the rhythm.

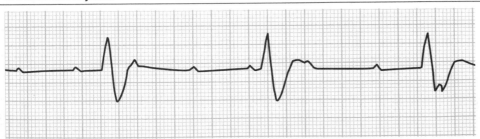

Characteristics

> Rate: Atrial rate is faster than the ventricular rate.

> Rhythm: Atrial and ventricular rhythms are usually regular.

> P waves: Consistently present, but not consistently followed by a QRS complex.

> PR interval: Inconsistent and no identifiable relationship between the P-wave and QRS complex.

> QRS complex: Usually consistent and can be wider than normal (greater than 0.12 seconds).

> Atrioventricular (AV) heart block: Cardiac electrical conduction transmission is blocked, not allowing any impulses to be conducted through the AV node. The atria and ventricles are beating independently from each other. Ventricular pacing is slow and unreliable.

Causes: Can be caused by medication (digitalis, beta blockers, calcium channel blockers), myocardial ischemia and infarction, cardiomyopathy, inflammatory heart disease, or valvular disorders.

Treatment: Depends on the cause but often requires the placement of a pacemaker.

7. Name the rhythm.

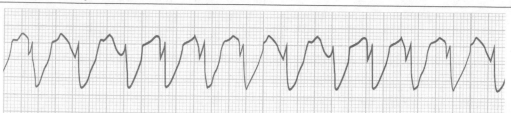

Characteristics

> Rate: Ventricular rate usually 140 to 180/min.

> Rhythm: Irregular.

> P waves: Not usually seen.

> PR interval: Not identifiable.

> QRS complex: Wide.

Causes: Similar to those for PVCs and more lethal if associated with myocardial infarction or low ejection fraction (percent of blood ejected from the heart with each contraction).

Treatment: If the client has a pulse, cardioversion is indicated as well as the administration of antidysrhythmic IV medications (procainamide, amiodarone). If the client does not have a pulse, the treatment is immediate defibrillation.

8. Name the rhythm.

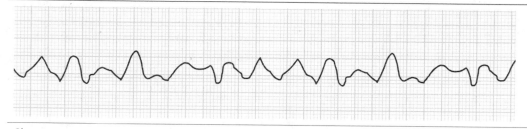

Characteristics: The electrical chaos in the heart causes the ventricles to fibrillate, resulting in a fibrillatory wave pattern. There are no recognizable waves or patterns. They do not contract and there is no pulse. There is no cerebral or systemic perfusion occurring. This rhythm is usually fatal if not reversed in 3 to 5 min.

Causes: Most commonly caused by myocardial infarction and is the most common dysrhythmia resulting in cardiac arrest.

Treatment: There is never a pulse with this rhythm. In addition to CPR, immediate defibrillation is critical to survival. The chance for survival decreases by 7% to 10% for every 1 min delay in defibrillation.

9. Name the rhythm.

Characteristics: There is no electrical activity in the heart. This results in a flat line with no identifiable waves or pattern. Because there is no electrical activity, there is no contraction, pulse, or perfusion occurring. The prognosis for these clients is usually poor.

Causes: Hypoxia, acidosis, severe electrolyte imbalances, drug overdose, hypovolemia, cardiac tamponade, tension pneumothorax, myocardial infarction, hypothermia, or trauma.

Treatment: High-quality CPR. Identify and treat cause. Medications such as epinephrine and vasopressin can be beneficial. If this does not correct the rhythm, resuscitation efforts are usually ceased.

Answer Key: 1. Normal sinus rhythm; 2. Sinus tachycardia; 3. Sinus bradycardia; 4. Atrial fibrillation; 5. Premature ventricular contractions; 6. Third-degree heart block; 7. Ventricular tachycardia; 8. Ventricular fibrillation; 9. Asystole

Genitourinary System Disorders

A. **Assessment of the Kidney and Urinary System**

1. Functions of the kidney

   a. Regulates acid-base balance

   b. Regulates fluid and electrolyte balance

   c. Excretes metabolic wastes (creatinine, urea)

   d. Regulates blood pressure: Renin (stimulated by decreased blood pressure or blood volume) stimulates the production of angiotensin I, which is converted to angiotensin II in the lungs; angiotensin II is a strong vasoconstrictor and stimulates aldosterone secretion; vasoconstriction and sodium reabsorption result in increased blood volume and increased blood pressure.

   e. Secretes erythropoietin

   f. Converts vitamin D to its active form for absorption of calcium

   g. Excretes water-soluble medications and medication metabolites

   h. Minimum urine output 0.5 ml/kg/hr

2. Contributing Factors

   a. History of genitourinary disorder

   b. History of hypertension

   c. History of diabetes

   d. Family history of renal disease, such as polycystic kidney disease (PKD)

   e. Incontinence, benign prostatic hyperplasia (BPH), cancer, or kidney stones

   f. Nephrotoxic medications

3. Manifestations

   a. Flank pain radiating to upper thigh, testis, or labium

   b. Changes in voiding: Hematuria, proteinuria, dysuria, frequency, urgency, burning, nocturia, incontinence, polyuria, oliguria, anuria

   c. Thirst, fatigue, generalized edema

B. **Diagnostic Tests**

1. **Urinalysis**

   a. Specific gravity

   b. Color: Yellow, amber, or clear

   c. Negative glucose, protein, nitrites, RBCs, and WBCs

   d. pH

   e. First voided morning sample preferred: 15 mL

   f. Sent to laboratory immediately or refrigerated

   g. If clean catch, get urine for culture prior to starting antibiotics.

      1) Cleanse labia or glans penis.

      2) Obtain midstream sample.

2. **Renal function tests** (several tests over a period of time are necessary)

   a. BUN

   b. Increased BUN can indicate

      1) Hepatic or renal disease

      2) Dehydration or decreased kidney perfusion

      3) High-protein diet

      4) Infection

      5) Stress

      6) Steroid use

      7) GI bleeding

   c. Creatinine

      1) Creatinine is the best measure of renal function.

   d. 24-hr creatinine clearance: 75 to 120 mL/min

      1) Have the client void and discard the first specimen.

      2) Obtain serum creatinine.

      3) Collect all urine from the client for the next 24 hr. (Refrigerate or keep container on ice.)

      4) At the completion of the 24 hr, the test is stopped following the client's last void.

   e. Uric acid (serum)

   f. Prostate-specific antigen: Greater than 10 indicates risk of prostate cancer

3. **Radiologic tests**

   a. Kidneys, ureters, bladder (x-ray): Shows the size, shape, and position of kidneys, ureters, and bladder. No preparation is necessary. (Verify that the client is not pregnant.)

   b. IV pyelography (contrast dye): Helps in visualization of the urinary tract.

      1) Collaborative Care

         a) **Nursing Interventions**

            (1) Verify that informed consent has been signed.

            (2) Verify the client's last creatinine level.

            (3) The client should remain NPO for 8 hr; fluids can be permitted.

            (4) Administer laxatives as prescribed.

            (5) Administer an enema or suppository on the morning of the test (as necessary).

            (6) Monitor for allergies to iodine or shellfish.

            (7) Inform the client of potential sensations during the exam (flushing, warmth, nausea, metallic or salty taste, incontinence).

            (8) Emergency equipment should be readily available during the test.

            (9) Encourage fluids to help flush out the dye.

4. **Renal angiography:** Visualization of renal arterial supply; contrast material injected through a catheter
   a. **Nursing Interventions** (preprocedure)
      1) Approach is through the femoral or brachial artery.
      2) Locate and mark peripheral pulses.
      3) Have the client void before the procedure.
      4) Explain that the procedure can create the feeling of warmth along the vessel.
   b. **Nursing Interventions** (postprocedure)
      1) Maintain bed rest for 6 to 8 hr.
      2) Monitor vital signs until stable.
      3) Observe for swelling and hematoma.
      4) Palpate peripheral pulses/vascular checks.
      5) Monitor I&O including urinary status.

5. **Cystoscopy:** An invasive procedure in which a scope is passed to view the interior of the bladder, urethra, or the position of urethral orifices to remove calculi from the urethra, bladder, and ureter to treat lesions of the bladder, urethra, and prostate.
   a. **Nursing Interventions** (preoperative)
      1) Maintain NPO if the client receives general anesthesia.
      2) Administer preoperative cathartics/enemas as prescribed.
      3) Reinforce teaching of deep breathing exercises to relieve bladder spasms.
      4) Monitor for postural hypotension.
      5) Inform the client that pink-tinged or tea-colored urine is common following the procedure, but bright-red urine or clots should be reported.
      6) Provide nonpharmacological pain management techniques following the procedure.
   b. **Nursing Interventions** (postoperative)
      1) Monitor for leg cramps due to lithotomy position.
      2) Monitor for back or abdominal pain.
      3) Offer warm sitz baths for comfort.
      4) Push fluids and provide analgesics.
      5) Monitor I&O.

6. **Renal biopsy**
   a. **Nursing Interventions** (preprocedure)
      1) Obtain bleeding, clotting, and prothrombin times.
      2) Obtain results of prebiopsy x-rays of kidney.
      3) Administer IV fluids.
      4) Maintain NPO status for 6 to 8 hr.
      5) Position the client with a pillow under the abdomen and shoulders on the bed.
      6) Verify that the informed consent form is signed.
      7) Remind the client to remain still during the procedure.
   b. **Nursing Interventions** (postprocedure)
      1) Maintain the client in the supine position. The client should remain in bed for 24 hr.
      2) Monitor vital signs every 5 to 15 min for 4 hr.
      3) Maintain pressure to the puncture site for 20 min.

      4) Observe for any pain, nausea, vomiting, and blood pressure changes.
      5) Encourage fluid intake.
      6) Monitor Hct and Hgb for 8 hr after procedure.
      7) Monitor urine output.
      8) Make sure the client avoids strenuous activity, sports, and heavy lifting for at least 2 weeks.

7. **Indwelling urinary catheterization:** A sterile procedure to empty the contents of the bladder, obtain a sterile specimen, determine residual urine, initiate irrigation of the bladder, or bypass an obstruction.
   a. Collaborative Care
      1) **Nursing Interventions**
         a) Maintain a closed system.
         b) Measure the client's output every shift.
         c) Provide meticulous perineal care.
         d) Keep a drainage bag below the level of the client's bladder.
         e) Increase daily fluid intake.
         f) Prevent dependent loops in the catheter tubing.
         g) Discontinue as soon as possible due to increased risk for urinary tract infection.

C. **Specific Disorders**
   1. **Cystitis:** Inflammation of the urinary bladder
      a. Contributing Factors
         1) Wiping back to front after toileting, secondary to ascending infection from *Escherichia coli*
         2) Prolonged baths with excessive soap (common in female clients)
         3) Benign prostatic hyperplasia (male clients)
         4) Indwelling urinary catheter
      b. Manifestations
         1) Frequency and urgency, and only voiding small amounts of urine each time
         2) Dysuria with hematuria
         3) Suprapubic tenderness; pain in the bladder region or flank pain
         4) Fever, malaise, chills
         5) Cloudy, foul-smelling urine
         6) Urinalysis: Increased protein and WBC, presence of leukoesterase, casts, and bacteria
      c. Collaborative Care
         1) **Nursing Interventions**
            a) Obtain a clean-catch urine sample for culture and sensitivity before initiating antibiotic therapy.
            b) Maintain acidic urine pH.
            c) Push fluids (greater than 3,000 mL/day).
            d) Encourage the client to drink cranberry juice.
            e) Apply heat to the perineum for comfort.

2) Medications

  a) Antimicrobial medications: Sulfonamides are the medications of choice unless the client is allergic (sulfamethoxazole-trimethoprim and nitrofurantoin macrocrystal).

  b) Urinary analgesics (phenazopyridine): Inform the client that the medication will temporarily turn urine orange.

  c) Antispasmodics: Hyoscyamine

3) Client Education and Referral

  a) Follow appropriate perineal care (such as wiping front to back).

  b) Wear cotton underwear.

  c) Avoid bubble baths. (They can irritate urethra.)

  d) Maintain an increased fluid intake.

  e) Void after sexual intercourse.

  f) Drink cranberry juice daily.

2. **Acute Glomerulonephritis:** An acute renal disease involving the renal glomeruli of both kidneys. Thought to be an antigen-antibody reaction that damages the glomeruli of the kidney. Can be a secondary response to infection in other areas of the body that usually occurs in children. The prognosis is good if treatment is implemented.

  a. Contributing Factors

    1) Beta-hemolytic streptococcal

    2) Can follow tonsillitis or pharyngitis

  b. Manifestations

    1) Hematuria (cola or tea-colored urine), with proteinuria

    2) Edema (especially facial and periorbital; ascites)

    3) Oliguria or anuria

    4) Hypertension with headache

    5) Azotemia

    6) Flank or abdominal pain

    7) Anemia

  c. Collaborative Care

    1) **Nursing Interventions**

      a) Maintain bed rest to protect the kidney.

      b) Restrict fluids.

      c) Increase calories, and reduce protein and sodium in the diet.

      d) Monitor daily weight.

    2) Medications

      a) Penicillin for streptococcal infection (substitute other antibiotics for clients allergic to penicillin)

      b) Corticosteroids for inflammatory disease

      c) Antihypertensives for increased blood pressure

3. **Nephrosis:** A disorder associated with protein wasting; secondary to diffuse glomerular damage

  a. Contributing Factors

    1) Can be autoimmune. The glomerular membrane is more permeable, especially to proteins.

  b. Manifestations

    1) Insidious onset of pitting edema (generalized edema is anasarca)

    2) Proteinuria

    3) Anemia

    4) Hypoalbuminemia

    5) Anorexia, malaise, and nausea

    6) Oliguria

    7) Ascites

  c. Collaborative Care

    1) **Nursing Interventions**

      a) Maintain bed rest (during severe edema only) to preserve renal function.

      b) Maintain a low-sodium, low-potassium, moderate-protein, high-calorie diet.

      c) Protect the client from infection.

      d) Monitor I&O.

      e) Weigh the client and measure abdominal girth daily.

    2) Medication therapy

      a) Loop diuretics: furosemide

      b) Steroids: prednisone

      c) Immunosuppressive agents: cyclophosphamide

4. **Urolithiasis (urinary calculi):** Stones in the urinary system

  a. Contributing Factors

    1) Obstruction and urinary stasis

    2) Uric acid stones (excessive purine intake)

    3) Immobilization

    4) More common in male clients ages 20 to 40 and tends to reoccur

  b. Manifestations (based on location and size of the stone)

    1) Pain: Severe renal colic (ureter); dull, aching (kidney); radiates to the groin

    2) Nausea, vomiting, diarrhea, or constipation

    3) Hematuria

    4) Manifestations of a urinary tract infection

  c. Collaborative Care (Goals: To eradicate the stone and prevent nephron destruction)

    1) **Nursing Interventions**

      a) Force fluids—at least 3,000 mL/day (IV or by mouth)

      b) Strain all urine

      c) Provide pain control

      d) Maintain proper urine pH (depends on type of stone)

2) Medications

  a) Opioids (morphine IV for rapid pain relief). NSAID ketorolac in acute phase.

  b) Administer allopurinol for uric acid stones.

3) Therapeutic Measures

  a) Lithotripsy to crush the stone through sound waves

4) Client Education

  a) Avoid foods high in oxalates (spinach, black tea, rhubarb, chocolate) if it is a calcium oxalate stone.

  b) Maintain fluid intake to maintain hydration.

5. **Acute renal failure:** An abrupt decrease in renal function; can be the result of trauma, allergic reactions, drug overdose, kidney stones, or shock

  a. Contributing Factors

    1) Prerenal: Disrupted blood flow to the kidneys; hypovolemic shock, dehydration, heart failure, burn injury, and anaphylaxis

    2) Renal: Renal tissue damage; trauma, hypokalemia, acute glomerulonephritis, hemolytic uremic syndrome (infection caused by *Escherichia coli*; common in children), substance abuse

    3) Postrenal: Urine flow from the kidney is compromised; kidney stones, prostate hyperplasia, tumors, and strictures

  b. Manifestations (four phases)

    1) Onset: Begins with the onset of the event and lasts for hours to days.

    2) Oliguric (1 to 3 weeks): Sudden onset, less than 400 mL in 24 hr, edema, elevated BUN, creatinine and potassium; increased specific gravity; acidosis; heart failure; dysrhythmias

    3) Diuretic: Urine output increases followed by diuresis of up to 4,000 to 5,000 mL/day, indicating recovery of damaged nephrons; decreased specific gravity; hypotension and fluid and electrolyte imbalances are a concern

    4) Recovery: Can take up to 1 year until renal function returns to normal (baseline); older adults are at increased risk for residual impairment

  c. Collaborative Care

    1) **Nursing Interventions**

      a) Eliminate or prevent cause.

      b) Correct metabolic acidosis, hyperkalemia, hyperphosphatemia, and hypocalcemia.

        (1) Kayexalate (an ion exchange resin given orally or by enema to treat hyperkalemia)

        (2) IV glucose and insulin (causes potassium to enter cells)

        (3) Calcium IV or sodium bicarbonate to stabilize cell membrane

      c) Implement dietary modifications.

        (1) For oliguric phase: low-protein, high-carbohydrate diet and restricted potassium intake

        (2) For diuresis phase: low-protein, high-calorie diet and restricted fluids as indicated

          (a) Encourage bed rest in the oliguric phase.

          (b) Monitor daily weight.

          (c) Monitor I&O.

          (d) Implement dialysis (as prescribed) until renal function returns.

          (e) Monitor for pericarditis (friction rubs).

    2) Medications

      a) Phosphate binders to lower phosphorus while replacing calcium (calcium acetate)

      b) Epogen to treat anemia

6. **Chronic Kidney Disease:** Progressive failure of kidney function that results in death unless hemodialysis or transplant is performed; irreversible

  a. Stages of chronic kidney disease

    1) Stage 1: Glomerular filtration rate (GFR) greater than 90 mL/min

    2) Stage 2: GFR 60 to 89 mL/min

    3) Stage 3: GFR 30 to 59 mL/min

    4) Stage 4: GFR 15 to 29 mL/min

    5) Stage 5: GFR less than 15 mL/min (end-stage renal disease [ESRD])

  b. Contributing Factors

    1) Diabetes mellitus (leading cause)

    2) Uncontrolled hypertension (second leading cause)

    3) Chronic glomerulonephritis

    4) Pyelonephritis

    5) Congenital kidney disease, such as PKD

    6) Ethnicity: African American, Native American, and Asian

  c. Manifestations (progressively worsen)

    1) Fatigue secondary to anemia

    2) Headache and hypertension

    3) Nausea, vomiting, diarrhea

    4) Irritability

    5) Edema

    6) Hypocalcemia, hyperkalemia

    7) Pruritus, uremic frost

    8) Pallid, gray-yellow complexion

    9) Metabolic acidosis; elevated BUN and creatinine; decreased GFR

    10) Convulsions, coma

d. Collaborative Care

1) **Nursing Interventions**

a) Maintain bed rest.

b) Implement a renal diet: low-protein, low-potassium, high-carbohydrate, vitamins and calcium supplements, low-sodium, low-phosphate.

c) Monitor for and treat hypertension as prescribed.

d) Strict I&O; fluid replacement: 500 to 600 mL more than previous 24-hr urine output.

e) Monitor electrolytes.

f) Do not administer antacids with magnesium or enemas with phosphorous.

g) Maintain dialysis.

h) Administer diuretics in early stages.

i) Provide meticulous skin care.

j) Provide emotional support to the client and family.

k) Monitor for bleeding tendencies.

2) Medications

a) Phosphate binders (aluminum hydroxide gel, calcium acetate, sevelamer hydrochloride)

b) Epoetin alfa/erythropoietin (for anemia to stimulate RBC formation and transfuse as necessary)

7. **Dialysis**

a. Goals

1) Remove end products of metabolism (urea and creatinine) from the blood.

2) Maintain safe concentration of serum electrolytes.

3) Correct acidosis.

4) Remove excess fluid from the blood.

b. **Hemodialysis:** The process of cleansing the blood of accumulated waste products and fluids; used for ESRD or clients who are acutely ill and require short-term treatment

1) Collaborative Care

a) **Nursing Interventions**

(1) Weigh the client before and after the procedure.

(2) Monitor blood pressure continuously during the procedure.

(3) Provide care to the access site to prevent clotting and infection.

(4) Monitor for presence of thrill and bruit.

(5) Provide adequate nutrition as prescribed.

(6) Post a sign above the bed that warns of no blood pressure readings or blood work on the side of the fistula.

(7) Maintain fluid restrictions.

(8) Withhold regular morning medications prior to dialysis.

(9) Instruct the client to notify the nurse of muscle cramps, headache, nausea, or dizziness during the procedure.

(10) Provide emotional support. Offer activities (books, magazines, music, cards, television) to occupy the client.

c. **Peritoneal dialysis:** An alternative method using the peritoneum to remove fluids, electrolytes, and waste products from the blood. Dialysis is accomplished via a catheter surgically placed into the peritoneal cavity.

1) Collaborative Care

a) **Nursing Interventions**

(1) Assist the client to void prior to the procedure.

(2) Weigh the client daily.

(3) Monitor vital signs and baseline electrolytes.

(4) Maintain asepsis.

(5) Sterile dressing changes per facility policy.

(6) Keep an accurate record of fluid balance.

(7) Procedure

(a) Warm dialysate (1 to 2 L of 1.5%, 2.5%, or 4.25% glucose solution).

(b) Allow to flow in by gravity.

(c) 5 to 10 min inflow time; close clamp immediately.

(d) 30 min of equilibration (dwell time).

(e) 10 to 30 min of drainage (should be clear and pale yellow).

(f) Monitor for complications (peritonitis, bleeding, respiratory difficulty, abdominal pain, bowel or bladder perforation).

d. **Continuous ambulatory peritoneal dialysis (CAPD):** Peritoneal dialysis performed by the client without the use of a machine (cycler)

1) Procedure (differs from acute peritoneal dialysis)

a) Permanent indwelling catheter inserted into peritoneum

b) Fluid infused by gravity (1.5 to 3 L)

c) Dwell time: 4 to 8 hr

d) Dialysate drains by gravity: 20 to 40 min

e) Four to five exchanges daily, 7 days/week (some clients elect to do at night with automatic cycling machines; 10 to 14 hr, 3 times/week); continuous cycling peritoneal dialysis (CCPD)

2) Collaborative Care

a) **Nursing Interventions**

(1) Monitor for complications.

(2) Monitor for peritonitis (rebound tenderness, fever, cloudy outflow).

(3) Monitor for bladder perforation (yellow outflow).

(4) Monitor for hypotension.

(5) Monitor for bowel perforation (brown outflow).

b) Advantages to CAPD

(1) More independence

(2) Clients can continue normal activities during CAPD.

(3) Free dietary intake and better nutrition

(4) Satisfactory control of uremia

(5) Least expensive dialysis

(6) Decreased likelihood of future transplant rejection

(7) More closely approximates normal renal function

8. **Renal and urinary tract surgery**

   a. Kidney transplantation

      1) For individuals who have ESRD

      2) Requires a well-matched donor

         a) Living donors (most desirable)

         b) Cadaver donors

      3) Preoperative management

         a) Interventions are prescribed to correct metabolic status.

         b) Administer immunosuppressive therapy.

         c) Schedule hemodialysis within 24 hr if the client currently requires dialysis

         d) Provide emotional support.

      4) **Nursing Interventions** (postoperative management)

         a) Monitor labs (CBC, electrolytes, BUN/creatinine).

         b) Administer immunosuppressive medications (azathioprine cyclosporine, steroids).

         c) Monitor for rejection (oliguria; edema; fever; tenderness over graft site; fluid and electrolyte imbalance; hypertension; elevated BUN, creatinine, or WBCs).

         d) Monitor for infection. Maintain protective isolation.

         e) Provide emotional support. Monitor for depression.

9. **Urinary diversion:** Removal of the bladder and surrounding structures to reroute urinary flow through a pouch and abdominal stoma

   a. Collaborative Care

      1) **Nursing Interventions**

         a) Monitor vital signs. (Hemorrhage and shock are frequent complications.)

         b) Monitor the stoma.

         c) Provide pain control.

         d) Observe for manifestations of paralytic ileus, which are very common.

         e) Provide adequate fluid replacement.

         f) Weigh the client daily.

         g) Maintain function and patency of the drainage tubes.

            (1) Indwelling urinary catheter (dependent position, tape tubing to the thigh)

            (2) Nephrostomy tube

               (a) Never clamp.

               (b) Irrigate only with prescription for 10 mL of 0.9% sodium chloride.

               (c) Monitor for leakage of urine.

(3) Ureteral catheters

   (a) Each catheter drains half of the urinary system.

   (b) Bloody drainage is expected after surgery, but should clear within 24 to 48 hr.

   (c) Never irrigate the surgical implant.

   (d) Aseptic technique is required.

10. **Benign prostatic hyperplasia:** Enlargement of the prostate that can accompany the aging process in males; exact cause is unknown.

    a. Manifestations

       1) Difficulty starting stream/dribbling

       2) Decrease in force of the urinary stream

       3) Frequent urinary tract infections

       4) Nocturia

       5) Hematuria

    b. Diagnosis

       1) Digital rectal exam or cystoscopy

       2) Prostate-specific antigen (PSA) for diagnosis

    c. Treatments

       1) Urinary antibiotics

       2) Alpha-blocker medications to promote urinary flow: terazosin, tamsulosin, alfuzosin, silodosin, doxazosin

       3) Enzyme inhibitors to decrease the size of the prostate gland: dutasteride, finasteride

       4) **Transurethral resection of prostate (TURP):** Enlarged portion of the prostate is removed through an endoscopic instrument.

          a) **Nursing Interventions** (preoperative)

             (1) Insert indwelling urinary catheter.

             (2) Administer antibiotics as prescribed.

          b) **Nursing Interventions** (postoperative)

             (1) Monitor for shock and hemorrhage.

             (2) Reinforce with the client to avoid heavy lifting, prolonged sitting, constipation, or straining (which could cause a rebleed).

             (3) Monitor for continuous bladder irrigation. (Expect bloody drainage. Monitor I&O carefully.)

             (4) Encourage fluid intake (at least 3,000 mL/day).

             (5) Monitor for TURP syndrome: A cluster of manifestations resulting from absorption of irrigating fluids through prostate tissue (hyponatremia, confusion, bradycardia, hypo/hypertension, nausea, vomiting, visual changes).

             (6) Medicate for pain control. The client can need medication and narcotics to decrease bladder spasm.

             (7) Keep the catheter taped tightly to the client's leg (for hemostasis at the surgical site by catheter balloon).

             (8) Reinforce teaching about Kegel exercises. (There can be temporary or permanent loss of sexual function or urinary control.)

11. **Prostate cancer:** A slow-growing cancer of the prostate gland
    a. Contributing Factors
       1) Males age 50 and older
       2) African American clients
       3) Family history
       4) Elevated testosterone levels
       5) High-fat diet
    b. Manifestations
       1) Asymptomatic in early stages
       2) Hematuria
       3) Prostate-specific antigen (PSA) greater than 10
       4) Rectal exam: Hard, pea-sized nodule
       5) Frequent UTIs
    c. Treatment
       1) Radical prostatectomy
       2) External radiation therapy
       3) Internal radioactive seeds
       4) Hormone therapy

12. **Testicular Cancer:** Rare cancer affecting one or both testes. Testicular self-examination (TSE) should begin during adolescence.
    a. Contributing Factors
       1) Males 20 to 54 years of age
       2) Higher risk in males who have an undescended testis
       3) Family history
    b. Manifestations
       1) Swelling or painless lump in one or both testes
       2) Possible heaviness or aching in lower abdomen or scrotum
    c. Treatment
       1) Offer sperm banking prior to surgery.
       2) Orchiectomy to remove affected testicle
       3) Chemotherapy
       4) Emotional support

13. **Incontinence**
    a. Types
       1) Urge: Cannot hold urine when stimulus to void occurs
       2) Functional: Cannot physically get to the bathroom or is not aware of the stimulus to void
       3) Stress: Pressure (coughing, straining, lifting, bearing down, laughing) causes incontinence; very common in middle-age females
    b. Collaborative Care
       1) **Nursing Interventions**
          a) Use adult incontinence devices.
          b) Decrease fluid intake after 6 p.m.
          c) Maintain a regular toilet schedule.
          d) Perform the Credé maneuver as needed.

    e) Monitor for signs of cystitis.
    f) Reinforce teaching about Kegel exercises to strengthen the sphincter.
    g) Ensure that the physical environment enhances the ability to get to the bathroom.
       2) Medications
          a) Urge incontinence
             (1) Anticholinergics: Tolterodine, oxybutynin
          b) Stress incontinence
             (1) Tricyclic antidepressant: Imipramine

14. **Urine retention:** Caused by a physical obstruction of the urethra from acute or chronic causes (edema, BPH, tumor, inflammation or inability of the bladder to work, postanesthesia, stroke); at risk for hydronephrosis
    a. Collaborative Care
       1) **Nursing Interventions**
          a) Stimulate relaxation of the urethral sphincter by providing privacy, placing the client's hands in warm water (or just turning on the water), and encouraging guided imagery.
          b) Administer bethanechol chloride.
          c) Position the client upright.
          d) Ensure adequate fluid intake.

Neurosensory Disorders

A. **Neurological Assessment**
   1. History of present illness
   2. Mental status
      a. Level of consciousness (alert, lethargic, obtunded, stuporous, comatose)
      b. Orientation (person, place, time)
      c. Affect
      d. Mood
      e. Speech (clarity, consistency, word-finding ability)
      f. Cognition (judgment and abstraction ability)
   3. Cranial nerves (I through XII)
      a. CN I, olfactory: Sensory, smell
      b. CN II, optic: Sensory, vision
      c. CN III, oculomotor: Motor, eye
      d. CN IV, trochlear: Motor, eye
      e. CN V, trigeminal: Sensory, face; motor, chewing
      f. CN VI, abducens: Motor, eye
      g. CN VII, facial: Sensory, face, and hands
      h. CN VIII, acoustic: Sensory, hearing, balance
      i. CN IX, glossopharyngeal: Sensory, posterior taste
      j. CN X, vagus: Sensory, throat; motor, swallow, speech; cardiac innervation (slows down)
      k. CN XI, accessory: Motor, throat, neck muscles, upper back
      l. CN XII, hypoglossal: Motor, tongue

4. Motor function
   a. Muscles
      1) Size
      2) Symmetry
      3) Tone
      4) Strength
   b. Coordination
   c. Movement
      1) Voluntary control/involuntary movements
      2) Tremors
      3) Twitches
      4) Balance and gait
   d. Posturing
      1) Decorticate (flexion): An abnormal posturing indicated by rigidity, flexion of the arms to the chest, clenched fists, and extended legs. Indicative of damage to the corticospinal tract (the pathway between the brain and the spinal cord).

DECORTICATE POSTURING

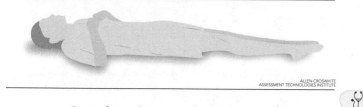

ALLEN CROSWHITE
ASSESSMENT TECHNOLOGIES INSTITUTE

      2) Decerebrate (extension): An abnormal body posturing indicated by rigid extension of the arms and legs, downward pointing of the toes, and backward arching of the head. Indicative of deterioration of structures of the nervous system, particularly the upper brain stem.

DECEREBRATE POSTURING

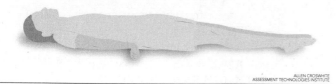

ALLEN CROSWHITE
ASSESSMENT TECHNOLOGIES INSTITUTE

5. Reflexes
   a. Deep tendon reflexes (DTRs)
      1) Biceps, triceps, brachioradial, quadriceps
   b. Superficial reflex
      1) Plantar, abdominal, Babinski
   c. Reflex activity
      1) Absent, no response = 0
      2) Weaker than normal = 1+
      3) Normal = 2+
      4) Stronger/more brisk = 3+
      5) Hyperactive = 4+

6. Glasgow Coma Scale: Neurologic assessment tool
   a. Rating: 3 (least responsive) to 15 (most responsive)

GLASGOW COMA SCALE

EYE OPENING RESPONSE (E)	VERBAL RESPONSE (V)	MOTOR RESPONSE (M)
4 = Spontaneous	5 = Normal conversation	6 = Normal
3 = To voice	4 = Disoriented conversation	5 = Localizes to pain
2 = To pain	3 = Words, but not coherent	4 = Withdraws to pain
1 = None	2 = No words, only sounds	3 = Decorticate posture
	1 = None	2 = Decerebrate
		1 = None
E Score	V Score	M Score

E + V + M = Total score

7. Pupil check: PERRLA
   a. **P**upils **E**qual in size, **R**ound and regular in shape, **R**eactive to **L**ight and **A**ccommodation
8. Vital signs
   a. Blood pressure or pulse changes can indicate increased intracranial pressure.

B. **Diagnostic Procedures**
   1. **Lumbar puncture:** Procedure that inserts a needle into the subarachnoid space to measure pressure, obtain cerebrospinal fluid (CSF) for analysis, and inject contrast, anesthetics, and certain medications.
      a. **Nursing Interventions**
         1) Verify that informed consent has been signed.
         2) Have the client empty the bladder and bowel.
         3) Position the client on the side with knees pulled toward the chest and chin tucked downward.
         4) Assist providers with measuring pressure and collecting fluid.
         5) Postprocedure
            a) Encourage fluid intake.
            b) Check puncture site for redness, swelling, and clear drainage.
            c) Monitor movement of extremities.
            d) Monitor for complications.
   2. **Computed tomography (CT) scan**
      a. **Nursing Interventions**
         1) Preprocedure
            a) Verify that informed consent has been signed.
            b) Check for any allergies to iodine, contrast dyes, or shellfish.
            c) Monitor BUN and creatinine.
            d) Instruct the client to lie still and flat.
         2) Postprocedure
            a) Increase fluids to clear dye from the client's system.
            b) Monitor dye injection site.
            c) Monitor for allergic reaction to dye.

3. **Cerebral arteriography:** Injection of dye usually via the femoral artery to allow visualization of the cerebral arteries

   a. **Nursing Interventions**

      1) Preprocedure

         a) Verify that informed consent has been signed.

         b) Check for allergies to iodine, contrast dyes, or shellfish.

         c) Monitor BUN and creatinine.

         d) Keep client NPO 4 to 6 hr before the procedure.

         e) Mark distal peripheral pulses.

         f) Reinforce teaching with the client that the face can feel warm during the procedure.

      2) Postprocedure

         a) Monitor for an altered level of consciousness and sensory or motor deficits.

         b) Check for bleeding or hematoma at the insertion site. Movement is restricted for 8 to 12 hr.

         c) Check peripheral pulses, color, and temperature of extremities.

4. **Electroencephalogram (EEG):** Noninvasive assessment of the electrical activity of the brain. Electrodes are placed over multiple areas of the scalp to detect and record patterns of electrical activity. They also check for abnormalities (seizure disorders, evaluation of head injuries, tumors, infections, degenerative diseases, metabolic disturbances) or to confirm brain death.

   a. **Nursing Interventions**

      1) Verify which medications should be administered before the EEG. Depressive, stimulant, and antiseizure medications are usually not given.

      2) Remind the client to avoid caffeine 8 hr before the test.

      3) Advise the client to wash hair before the test, because it must be free of oils, sprays, and conditioners.

      4) Verify if the test is to be done awake, asleep, or sleep-deprived.

5. **Magnetic resonance imaging (MRI):** A noninvasive procedure that uses a magnetic field to construct clear, detailed, cross-sectional images of the body

   a. **Nursing Interventions**

      1) Verify that informed consent has been signed.

      2) Monitor for claustrophobia.

      3) Remove all metal objects (body piercings, jewelry, credit cards, watches).

      4) No specific test, diet, or medications are required.

C. **Disorders**

1. **Head injury:** Any trauma that leads to injury of the scalp, skull, or brain, ranging from concussion to skull fracture; classified as either closed or open (scalp, skull, and dura open).

   a. **Closed-head injury**

      1) Head sustains blunt force trauma

      2) Concussion (temporary loss of neurological function with no apparent structural damage)

      3) Contusion (brain is damaged; characterized by loss of consciousness and confusion)

      4) Diffuse axonal injury (shearing and rotational forces produce brain damage)

   b. **Basilar skull fracture**

      1) Manifestations

         a) Bleeding from the nose and ears

         b) Otorrhea, rhinorrhea: CSF from the ears or nose; differentiate between CSF and mucus by assessing glucose content of the drainage

         c) Raccoon eyes (periorbital edema and ecchymosis)

         d) Battle's sign (postauricular ecchymosis) noted on mastoid bone

   c. **Hematomas**

      1) Epidural hematoma: Bleeding into the space between the skull and the dura

         a) Commonly involves the middle meningeal artery

         b) Typical presentation: Client sustains the injury, followed by a brief loss of consciousness; this is followed by a lucid interval, then rapid deterioration

         c) Emergency management: Burr holes and placement of drain to relieve increasing intracranial pressure

      2) Subdural hematoma: Bleeding below the dura

         a) Usually venous

         b) Can be acute, subacute, or chronic

         c) Manifestations

            (1) Acute: Symptoms develop over 24 to 48 hr and include change in LOC, pupillary changes, and hemiparesis.

            (2) Subacute: Symptoms develop from 48 hr to 2 weeks after injury.

            (3) Chronic: Seen frequently in the elderly; symptoms can mimic CVA.

            (4) Management: Surgical evacuation of hematoma and/or burr holes and drain placement.

      3) **Nursing Interventions**

         a) Monitor frequently for signs of increased intracranial pressure (ICP).

         b) Prevent or minimize increased ICP.

2. **Increased ICP:** A rise in pressure within the skull that can result from or cause a brain injury

   a. Contributing Factors

      1) Head injury with subdural or epidural hematoma

      2) Cerebrovascular accident or cerebral edema

      3) Brain tumor

      4) Hydrocephalus

      5) Ruptured aneurysm and subarachnoid hemorrhage

      6) Meningitis, encephalitis

   b. Manifestations (vary depending on cause and location; will affect level of consciousness)

      1) Earliest sign: Changes in LOC (restlessness, confusion, drowsiness, lethargy, stupor); motor and sensory changes

      2) Headache, diplopia, irritability

      3) Nausea and vomiting, often projectile

      4) Pupil changes: Dilated, unequal, nonreactive

     5) Changes in vital signs

       a) Cushing's triad: Hypertension with widening pulse pressure, bradycardia, and irregular breathing (Cheyne-Stokes respirations)

       b) Ineffective thermoregulation

  c. Collaborative Care

    1) **Nursing Interventions**

      a) Monitor vital signs and neurological function.

      b) Keep head of bed elevated 30° to 45°.

      c) Keep the client's head in a neutral position to enhance drainage.

      d) Avoid coughing, sneezing, straining, and suctioning.

      e) Maintain maximum respiratory exchange. (Hypercapnia causes vasodilation, thus increasing ICP.)

      f) Administer oxygen to increase the supply to the brain.

      g) Monitor fluid I&O. Can restrict fluids to prevent increased cerebral edema.

      h) Administer medications as prescribed.

      i) Use hypothermia as prescribed to decrease ICP.

      j) Decrease environmental stimuli.

      k) Intensive care is required when monitoring ICP (ventriculostomy).

    2) Medications

      a) Avoid opiates and sedatives unless ventilated (will restrict neurological assessment).

      b) Barbiturates to place the client into a therapeutic coma with ventilator support and close monitoring of cardiac status.

      c) Acetaminophen can be used for fever.

      d) Osmotic diuretics (such as mannitol) and steroids (such as dexamethasone) can be used to decrease cerebral edema.

3. **Hyperthermia**: Elevated temperature can be caused by infection or damage to the hypothalamic temperature regulating center. This increases cerebral oxygen demand.

  a. Contributing Factors

    1) Infections

    2) Cerebral edema

    3) Environmental heat

  b. Manifestations

    1) Temperature elevation, shivering

    2) Hypoxia

  c. Collaborative Care

    1) **Nursing Interventions**

      a) Monitor neurologic status and vital signs.

      b) Use a hypothermia blanket or cool sponge bath.

      c) Monitor ECG for tachycardia and dysrhythmias.

      d) Monitor for manifestations of dehydration by checking I&O and weighing the client daily.

      e) Initiate seizure precautions (can be prescribed benzodiazepines to suppress seizure activity).

      f) Prevent shivering (which can occur if temperature is reduced quickly) to decrease risk of increased ICP and oxygen consumption

        (1) Chlorpromazine

        (2) Benzodiazepines: diazepam

4. **Seizure disorders**: Abnormal, sudden, uncontrolled, excessive discharge of electrical activity within the brain

  a. Contributing Factors

    1) Drug or alcohol withdrawal

    2) Trauma

    3) Brain tumors

    4) Toxicity or infection

    5) Fever

  b. Classifications

    1) Generalized seizures

      a) Tonic-clonic (formerly grand mal)

      b) Absence (formerly petit mal)

      c) Myoclonic

      d) Atonic or akinetic (drop attacks)

    2) Partial seizures

      a) Complex (usually with impairment of consciousness)

      b) Simple (usually without alteration of consciousness)

  c. Collaborative Care

    1) **Nursing Interventions**

      a) Maintain patent airway. (Position side-lying.)

      b) Monitor respiratory status and loosen constrictive clothing.

      c) Protect the client from injury.

      d) Do not restrain the client.

      e) Do not put anything in the client's mouth.

      f) Turn the client's head to the side to prevent aspiration.

      g) Document observations before, during, and after a seizure.

      h) Observe for prodromal signs of an aura (a sensory warning that the seizure is about to occur).

      i) Document how long the client remains unconscious.

      j) Determine if there is any incontinence.

      k) Identify precipitating factors.

      l) Monitor and document behavior during the postictal phase (period following seizure).

      m) Initiate seizure precautions.

        (1) Bed rest should include padded side rails.

        (2) Ensure that immediate access is available for oxygen administration and suction.

2) Medications
   a) Phenytoin
   b) Carbamazepine
   c) Valproic acid
   d) Phenobarbital
   e) Levetiracetam
   f) Topiramate
3) Client Education
   a) Take medications consistently. Never stop abruptly.
   b) Teach manifestations of medication toxicity.
   c) Get adequate rest to minimize fatigue.
   d) Avoid alcohol.
   e) Wear a medical alert bracelet.
   f) Follow state laws regarding operating vehicles and machinery.
   g) Keep all follow-up appointments.
   h) Identify seizure triggers.

5. **Status epilepticus**: A life-threatening condition characterized by a series of generalized seizures without full recovery of consciousness between; can be caused by a sudden withdrawal of anticonvulsant medications; can lead to brain damage or death.
   a. Collaborative Care
      1) **Nursing Interventions**
         a) Initiate seizure precautions.
      2) Medications
         a) Lorazepam is the medication of choice.
         b) Diazepam
         c) Phenytoin: Administer IV slowly, giving no more than 50 mg/min.
            (1) Do not mix with glucose. Administer in 0.9% sodium chloride.
            (2) Monitor for bradycardia and heart block.
         d) Fosphenytoin

6. **Transient ischemic attack (TIA)**: Sudden temporary episode of neurological dysfunction lasting usually less than 1 hr secondary to decreased blood flow to the brain; can be a warning sign of an impending stroke.
   a. Contributing Factors
      1) Nonmodifiable
         a) Advanced age
         b) Male sex
         c) Genetics
      2) Modifiable
         a) Hypertension
         b) Hyperlipidemia
         c) Diabetes mellitus
         d) Smoking
         e) Atrial fibrillation
   b. Manifestations
      1) Sudden change in visual function
      2) Sudden loss of sensory or motor functions

c. Diagnostic Procedures
   1) Carotid ultrasound
   2) CT scan and/or MRI
   3) Arteriography
   4) 12-lead ECG
d. Collaborative Care
   1) **Nursing Interventions**
      a) Encourage the client to stop smoking and limit alcohol intake.
      b) DASH diet (high in fruits and vegetables, moderate in low-fat dairy products, and low in animal protein)
      c) Stress the importance of maintaining ideal body weight with regular exercise.
   2) Medications
      a) Antiplatelet medications
         (1) Clopidogrel
         (2) Dipyridamole plus aspirin
         (3) Ticlopidine
      b) Anticoagulant medications
         (1) Warfarin
      c) Lipid-lowering agents
   3) Therapeutic Measures
      a) Angioplasty
      b) Carotid endarterectomy (removal of plaque from one or both carotid arteries)

7. **Cerebrovascular accident (CVA)**: Commonly referred to as a stroke or "brain attack"; the sudden loss of brain function resulting from a disruption of blood supply to the involved part of the brain; causes temporary or permanent neurological deficits.
   a. Contributing Factors
      1) Hypertension and obesity
      2) Smoking or cocaine use
      3) Hyperlipidemia
      4) Diabetes mellitus
      5) Peripheral vascular disease
      6) Aneurysm or cranial hemorrhage
   b. Manifestations: The severity of the neurological deficit is determined by location and the extent of tissue ischemia. Physical manifestations occur on the side opposite of damage to the brain.
      1) Change in mental status
      2) Slurred speech, aphasia, dysphagia
      3) Numbness or weakness of the face or extremities, especially on one side of the body
      4) Visual disturbance
      5) Cranial nerve disturbance
      6) Loss of balance or coordination
      7) Sudden severe headache

c. Collaborative Care

1) **Nursing Interventions**

   a) Maintain airway.

   b) Monitor neurological function and vital signs.

   c) Establish baseline level of function and Glasgow coma scale.

   d) Maintain fluid and electrolyte balance.

   e) Monitor for aspiration due to risk of dysphagia. Feed the client slowly, placing food in the back of the mouth and to the unaffected side.

   f) Provide psychological support to the client and family.

   g) Establish means of communication with a client who is experiencing aphasia (expressive, receptive, global).

   h) Encourage slow, deliberate speech.

   i) Range of motion: To prevent flexion contractures, keep extremities in a position of extension or neutrality.

   j) Maintain skin integrity.

   k) Hemiparesis, hemiplegia: Will cause safety issues in the client.

   l) Help the client achieve bowel and bladder control.

   m) Hemianopsia: Place articles within the client's visual range.

2) Therapeutic measures

   a) Thrombolytic therapy (ischemic CVA); Contraindicated if longer than 4.5 hr

   b) Surgical management (usually hemorrhagic CVA)

   c) Endovascular interventions (embolectomy and carotid artery angioplasty/stent)

3) Client Education and Referral

   a) Occupational and physical therapy

   b) Speech therapy

8. **Spinal cord injury**: Partial or complete disruption of nerve tracts and neurons; resulting in paralysis, sensory loss, altered activity, and autonomic nervous system dysfunction.

a. Contributing Factors

1) Males age 16 to 30 years

2) Motor vehicle accidents

3) Falls

4) Violence

5) Sporting activities

b. Types

1) Contusion

2) Laceration

3) Compression of the cord

4) Complete transection (paralyzed below the level of injury)

c. Manifestations (determined by the level of injury)

1) Cervical: Partial or complete quadriplegia/ tetraplegia

   a) Respiratory dysfunction (client can be ventilator-dependent)

   b) Partial or complete paralysis of all four extremities

   c) Loss of bladder and bowel control, alteration in sexual function

2) Thoracic injury: Partial or complete paraplegia

   a) Loss of bladder and bowel control, alteration in sexual function

   b) Partial or complete paralysis of lower extremities and major control of body trunk

   c) Potential complication of autonomic dysreflexia (injury above T6)

   d) Respiratory complications

3) Lumbar

   a) Partial or complete paralysis of lower extremities

   b) Loss of bladder and bowel control, alteration in sexual function

d. Collaborative Care

1) **Nursing Interventions**

   a) Immobilize the client.

     (1) Spinal board

     (2) Halo traction

     (3) Gardner-Wells traction or Crutchfield tongs

     (4) Cervical collar

   b) Maintain and monitor respiratory function.

   c) Monitor for spinal shock (loss of sensation, flaccid paralysis, reflexes below the level of injury).

   d) Monitor for neurogenic shock (decreased blood pressure, heart rate, and cardiac output; venous pooling).

   e) Monitor for autonomic dysreflexia (a life-threatening syndrome with sudden, severe hypertension triggered by noxious stimuli below damage of cord), which can be caused by impaction, bladder distension, pressure points or ulcers, or pain.

     (1) Manifestations

       (a) Hypertension with bradycardia

       (b) Headache, flushing

       (c) Piloerection (goose bumps), sweating

       (d) Nasal congestion

     (2) **Nursing Interventions**

       (a) Place the client in the high-Fowler's position to help decrease blood pressure.

       (b) Determine and remove causative stimuli.

       (c) Reinforce teaching about bowel and bladder management.

       (d) Administer medications as prescribed.

     (3) Therapeutic measures

       (a) Surgical management

     (4) Client Education and Referral

       (a) Occupational and physical therapy

9. **Multiple sclerosis (MS)**: Chronic, progressive immune-mediated disease of the CNS, characterized by patches of demyelination in the brain and spinal cord in which symptoms occur in relapse and remission type pattern (exact cause unknown)

   a. Contributing factors

      1) Age 20 to 40 years

      2) Female sex

      3) Geographic: Europe, New Zealand, southern Australia, northern U.S., southern Canada

      4) Genetic predisposition

   b. Manifestations vary in relation to location of lesion (plague).

      1) MRI shows sclerotic patches through the brain and spinal cord

      2) Fatigue

      3) Visual disturbances (nystagmus, blurred vision, diplopia)

      4) Slurred speech

      5) Spasticity and/or weakness of extremities, paresthesia, numbness, and pain

      6) Emotional lability, depression

      7) Intention tremors

      8) Spastic bladder

   c. Management

      1) Currently there is no cure. Treatment is aimed at relieving symptoms and decreasing the frequency and severity of relapses.

      2) During exacerbation, administer corticosteroids as prescribed.

      3) Stress management techniques can be helpful to prevent exacerbations.

   d. Collaborative Care

      1) **Nursing Interventions**

         a) Promote independence and maintaining an active, normal lifestyle as possible.

         b) Reinforce self-catheterization techniques, if needed.

         c) Promote daily exercise with fall precautions.

         d) Remind the client to avoid stressors that exacerbate the condition (infections).

         e) Reinforce the self-injection technique.

         f) Prevent injury.

      2) Medications

         a) Immunosuppressants to reduce the frequency and duration of relapses: interferon beta-1a (IM weekly), interferon beta-1b (subcutaneously), glatiramer acetate (subcutaneously daily)

         b) Muscle spasticity and tremors: baclofen, gabapentin, clonazepam

         c) Urinary problems and constipation: oxybutynin, tolterodine, propantheline, psyllium

         d) Depression: amitriptyline, sertraline, fluoxetine

         e) Sexual difficulties: sildenafil

         f) Fatigue: amantadine, modafinil

      3) Client Education and Referrals

         a) Referrals to occupational, physical, and speech therapy

         b) Proper medication administration to include self-injection

         c) Prevention of relapse

         d) Self-catheterization, if needed

10. **Parkinson's disease**: Chronic, progressive neurological disorder caused by loss of pigmented cells of substantia nigra and depletion of dopamine

    a. Manifestations

       1) Bradykinesia with rigidity

       2) Resting tremor

       3) Postural and gait disturbances

       4) Expressionless, fixed gaze; masklike

       5) Depression

       6) Drooling and slurred speech

    b. Collaborative Care

       1) **Nursing Interventions**

          a) Reinforce teaching about fall precautions.

          b) Encourage clothing that fosters independence (no snaps, buttons, or zippers).

          c) Encourage a high-fiber diet.

       2) Medications

          a) Antiparkinsonian agent: levodopa

          b) Dopamine agonist: bromocriptine mesylate

          c) Anticholinergic: benztropine

          d) Antiviral: amantadine hydrochloride (side effects include tremor, rigidity, and bradykinesia)

          e) Antihistamine: diphenhydramine

       3) Therapeutic measures

          a) Thalamotomy and pallidotomy

          b) Neural transplantation

          c) Deep brain stimulation

       4) Client Education and Referral

          a) Injury prevention

          b) Medication regimen

          c) Promotion of adequate nutrition (can need supplementation)

          d) Strategies to improve bowel and bladder function

          e) Use of assistive devices

          f) Referral to occupational, physical, and speech therapy

11. **Amyotrophic lateral sclerosis (ALS)**: Progressive, invariably fatal neurological disease that attacks nerve cells (neurons) that control voluntary muscles; also known as Lou Gehrig's disease

    a. Manifestations

       1) Fasciculations (twitching), cramping, and muscle weakness

       2) Fatigue

       3) Slurred or nasal speech with difficulty forming words (dysarthria)

4) Difficulty chewing and swallowing (dysphagia)

5) Overactive deep tendon reflex

6) Fatigue

7) Some experience cognitive impairment.

8) Eventual respiratory compromise. Death usually occurs from respiratory failure, infection, or aspiration.

b. Etiology unknown; no known cure; treatment is symptomatic

c. Collaborative Care

1) **Nursing Interventions**

a) Reinforce education.

b) Provide information and support. Verify home support systems.

c) Implement aspiration precautions and alternate methods of communication if needed.

d) Support respiratory function (mechanical ventilation or noninvasive positive-pressure ventilation).

e) Administer medications to provide relief from excessive salivation, pain, muscle cramps, constipation, and depression.

f) Provide supportive services to the client and family with anticipatory grieving.

2) Medications

a) Glutamate antagonist: Riluzole can have a neuroprotective effect in early stages.

b) Manage spasticity: baclofen, dantrolene sodium, diazepam

c) Client Education and Referral

(1) Disease progression and prognosis

(2) Complete advance directive

(3) Interventions to maximize respiratory function and prevent infection

(4) Strategies to prevent aspiration

(5) Alternate communication methods

(6) Referral to occupational, physical, speech therapy, home care, and hospice as needed

12. **Myasthenia gravis**: Autoimmune disorder in which antibodies attack acetylcholine receptors in the muscles, causing impaired nerve impulse transmission. This results in voluntary muscle weakness that increases with activity, improves with rest, and is characterized by periods of exacerbation and remission.

a. Manifestations

1) Muscular weakness that increases with activity and improves with rest

2) Early manifestations involve the ocular muscles leading to an increased risk of aspiration. Symptoms include diplopia, ptosis, dysphagia, and dysphonia.

3) Progressive deterioration, particularly the respiratory system, and muscle wasting

b. Diagnostic Procedures

1) Edrophonium chloride: An acetylcholinesterase inhibitor is injected IV; immediate improvement of symptoms that lasts approximately 5 min is considered a positive test and diagnostic of myasthenia gravis. Can be used to differentiate between cholinergic and myasthenic crisis. The antidote atropine should be available to counteract possible adverse effects (bradycardia, sweating, cramping).

2) Serum acetylcholine receptor antibodies

3) MRI of thymus gland

4) EMG

c. Types of Crisis

1) Cholinergic: Usually from overmedication; muscle fasciculations, which can lead to respiratory distress, increased GI motility, hypersecretion, hypotension. No improvement or worsening of symptoms with Tensilon test.

2) Myasthenic: Can be caused by an exacerbation trigger or inadequate medication. It is characterized by varying degrees of respiratory distress, dysphagia, dysarthria, ptosis, diplopia, hypertension, and increased muscle weakness. Symptoms improve during Tensilon test.

d. Factors contributing to exacerbations

1) Infections

2) Pregnancy

3) Stress, emotional distress, fatigue

4) Increases in body temperature

5) Inconsistency with medication administration

e. Collaborative Care

1) **Nursing Interventions**

a) Maintain patent airway.

(1) Prevent aspiration.

(2) Keep suction and manual ventilation equipment at bedside.

b) Plan activities for the client early in the day to avoid fatigue.

c) Provide small, frequent, high-calorie meals during the peak time for medications (within 45 min of administration).

d) Administer medications on time.

e) Provide eye care (instilling artificial tears and/or taping the eye shut at intervals as prescribed).

2) Medications

a) Anticholinesterase medications increase the amount of acetylcholine in the neuromuscular function.

(1) Pyridostigmine: First-line therapy

(2) Atropine is the antidote for anticholinesterase medications

b) Immunosuppressants

(1) Steroids: prednisone

(2) Cytotoxic medications: azathioprine

3) Therapeutic Measures

  a) Thymectomy (excision of the thymus)

  b) Intravenous immunoglobulin (IVIG)

  c) Plasmapheresis

4) Client Education and Referral

  a) Importance of appropriate medication administration

  b) Prevention of aspiration (meals need to be timed with peak action of medication, head flexed forward, foods with thickened consistency, suction available in home)

  c) Energy conservation; mobility strategies

  d) Factors that contribute to exacerbations and actions to take if an exacerbation occurs

  e) Referral to speech therapy and Myasthenia Gravis Foundation of America

13. **Guillain-Barré syndrome**: Acute, autoimmune attack on the peripheral nerve and some cranial nerve myelin.

  a. Manifestations

    1) Usually preceded by an infection (respiratory, gastrointestinal)

    2) Usually presents with ascending weakness, which can progress to paralysis, leading to acute respiratory failure

    3) Hyporeflexia

    4) Recovery takes several months to 2 years

    5) Paresthesia and pain

  b. Collaborative Management

    1) **Nursing Interventions**

      a) Monitor respiratory status, and provide respiratory support as indicated.

      b) Monitor vital signs and ECG.

      c) Provide nutrition and prevent aspiration (can need parenteral supplementation).

      d) Manage bowel and bladder problems.

      e) Collaborate with physical therapy to maintain muscle strength, flexibility, and contractures.

      f) Prevent complications of immobility (pneumonia, deep-vein thrombosis, urinary tract infection atelectasis, skin breakdown).

      g) Decrease anxiety by providing information and support.

    2) Therapeutic Measures

      a) Respiratory support (can need mechanical ventilation)

      b) Plasmapheresis

      c) Intravenous immunoglobulin (IVIG)

    3) Client Education and Referral

      a) Refer to occupational, physical, speech, and respiratory therapy.

      b) Use strategies to prevent complications of immobility.

      c) Recovery can take up to 2 years.

D. **Common Surgical Procedures**

1. **Laminectomy**: A surgical procedure to remove a portion of vertebrae for the treatment of severe pain and disability resulting from compression of spinal nerves by a ruptured disk or bony compression; also an option to relieve persistent pain or to treat progressive neurological problems due to nerve compression

2. **Discectomy**: Surgical procedure to remove a herniated disk

3. **Spinal Fusion**: Surgical fusion of the vertebral spinous process with a bone graft (autologous or banked), which provides stabilization of the spine and decreases the risk of recurrence

  a. Collaborative Care (interventions for all procedures)

    1) Monitor vital signs.

    2) Monitor for neurological deficits.

    3) Monitor the dressing for spinal fluid, bleeding, or signs of infection.

    4) Log roll the client. Reinforce with client to maintain proper alignment and decrease stress on the spine.

    5) Address sexual concerns.

    6) Manage pain.

    7) Refer for rehabilitation if indicated.

E. **Sensory Assessment**

1. Ocular assessment

  a. Assessment of visual acuity with the use of the Snellen chart. The client stands 20 feet from the chart and is asked to read the smallest line. Corrective lenses for distance vision should be worn during test.

    1) Manifestation

      a) Myopia (nearsightedness): Distant objects appear blurred.

      b) Hyperopia (farsightedness): Close objects appear blurred.

      c) Presbyopia (farsightedness associated with aging): A progressive condition in which the lens of the eye loses its ability to focus.

      d) Macular degeneration: A progressive disorder of the retina causing the loss of central vision.

      e) Legal blindness is when the vision in the better eye does not exceed 20/200 with correction or whose widest visual field diameter is 20° or less.

  b. External eye exam

  c. Direct and indirect ophthalmoscopy

  d. Tonometry: Measures intraocular pressure

2. Treatment of visual acuity problems

  a. Abnormal refractory findings are typically treated with corrective lenses.

  b. Laser eye surgery (Lasik): This procedure changes the shape of the cornea with the goal of 20/20 vision.

3. Common optical problems

a. **Detached retina:** Occurs when the sensory retina separates from the pigment epithelium of the retina; vitreous humor fluid flows between the layers when a tear occurs in the retina; can be related to age or trauma

   1) Manifestations

      a) Sudden visual disturbances

      b) Flashes of light

      c) Blurred vision with floaters

      d) Curtain or shadow over visual field across one eye

   2) **Nursing Interventions** (preoperative)

      a) Maintain bed rest with patch to affected eye.

      b) Remind the client to avoid coughing, sneezing, and straining.

      c) Surgical intervention includes scleral buckling, photocoagulation, cryosurgery, vitrectomy, and pneumatic retinopexy.

   3) **Nursing Interventions** (postoperative)

      a) Maintain bed rest in prescribed position with eye patch and shield in place

      b) Avoid jarring, bumping head, straining, or coughing.

      c) Administer medications as prescribed (antiemetic, antibiotic, anti-inflammatory).

      d) Reinforce regular self-administration of eye drops on schedule.

b. **Cataract:** Slow, progressive clouding of the lens

   1) Manifestations

      a) Painless diplopia and/or blurred vision

      b) Decreased visual acuity; frequent change in eyeglasses prescription

      c) Can perceive surroundings being dimmer

   2) **Nursing Interventions** (preoperative—dilate the eye)

      a) Administer medications as prescribed.

         (1) Mydriatics

         (2) Antibiotics

         (3) Corticosteroids

   3) **Nursing Interventions** (postoperative)

      a) Keep the operative eye covered.

      b) Elevate head of bed 30° to 45°. Do not turn the client onto the operative side.

      c) Reinforce with the client to avoid bending at the waist, lifting, sneezing, and coughing, and to not touch the eye area.

      d) Prevent vomiting or straining.

      e) Report severe pain immediately.

   4) Therapeutic Measures

      a) Surgical treatment: Removal of the lens usually under local anesthesia, with intraocular lens implant

c. **Glaucoma:** Group of ocular conditions characterized by optic nerve damage, which can be caused by increased intraocular pressure (IOP)

   1) Manifestations

      a) Acute (closed-angle) ocular emergency

         (1) Results from an obstruction to the outflow of aqueous humor, resulting in increased IOP

         (2) Rapidly progressive visual impairment

         (3) Severe pain in and around the eye

         (4) Blurred vision with dilated pupils

         (5) Nausea and vomiting

      b) Open angle

         (1) Insidious onset with slowly decreasing visual acuity

         (2) Usually bilateral, but one eye can be more affected

         (3) Halos around lights and loss of peripheral vision (late manifestations)

         (4) Fluctuating intraocular pressures

         (5) Can have no symptoms

   2) Collaborative Care

      a) **Nursing Interventions**

         (1) Administer medications consistently on time.

         (2) Avoid anticholinergic medications.

      b) Medications to promote pupils to contract

         (1) Cholinergics: miotics (pilocarpine, carbachol)

         (2) Adrenergic agonists: dipivefrin, epinephrine

         (3) Beta blockers: betaxolol, timolol

         (4) Carbonic anhydrase inhibitors: acetazolamide

         (5) Prostaglandin analogues: latanoprost, bimatoprost

         (6) Alpha-adrenergic agonists: apraclonidine, brimonidine

      c) Therapeutic Measures

         (1) Laser trabeculoplasty

         (2) Iridotomy

         (3) Drainage implants or shunts

      d) Client Education

         (1) Appropriate administration of medications

         (2) Avoiding activities that can increase IOP

         (3) Adherence to follow-up appointments

F. **Auditory Assessment**

1. Auditory Assessment

    a. Inspection of external ear

    b. Otoscopic examination

    c. Evaluation of gross auditory acuity

    d. Audiometry

2. Disorders

    a. **Ménière's disease**: Abnormal inner ear fluid balance, which can lead to disabling symptoms

        1) Manifestations

            a) Vertigo

            b) Tinnitus

            c) Pressure in the ear

3. Collaborative Care

    a. **Nursing Interventions**

        1) Provide small, frequent meals low in sodium.

        2) Initiate and reinforce teaching of fall precautions.

        3) Maintain a quiet environment.

    b. Medications

        1) Antihistamines: meclizine

        2) Tranquilizers to control acute vertigo: diazepam

        3) Antiemetics to control nausea, vomiting, and vertigo: promethazine

        4) Diuretics to reduce pressure from fluid

    c. Client Education

        1) Follow a low-sodium diet.

        2) Drink plenty of fluids, but avoid caffeine and alcohol.

        3) Avoid monosodium glutamate (MSG), aspirin, and aspirin-containing medications, which can increase symptoms.

NEUROSENSORY END-OF-SECTION REVIEW

1. It is important to monitor _____ function and allergies to shellfish prior to a client receiving contrast dye.

2. Preprocedure instructions for a client scheduled for an electroencephalogram (EEG) would include avoiding _____, holding _____ and depressant medications, and _____ hair prior to procedure.

3. One of the earliest indicators of increased intracranial pressure is a change in _____. Cushing's triad is a late sign of increasing intracranial pressure characterized by _____ (with widening pulse pressure), _____, and _____.

4. The best position for a client who has intracranial pressure would be with the head of bed _____ 30° to 45°, with the head positioned _____. This client should be suctioned as determined by _____.

5. Seizure precautions would include placing the bed in the _____ position, _____ side rails, and ensuring that _____ and _____ equipment is at bedside. The medication of choice for acute seizures is _____.

6. The client who has experienced a stroke is at risk for _____. Strategies to prevent this include feeding slowly, placing food on the _____ side, with the head slightly flexed _____.

7. The client who has a spinal cord injury at T6 or above is at risk for a potentially life-threatening condition called _____, which is caused by noxious _____ below the level of injury. This condition is characterized by severe hypertension. Priority interventions include elevating the _____, identifying and _____ the stimuli, and administering _____ medications as prescribed.

8. It is important to time meals with the administration of medications (usually given within 45 min of meals) for the client who has _____ to prevent aspiration.

9. Acute glaucoma is considered an optical emergency. The client experiencing this disorder can experience _____ and _____ vision. Medication to reduce intraocular pressure can include _____ and _____.

10. The client who has Ménière's disease should be advised to follow a low-_____ diet. Due to the client potentially experiencing vertigo, it is important to reinforce with the client about _____ precautions.

WORD BANK	
acetazolamide	lowest
antihypertensive	midline
aspiration	myasthenia gravis
assessment	oxygen
autonomic dysreflexia	padding
blurred	pain
bradycardia	pilocarpine
bradypnea	removing
caffeine	renal
elevated	sodium
fall	stimulant
forward	suction
head of bed	stimuli
hypertension	unaffected
level of consciousness	washing
lorazepam	

Answer Key: 1. Renal; 2. Caffeine, stimulant, washing; 3. Level of consciousness, hypertension, bradycardia, bradypnea; 4. Elevated, midline, assessment; 5. Lowest, padding, oxygen, suction, lorazepam; 6. Aspiration, unaffected, forward; 7. Autonomic dysreflexia, stimuli, head of bed, removing, antihypertensive; 8. Myasthenia gravis; 9. Pain, blurred, pilocarpine, acetazolamide; 10. Sodium, fall

Oncology Nursing

A. **Overview of Cancer**

1. Healthy cells transform into malignant cells upon exposure to certain etiological agents (viruses, chemicals, physical agents).

2. Malignant cells metastasize and extend directly into adjacent tissue, moving through the lymph system, entering the blood circulation, and diffusing into body cavities.

B. **Risk Factors**

1. Age

   a. Older adult women most commonly develop colorectal, breast, lung, pancreatic, and ovarian cancers.

   b. Older adult men most commonly develop lung, colorectal, prostate, pancreatic and gastric cancers.

2. Race

3. Genetic disposition

4. Exposure to chemicals, viruses, tobacco, alcohol

5. Exposure to some viruses, bacteria

6. Sun exposure

7. Diet high in red meat and fat, and low in fiber

C. **General Disease-Related Consequences of Cancer**

1. Decreased immunity and blood-producing function

   a. Occurs most often with leukemia and lymphoma or any cancer that invades the bone marrow and reduces the production of WBCs, RBCs, and platelets, causing thrombocytopenia.

   b. Clients are at increased risk for infection.

   c. Changes are caused by either the cancer or chemotherapy.

   d. Clients can experience weakness, fatigue, and bleeding.

2. Altered GI structure and function

   a. Impaired absorption and elimination related to tumor obstruction or compression.

   b. Tumors increase the metabolic rate, increasing the need for proteins, fats, and carbohydrates.

   c. Liver tumors reduce function and lead to malnutrition.

3. Motor and sensory deficits

   a. Occur when cancers invade the bone or brain or compress nerves.

   b. Bone metastases cause pain, fractures, spinal cord obstruction, and hypercalcemia, which decreases mobility.

   c. Sensory changes occur if the spinal cord is damaged by tumor pressure or compression.

   d. Sensory, motor, and cognitive functions are impaired when cancer is in the brain.

   e. Pain is often significant, especially in the terminal stages of the disease process.

4. Decreased respiratory function

   a. Disrupts respiratory function and gas exchange. (Tumors in an airway cause an obstruction.)

   b. Lung capacity is decreased. Gas exchange is impaired.

   c. Tumors can compress blood and lymph vessels in the chest, blocking blood flow through the chest and lungs, causing pulmonary edema and dyspnea.

D. **Cancers/Tumors**

1. Classified according to type of tissue from which they evolve.

2. Carcinomas begin in epithelial tissue (skin, gastrointestinal tract lining, lung, breast, uterus).

3. Sarcomas begin in nonepithelial tissue (bone, muscle, fat, lymph system).

4. Adenocarcinomas arise from glandular organs.

5. Leukemias are malignancies of the blood-forming cells.

6. Lymphomas arise from the lymph tissue.

7. Multiple myeloma arises from plasma cells and affects the bone.

E. **Manifestations Suggesting Malignant Disease**

1. American Cancer Society Seven Warning Signs

   a. **C** – Changes in bowel or bladder habits

   b. **A** – A sore that does not heal

   c. **U** – Unusual bleeding or discharge

   d. **T** – Thickening or lumps in breast or elsewhere

   e. **I** – Indigestion or difficulty swallowing

   f. **O** – Obvious change in wart or mole

   g. **N** – Nagging cough or hoarseness

2. Other manifestations

   a. Weight loss

   b. Fatigue/weakness

   c. Pain (might not occur until late in the disease process)

   d. Nausea/anorexia

F. **Cancer Management:** Systemic or local medications used to cure and/or increase survival rate by damaging cell DNA and interfering with cell mitosis. Rapid growth tumors are more sensitive to chemotherapy.

1. **Chemotherapy**

   a. Systemic or local cytotoxic medications that damage a cell's DNA or destroy rapidly dividing cells. Combination of medications usually given.

   b. Classification (all cause bone marrow depression)

      1) Alkylating agents: mechlorethamine cyclophosphamide, cisplatin

      2) Antimetabolite: fluorouracil, methotrexate

      3) Antibiotics: doxorubicin hydrochloride, bleomycin, dactinomycin

      4) Antimitotics: vincristine, vinblastine

      5) Hormones: estrogen, progesterone, tamoxifen citrate, peclitaxel

      6) Biological modifiers: epoetin alfa, filgrastim

c. Common side effects and interventions to counteract

1) Bone marrow suppression: neutropenia and leukopenia (WBC less than 1,000 mm³)

   a) Interventions to enhance the immune system include a balanced diet, rest, and handwashing.

   b) Interventions to avoid infections include

      (1) Limit visitors who might be ill.

      (2) Avoid fresh fruits, vegetables, and live plants.

   c) Monitor temperature. Consider any temperature elevation in a client who has neutropenia a possible sign of infection and report to provider.

2) Anemia (Hgb less than 10 g/dL)

   a) Administer oxygen therapy. Provide iron-rich foods.

   b) Monitor CBCs and administer blood transfusions as needed.

   c) Administer erythropoietin and epoetin alfa to increase RBCs.

3) Thrombocytopenia

   a) Administer prescribed platelet transfusions; oprelvekin to increase platelets.

   b) Implement bleeding precautions. Avoid use of aspirin.

4) Alopecia (Hair loss 2 weeks after start of treatment. Regrowth occurs 1 month after last chemotherapy treatment.)

   a) Apply ice to the client's scalp during chemotherapy to slow hair loss. Use gentle shampoo, hats, scarves, and sunscreen.

   b) Refer the client to the American Cancer Society, which provides wigs and supportive services.

5) Anorexia, nausea, vomiting, and GI issues

   a) Administer antiemetic (ondansetron, dolasetron) prior to therapy.

   b) Administer loperamide to manage diarrhea.

   c) The client should drink cool beverages and eat small, favorite meals high in potassium with high-calorie supplements. Avoid unpleasant odors.

   d) Provide soft, bland, high-protein foods at room temperature for stomatitis, and use a straw for fluids. Rinse mouth with a topical anesthetic. Can need topical steroids and zinc supplements.

6) Elevated uric acid, crystal, and urate stone formation

   a) Administer allopurinol. Increase fluid intake.

7) Mucositis: Often develops in the GI tract, especially in the mouth (stomatitis). Mucous membranes, because they undergo rapid cell division, are killed more rapidly than the cells are replaced.

   a) Provide frequent mouth assessment and oral hygiene (teeth cleaning, mouth rinsing).

   b) Avoid traumatizing oral mucosa due to risk of bleeding. Use soft-bristled toothbrush or swabs.

   c) Use plain water or saline for oral rinses.

8) Specific medications have specific toxic effects.

   a) Doxorubicin hydrochloride: Irreversible cardiomyopathy

   b) Anzemet, methotrexate: Renal toxicity

   c) Vincristine sulfate: Peripheral neuropathy

9) Cognitive Function

   a) Reduced ability to concentrate, recall information, and learn new information during treatment and for months to 3 years following treatment.

   b) Referred to as "chemo brain," most common in female clients treated for breast cancer.

2. **Radiation:** Therapy destroys cancer cells with minimal exposure of normal cells to the damaging actions of radiation. Cells damaged by radiation either die or become unable to divide. Gamma rays are used most commonly because of their ability to penetrate tissues and damage cells.

   a. Radiation Delivery

      1) Teletherapy: Distance treatment; the radiation source is external to the client.

      2) Brachytherapy: Short or close therapy; radiation comes into direct, continuous contact with the tumor tissues. Provides a high dose of radiation with a limited amount to surrounding tissues. (With brachytherapy, the radiation source is within the client who emits radiation and is a hazard to those around for a period of time.)

   b. **Nursing Interventions**

      1) Ensure precise client position with each radiation treatment to align with fixing devices and markings.

      2) Monitor condition of skin, and cleanse the area gently each day with water or mild soap.

      3) Wet reaction: Skin's response to radiation; skin becomes dry or develops blisters that can break, causing pain and the potential for infection. If dry reaction, keep clean and lubricated. If wet reaction, clean and cover to prevent infection.

      4) Reinforce with the client to not remove skin markings. Avoid powders, lotions, and creams unless prescribed.

      5) Reinforce with the client to wear soft, loose clothing and avoid exposure to the sun.

      6) Advise the client to avoid prolonged sun exposure during treatment and for 1 year after completing radiation therapy.

      7) For clients who have sealed implants of radioactive sources

         a) Assign the client to a private room.

         b) Place "Caution: Radioactive Material" sign on the client's door in the hospital setting.

         c) Wear a lead apron while providing care. Nurses who are pregnant should not care for these clients.

         d) Limit visitors to ½ hr each day, and instruct them to remain at least 6 feet from the source.

e) Do not touch the radioactive source with bare hands.

f) Save all radioactive dressings and linens until the radioactive source is removed.

g) Follow institution guidelines for radiation containment.

8) Managing Cancer Pain

a) Provide effective pain management and monitor client response. (See Opioid Analgesics in Unit Four: Pharmacology in Nursing.)

b) Monitor body image disturbance, coping mechanisms, and support system. Make appropriate referrals.

KEY POINT: The Centers for Disease Control and Prevention (CDC) is the best source for the most up-to-date information regarding HIV and AIDS.

A. Acquired Immune Deficiency Syndrome (AIDS)

1. Human immunodeficiency virus (HIV) can progress to acquired immune deficiency syndrome (AIDS). HIV is a viral infection that is transmitted via blood and other body fluids. It affects the ability of the immune system to fight infection—specifically, CD4+T cells. (A healthy adult has 800 to 1,000 cells/mm³ of blood.)

   a. HIV infection is divided into four stages.

      1) *Stage 1, Acute infection*: Described as the "worst flu ever," retroviral syndrome usually occurs 2 to 4 weeks after the infection is acquired. CD4+T cells greater than 500 cells/mm³.

      2) *Stage 2, Latency*: Sometimes called asymptomatic HIV infection or chronic HIV infection. CD4+T cell count between 200 and 499 cells/mm³. This stage can last for 8 years or longer.

      3) *Stage 3, AIDS*: CD4+T cell counts drop below 200 cells/mm³. The body becomes susceptible to opportunistic infections. Survival in this stage is usually 1 to 3 years.

      4) *Stage 4, HIV Infection, Stage Unknown*: No information available on CD4+T-lymphocyte count or percentage and no information available on AIDS-defining conditions.

2. Contributing Factors

   a. Unprotected sexual contact

   b. IV drug use; use of contaminated needles

   c. Multiple sexual partners

   d. Pregnancy and breastfeeding: transmission from mother to baby

   e. Blood transfusion (very small risk: 0.02%)

3. Manifestations

   a. Stages

      1) Stage 1: Acute infection

         a) Fever

         b) Lymph adenopathy

         c) Pharyngitis

         d) Rash

         e) Arthralgia, myalgia

         f) HIV viral load is high; may or may not test positive for antibodies.

         g) CD4+T cell count is greater than 500 cells/mm³

         h) Virus is transmissible to others

      2) Stage 2: Latency

         a) Lymphadenopathy, but can be asymptomatic

         b) Will test positive for HIV antibodies

         c) CD4+T cell count is between 200 and 499 cells/mm³

      3) Stage 3: AIDS

         a) Opportunistic infections occur

            (1) Respiratory: Pneumocystis carinii pneumonia, tuberculosis; Kaposi's sarcoma

            (2) GI: Cryptosporidiosis, candida, cytomegalovirus (CMV), isosporiasis, Kaposi's sarcoma

            (3) Neurological: Cytomegalovirus, toxoplasmosis, cryptococcosis, non–Hodgkin's lymphoma, varicella zoster (shingles), herpes simplex

            (4) Skin: Shingles, herpes simplex, Kaposi's sarcoma

KAPOSI'S SARCOMA

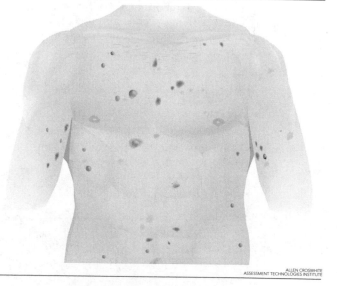

ALLEN CROSWHITE
ASSESSMENT TECHNOLOGIES INSTITUTE

         b) Wasting syndrome

         c) AIDS dementia

         d) Weakness and malaise

         e) Psychosocial: anxiety, depression, poor self–image

         f) CD4+T cell count drops below 200 cells/mm³

4. Diagnostic Procedures

 a. ELISA (antibody assay): Positive within 3 weeks to 3 months following infection. Most common and least expensive.

 b. Western Blot blood test used when ELISA is positive to confirm or rule/out infection.

 c. Plasma HIV-1 RNA viral load is greater than 1,500 copies.

 d. CD4+T cell count: Decreased less than 750 cells/mm^3. Clients with values less than 200 cells/mm^3 have an 85% likelihood of progressing to AIDS within 3 years.

 e. CBC and platelets are decreased.

 f. Brain, lung, or CT scans can be abnormal.

5. Collaborative Care

 a. **Nursing Interventions**

  1) Prevention

   a) Reinforce teaching about transmission routes.

   b) Emphasize the need to use condoms with sexual encounters.

   c) Explain that risk is reduced by limiting sexual partners.

   d) Reinforce teaching to IV drug users to use clean needles or, if they reuse, to clean between each use with water and bleach.

   e) Emphasize need for pregnant clients who are HIV-positive to begin or remain on antiviral therapy; infants should NOT be breastfed.

   f) Ensure consistent use of standard precautions by health care workers in clinical settings.

  2) Stages 1 and 2

   a) Reinforce teaching about risk of transmission of HIV to others and ways to prevent.

   b) Emphasize importance of adherence with antiviral therapy, once initiated.

   c) Encourage healthy lifestyle habits.

   d) Provide psychological support.

  3) Stage 3

   a) Prevent infection.

   b) Enhance oxygenation.

   c) Provide comfort measures.

   d) Monitor weight, I&O and calorie count; encourage high-calorie foods.

   e) Perform frequent oral care.

   f) Provide scrupulous skin care.

   g) Monitor mental status; reorient PRN; maintain consistent environment.

   h) Provide psychosocial support; include significant others.

 b. Medications

  1) Medication therapy: highly active antiretroviral therapy guidelines (HAART) are devised by the World Health Organization and are updated as new research findings become available.

KEY POINT: It is crucial that once a client begins HAART therapy, doses must NOT be missed. Doing so contributes to medication resistance and reduces medication treatment options.

  2) Efavirenz, azidothymidine, and lamivudine

   a) Common adverse effects: neutropenia, gastrointestinal distress, anemia, insomnia

  3) Zidovudine recommended for protecting the unborn fetus of clients who are HIV-positive

  4) Interferon

  5) Pneumocystis pneumonia prophylaxis: pentamidine

  6) Antifungals: metronidazole and amphotericin B

  7) Antituberculosis medications as needed

  8) Acyclovir herpes treatment

  9) Protease inhibitors: saquinavir, ritonavir

  10) Antivirals: zalcitabine, dideoxycytidine

 c. Client Education

  1) Transmission, control measures, and safe sex practices

  2) Nutritional needs, self-medication of prescribed medications, and potential adverse effects

  3) Symptoms that need to be reported immediately (infection, bleeding)

  4) Need for follow-up monitoring CD4+T cell and viral load counts

B. **Systemic Lupus Erythematosus (SLE):** A chronic inflammatory disease that occurs when the body's immune system attacks the tissues and organs. Inflammation caused by lupus can affect multiple organ systems (joints, skin, kidneys, blood cells, heart, lungs).

 1. Contributing Factors

  a. Female sex

  b. Age between 15 and 40 years

  c. African American, Latino, or Asian ethnicity

  d. Exposure to sunlight

  e. Long-term use of certain medications

   1) Chlorpromazine

   2) Hydralazine

   3) Isoniazid

   4) Procainamide

  f. Exposure to mercury and/or silica

2. Manifestations
   a. Insidious onset characterized by remissions and exacerbations
   b. Erythematosus "butterfly rash" on both cheeks and across the bridge of the nose; rash deepens on exposure to sunlight

ERYTHEMATOSUS "BUTTERFLY RASH"

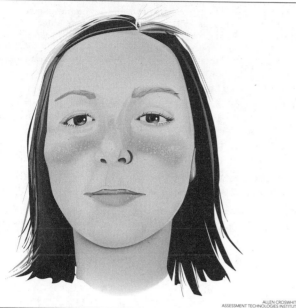

ALLEN CROSWHITE
ASSESSMENT TECHNOLOGIES INSTITUTE

   c. Polyarthralgia
   d. Fever, malaise, and weight loss
   e. Alopecia
   f. Anemia, lymphadenopathy
   g. Positive for antinuclear antibodies
   h. Depression
   i. Coin-like lesions (in discoid lupus)
   j. Pleural effusion, pneumonia
   k. Pericarditis
   l. Raynaud's phenomenon
   m. Neurological: Psychosis, paresis, seizures, migraines
   n. Abdominal pain
   o. Edema
   p. Nephritis
3. Collaborative Care
   a. **Nursing Interventions**
      1) Monitor vital signs, especially related to cardiovascular function.
      2) Monitor urinary function.
      3) Provide comfort measures.
      4) Instruct to use sunscreen and cover skin and head when exposed to sunlight.
      5) Encourage rest periods during the day.
      6) Provide measures that promote restful sleep.
      7) Cleanse skin with mild soap and pat to dry; apply moisturizer.
      8) Monitor for infection and teach measures to avoid.

   b. Medications
      1) NSAIDs to reduce inflammation: Contraindicated for clients who have renal compromise
      2) Corticosteroids for immunosuppression and to reduce inflammation
      3) Immunosuppressant agents: Methotrexate, azathioprine
      4) Antimalarial (hydroxychloroquine) for suppression of synovitis, fever, and fatigue
   c. Client Education and Referral
      1) Use sunscreen and wear protective clothing.
      2) Consume small, frequent meals if anorexia is present.
      3) Limit salt intake for fluid retention secondary to steroid therapy and renal involvement.
      4) Refer to support groups as appropriate.

SECTION 13

Burns

A. **Overview**
1. Thermal, chemical, electrical, and radioactive agents can cause burns, resulting in cellular destruction of the skin layers and underlying tissue. The type and severity of the burn impact the treatment plan.
2. Burn injuries can result in the loss of temperature regulation, sweat and sebaceous gland function, and sensory and organ function.
3. Assessment and severity of the burn is based upon the following.
   a. Percentage of total body surface area (TBSA)
   b. Depth of the burn
   c. Body location
   d. Client's age
   e. Causative agent
   f. Presence of other injuries
   g. Respiratory involvement and overall health of the client

B. **Burn Assessment**
1. Extent of body surface
2. Depth of burn and manifestations

C. **Maintain cardiac output and provide IV fluid replacement using Parkland formula**
1. Give 4 mL/kg/% burn.
2. Give half of total fluids in first 8 hr.
3. Give second half over remaining 16 hr.
4. Deduct any fluid given prehospital from the amount to be infused in the first 8 hr.

! Point to Remember

The Rule of Nines assesses the percentage of burn and is used to help guide treatment decisions including fluid resuscitation. It is part of the guidelines to determine burn management.

RULE OF NINES

Estimating TBSA Affected by Burns

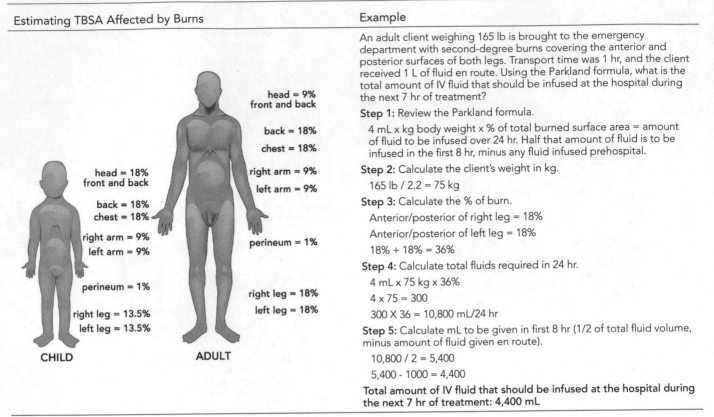

CHILD

head = 18% front and back
back = 18%
chest = 18%
right arm = 9%
left arm = 9%
perineum = 1%
right leg = 13.5%
left leg = 13.5%

ADULT

head = 9% front and back
back = 18%
chest = 18%
right arm = 9%
left arm = 9%
perineum = 1%
right leg = 18%
left leg = 18%

Example

An adult client weighing 165 lb is brought to the emergency department with second-degree burns covering the anterior and posterior surfaces of both legs. Transport time was 1 hr, and the client received 1 L of fluid en route. Using the Parkland formula, what is the total amount of IV fluid that should be infused at the hospital during the next 7 hr of treatment?

Step 1: Review the Parkland formula.

4 mL x kg body weight x % of total burned surface area = amount of fluid to be infused over 24 hr. Half that amount of fluid is to be infused in the first 8 hr, minus any fluid infused prehospital.

Step 2: Calculate the client's weight in kg.

165 lb / 2.2 = 75 kg

Step 3: Calculate the % of burn.

Anterior/posterior of right leg = 18%

Anterior/posterior of left leg = 18%

18% + 18% = 36%

Step 4: Calculate total fluids required in 24 hr.

4 mL x 75 kg x 36%

4 x 75 = 300

300 X 36 = 10,800 mL/24 hr

Step 5: Calculate mL to be given in first 8 hr (1/2 of total fluid volume, minus amount of fluid given en route).

10,800 / 2 = 5,400

5,400 - 1000 = 4,400

Total amount of IV fluid that should be infused at the hospital during the next 7 hr of treatment: 4,400 mL

BURN DESCRIPTIONS

CLASSIFICATION	DEGREE (OLD TERM)	LAYER INVOLVED	APPEARANCE	EXAMPLES	PAIN
Superficial	First degree	Epidermis	Pink to red, tender, no blisters, mild edema, no eschar	Sunburn, flash burns	Yes
Superficial Partial Thickness	Second degree	Epidermis and parts of dermis	Red to white with blisters, mild to moderate edema, no eschar	Flame or burn scalds	Yes
Deep Partial Thickness	Third degree	Epidermis and deep into dermis	Red to white with moderate edema, no blisters, soft/dry eschar	Flame and burn scalds; Grease, tar, or chemical burns; Exposure to hot objects for prolonged time	Yes
Full-Thickness	Third degree	Same as partial (can extend into subcutaneous tissue; nerve damage)	Red to tan, black, brown, white; No blisters, severe edema, hard inelastic eschar	Burn scalds; Grease, tar, chemical, or electrical burns; Exposure to hot objects for prolonged time	Can be painful
Deep Full-Thickness	Fourth degree	All layers plus muscles, tendons, bones	Black with no edema	Chemical	None

5. Diagnostic testing
   a. CBC, serum electrolytes, BUN, ABGs, fasting blood glucose, liver studies, urinalysis, clotting studies, and chest x-ray. Add creatinine and myoglobin for deep burns.
      1) Initial fluid shift (first 24 hr after injury)
         a) Hct/Hgb elevated due to fluid shifts into interstitial spacing and fluid loss
         b) Sodium decreased secondary to third spacing
         c) Potassium increased due to disruption of sodium-potassium pump, tissue destruction, and RBC hemolysis
      2) Fluid mobilization (48 to 72 hr after injury)
         a) Hct/Hgb decrease due to fluid shift from interstitial back into vascular fluid
         b) Sodium remains decreased; potassium increases due to renal loss and movement back into the cells
   b. WBC count: Initial increase then decrease with a shift to the left (an increase in the percentage of neutrophils having only one or a few lobes)
      a) Blood glucose: Elevated due to stress response
      b) ABGs: Slight hypoxemia and metabolic acidosis
      c) Total protein and albumin: Low due to fluid loss

D. **Collaborative Care**
   1. **Nursing Interventions** for moderate and major burns
      a. Maintain airway and ventilation.
      b. Provide humidified oxygen as prescribed.
      c. Monitor vital signs.
      d. Maintain cardiac output and provide IV fluid replacement using Parkland formula.
         1) Give 4 mL/kg/% burn.
         2) Give half of total fluids in first 8 hr.
         3) Give second half over remaining 16 hr.
         4) Deduct any fluid given prehospital from the amount to be infused in the first 8 hr.
      e. Maintain urine output of 30 to 50 mL/hr for a burn client.
      f. Monitor for manifestations of shock.
      g. Provide pain management.
      h. Monitor for and prevent infection.
      i. Provide nutritional support.
         1) Client who has a large burn injury will be in a hypermetabolic state and can exceed 5,000 calories/day.
         2) Increase protein intake to prevent tissue breakdown and promote healing.
         3) Enteral or total parenteral therapy is often necessary.
      j. Promote restoration of mobility.
      k. Provide psychological support to the client and family.

2. Medications
   a. Antimicrobial creams
      1) Silver nitrate 0.5% soaks
      2) Silver sulfadiazine 1% cream: Broad-spectrum coverage; water soluble
      3) Mafenide acetate cream: Broad-spectrum coverage; penetrates tissue wall; painful. Never use a dressing. Breakdown of medication causes a heavy acid load, which can cause acidosis.
      4) Bacitracin
   b. Pain management
      1) PCA infusion pump for continuous dosing
      2) Intravenous opioid analgesics (morphine sulfate, hydromorphone, fentanyl)
3. Treatments
   a. Wound care
   b. Biologic skin coverings
   c. Permanent skin coverings
4. Methods of Treating Burns
   a. Open-exposure method
      1) Allows for drainage of burn exudate
      2) Eschar forms hardened crust (can constrict circulation, requiring escharotomy)
      3) Use of topical therapy; asepsis crucial
      4) Skin easily visualized and assessed
      5) Range of motion easier
      6) Disadvantages
         a) Increases pain and heat loss
         b) Difficult to manage burns of hands and feet
   b. Closed method
      1) Gauze dressing wrapped distal to proximal
      2) Decreased fluid and heat loss
      3) Limited mobility can result in contractures
      4) Wound assessment only during dressing changes
   c. Topical antimicrobials
   d. Biologic dressings and tissue grafts
      1) Homograft or allograft (human tissue donors)
      2) Xenograft or heterograft (animal sources)
      3) Amniotic membrane
      4) Biosynthetic or synthetic (transparent film)
5. Client Education
   a. Skin care following discharge
      1) Wear pressure garment 23.5 hr/day to reduce scarring and control swelling.
      2) Engage in regular exercise per physical therapy.
      3) Elevate affected areas as much as possible.
      4) Keep skin moisturized.
      5) Control itching with cool baths and loose cotton fabric.
      6) Avoid sun exposure.
      7) Change in appearance of skin as scars fade from red to near natural coloration.
      8) Encourage the client to consume extra calories and protein.

End-of-Life Care

A. **Definition:** Care and management of the client and caregivers facing end-of-life care issues with the outcome of providing "good death." A good death is free from avoidable suffering for patients and families in consideration with their preferences and consistent with practice standards.

B. **Contributing Factors**

1. Age
2. Chronic terminal illness
3. Hospice care
4. Palliative care

C. **Manifestations**

1. Anorexia
2. Decreased peripheral circulation (mottled skin)
3. Disorientation and somnolence
4. Change in breathing pattern; Cheyne-Stokes respirations
5. Increased respiratory secretions
6. Decreased metabolic function
7. Incontinence
8. Restlessness
9. Weakness and fatigue

D. **Collaborative Care**

1. **Nursing Interventions**

   a. Determine if the client has an end-of-life care plan, advanced directives, and caregiver support.
   b. Do not force the client to eat or drink.
   c. Talk to the client even if the client does not respond.
   d. Keep the perineal area clean and dry.
   e. Position the client for comfort.
   f. Elevate the head of the bed.
   g. Administer medications to manage symptoms of pain, restlessness, and excess secretions.
   h. Avoid noxious stimuli.

2. Symptom Management

   a. Pain is the symptom dying clients fear the most.
      1) Long-acting opioid narcotics (morphine 20 mg/mL)
      2) Massage
      3) Music therapy
      4) Aromatherapy
   b. Dyspnea and gurgling are the most distressing symptoms noted by caregivers.
      1) Morphine elixir
      2) Scopolamine, atropine sulfate ophthalmic drops 1% (oral or sublingual) or hyoscyamine drops (oral)
      3) Oxygen via nasal cannula (Offer oxygen for comfort, regardless of O_2 saturation.)
      4) Avoid deep suctioning.

   c. Restlessness and agitation
      1) Lorazepam
      2) Haloperidol
   d. Nausea and vomiting
      1) Prochlorperazine
   e. Incontinence
      1) Keep perianal area clean and dry.
      2) Use disposable underpads or paper undergarments.
      3) The client can be more comfortable with a urinary catheter.

E. **Referral and Follow-up**

1. Hospice care
2. Chaplain
3. Social services

F. **Postmortem Care**

1. Notify provider, chaplain, and mortuary as defined by end-of-life care plan.
2. If no autopsy is planned, remove any tubes or lines.
3. Clean and prepare the client for immediate viewing as desired by family or significant others.
4. Provide family or significant others the opportunity to participate in care as desired.
5. Be aware that clients differ in their needs at end of life based on factors such as gender and ethnicity.
6. Identify cultural values and religious beliefs of the patient and family for their influence on the dying experience.
7. Verify the completion of death certificate and required facility documents.
8. Prepare client for transport to morgue, funeral home, or mortuary per facility protocol. (Ensure client identification tags are present.)

Nutrition: Therapeutic Diets

Overview

A. To a large degree, nutrients absorbed and used by the body determine the health of the body.

B. The process of ingestion, digestion, absorption, and metabolism of food and fluids is essential for life. Disease processes and altered clinical conditions involving the GI tract can prevent all or some of these processes from taking place.

C. The nurse reviews the medical history and conducts a nutritional assessment to determine the possibility of increased metabolic needs, and sources of potential problems with ingestion, digestion, or absorption.

D. Contributing factors can include chronic disease, trauma, recent surgery of the GI tract, drug and alcohol use, and altered cognitive and functional processes that can affect nutritional status.

E. The nurse monitors for
1. Decreased appetite; weight loss
2. History of recent illness
3. Poor-fitting or no dentures; poor dental health; poor eyesight; dry mouth or mucous membranes
4. Cognitive or functional decline; chronic physical illness
5. Acute or chronic pain; history of substance abuse
6. Altered mental health conditions, economic, or environmental factors that can affect nutritional requirements
7. Weight gain or subjective complaints of lack of satiety

F. Older adult clients in any health care or community setting are at increased risk for altered nutrition due to the physiologic changes of aging, cognitive and functional decline, environmental factors, and social isolation.

II Guidelines for Healthy Eating

A. **Protein:** 10% to 35% of total kcal/day
B. **Fat:** 20% to 35% of total kcal/day
C. **Carbohydrates:** 40% to 65% of total kcal/day
D. **Fluid recommendations:** 2 to 3 L/day for females; 3 to 4 L/day for males
E. **Fiber recommendations:** 25 g/day for females; 38 g/day for males.
F. **Sodium recommendations:** Less than 2,300 mg for people younger than age 50; 1,500 mg/day or less for people older than 50 years, African American clients, or clients who have a history of diabetes mellitus, hypertension, or chronic kidney disease.
G. Recommendations differ for children, teens, and pregnant/lactating clients.
H. Consider cultural and religious influence on food preferences when planning diet.
I. **Older adult recommendations:** Drink 8 glasses of water. Eat plenty of fiber. Take daily calcium and vitamin D and B_{12} supplements. Consume a diet low in sodium and cholesterol.

FOODS WITH INCREASED LEVELS OF FAT AND WATER-SOLUBLE VITAMINS

Foods Rich in Fat-Soluble Vitamins

Vitamin A	Liver, egg yolk, whole milk, butter, green and yellow vegetables
Vitamin D	Fish oils, fortified milk and margarine, sunlight
Vitamin K	Egg yolks, liver, cheese, green leafy vegetables

Foods Rich in Water-Soluble Vitamins

Vitamin C	Citrus fruits, tomatoes, broccoli, cabbage
Thiamine (B_1)	Lean meats (beef, pork, liver), whole grain cereals, legumes
Riboflavin (B_2)	Milk, organ meats, enriched grains, green leafy vegetables
Niacin (B_3)	Meat, beans, peas, peanuts, enriched grains
Pyridoxine (B_6)	Products containing yeast, wheat, corn, organ meats
Cobalamin (B_{12})	Lean meats, liver, kidneys
Folic acid (B_9)	Leafy green vegetables, eggs, liver

III Therapeutic and Modified Diets

A. **Overview**
1. Therapeutic nutrition is often an essential component in the treatment of disease and clinical disorders.
2. The diet becomes therapeutic when modifications are made to meet client needs. Modifications can include increasing or decreasing caloric intake, fiber, or other specific nutrients; omitting specific foods; and modifying the consistency of foods.
3. Nurses often collaborate with or refer clients to a dietitian for nutritional or dietary concerns.

B. **Clear–Liquid Diet**
1. Indications
   a. Resting the GI tract
   b. Maintaining fluid balance
   c. Immediate postoperative period
   d. Nausea, vomiting, diarrhea
   e. Preparation for diagnostic testing
   f. Short-term basis only; nutritionally inadequate
2. Consists of products that are liquid at room temperature
   a. Primarily water
   b. Tea and coffee
   c. Broth
   d. Carbonated beverages
   e. Clear juices
   f. Gelatin
   g. Limited caffeine due to risk of dehydration

C. **Full–Liquid Diet**
1. Indications
   a. Advanced to this if tolerates clear liquids
   b. Intolerance to solid foods
   c. Febrile illness
   d. Acute gastritis
2. Consists of
   a. Clear liquids
   b. Milk products
      1) Milk
      2) Custard
      3) Pudding
      4) Creamed soups
      5) Ice cream/sherbet
   c. Strained fruits, vegetables, and cereal

D. **Pureed Diet**
1. Indications
   a. Transition from full liquid to regular diet
   b. Swallowing or chewing difficulties; oral/facial surgery
2. Consists of
   a. Food and fluids that have been pureed to a thick liquid form (scrambled eggs; pureed meats, vegetables, fruits).
   b. Consistency varies with client needs.
   c. Nutritional content varies with client needs.

E. **Soft Diet (Bland or Low-Fiber)**

  1. Indications

     a. Transition from liquid to regular diet

     b. Acute infections

     c. Chewing difficulties

     d. Gastric or duodenal ulcers by eliminating irritating foods

  2. Consists of the following foods

     a. Low-fiber

     b. Lightly seasoned

     c. Easily digested

     d. Smooth and creamy

     e. Non-gas-forming (Avoid cereals, beans, fruits and vegetables.)

F. **Mechanical Soft Diet**

  1. Indications

     a. Chewing or swallowing difficulty

     b. Head, neck, or mouth surgery

     c. Intestinal stricture

     d. Following CVA

  2. Consist of foods that require minimal chewing

     a. Ground or finely diced meat

     b. Canned fruits

     c. Softly cooked vegetables

     d. Cheese

     e. Rice

     f. Light bread

  3. Foods to exclude

     a. Dried fruits

     b. Most raw fruits and vegetables

     c. Nuts and food with seeds

G. **Low-Protein Diet**

  1. Indications

     a. Hepatic encephalopathy

     b. Hepatic coma

     c. Renal impairment

  2. Limit high-protein foods.

     a. Meats

     b. Eggs

     c. Milk and milk products

     d. Beans

  3. Other dietary considerations

     a. Increase carbohydrates to meet nutritional needs.

     b. Limit sodium in presence of edema or ascites.

H. **High-Protein Diet**

  1. Indications

     a. Tissue repair and building

     b. Burns

     c. Malabsorption syndromes

     d. Pregnancy

  2. Encourage high biological value (HBV) protein

     a. Egg whites (gold standard)

     b. Soy products

     c. Milk products

     d. Fish and fowl

     e. Organ and meat sources

  3. Encourage oral fluids to decrease damage to renal capillaries as a result of increased protein.

I. **Diet for Alteration in Amino-Acid Metabolism**

  1. Use for phenylketonuria (PKU), galactosemia, and lactose intolerance.

  2. Dietary restrictions are aimed at reducing or eliminating the offending enzyme.

  3. Avoid milk and milk products for all three diets; include soy-based supplements.

  4. For PKU, avoid high-protein foods (meats, dairy products, eggs). Also avoid aspartame, as it contains phenylalanine.

  5. For galactosemia, the simple sugar in lactose must be avoided. Educate families to read labels carefully, as galactosemia can be life-threatening.

  6. Supplement calcium and vitamin D in those who have lactose-restricted or -eliminated diets.

J. **Low-Cholesterol Diet**

  1. Indications

     a. Cardiovascular disease

     b. Diabetes mellitus

     c. Hyperlipidemia

  2. Limit animal products that are high in low-density lipoproteins, saturated fats, and trans fats

     a. Egg yolks

     b. Organ meats

     c. Fatty meats (such as bacon)

     d. Whole milk, butter

  3. Encourage HDLs, omega-3 fatty acids, and unsaturated fats.

     a. Sardines and salmon

     b. Olive and flaxseed oils

     c. Shellfish

     d. Walnuts

     e. Fruits and vegetables

     f. Lean meats

     g. Skinless fowl

K. **Modified-Fat Diet**
  1. Indications
     a. Gallbladder disease
     b. Hepatic disorders
     c. Cystic fibrosis
     d. Malabsorption syndrome
  2. Avoid the following foods.
     a. Whole-milk products
     b. Gravies, creams
     c. Fatty meat and fish
     d. Nuts and chocolate
     e. Polyunsaturated oils
  3. Foods allowed
     a. Two to three eggs per week
     b. Lean meat, fowl, fish
     c. Fruits and vegetables
     d. Bread and cereal

L. **Potassium-Modified Diets**
  1. High-potassium foods
     a. Bananas
     b. Oranges
     c. Milk
     d. Spinach
     e. Apricots and prunes
     f. Soy, lima, and kidney beans
     g. Baked potatoes (white and sweet)
  2. Low-potassium foods
     a. Breads
     b. Cereals
     c. Asparagus
     d. Cabbage
     e. Cherries
     f. Blackberries and blueberries

M. **Sodium-Restricted Diets**
  1. Indications
     a. Hypertension
     b. Heart failure
     c. Myocardial infarction
     d. Adrenal cortical diseases
     e. Kidney disease
     f. Liver cirrhosis
     g. Pre-eclampsia

  2. High-sodium foods
     a. Salty snack foods (such as potato chips)
     b. Canned soups and vegetables
     c. Baked goods that contain baking powder or baking soda
     d. Processed meats (bologna, ham, bacon)
     e. Dairy products, especially cheese
     f. Pickles, olives
     g. Soy sauce, steak sauce
     h. Salad dressings
  3. Encourage clients to become label-savvy for sodium.

N. **Iron Alterations**
  1. Increased iron intake is indicated for correction or prevention of iron deficiency anemia, which is most likely to occur in infants, toddlers, adolescents, and pregnant clients.
  2. Food sources high in iron include fish, meats (particularly organ meats), green leafy vegetables, enriched breads, cereals and macaroni products, whole-grain products, dried fruits (raisins, apricots), and egg yolks.
  3. Vitamin C enhances absorption of iron from the gastrointestinal tract.
  4. Oral iron supplementation can cause constipation and GI distress, so adequate iron intake through foods is ideal.

O. **Calcium Alterations**
  1. Increased calcium intake is indicated for growing children and adolescents, pregnant and lactating clients, and postmenopausal clients (to help prevent osteoporosis and osteopenia).
  2. Food sources high in calcium include milk and milk products (yogurt, cheese); dark green vegetables (collard greens, kale, broccoli); dried beans and peas; shellfish and canned salmon; and antacids.
  3. No more than 600 mg calcium can be absorbed at one time, so supplements should be taken three times daily. No more than 2,500 mg of calcium should be consumed per day.
  4. Vitamin D is required for absorption of calcium from the gastrointestinal tract.

"Need to Know" Laboratory Values

I Serum Electrolytes

A. **Sodium (Na⁺):** 136 to 145 mEq/L
B. **Potassium (K⁺):** 3.5 to 5 mEq/L
C. **Calcium total (Ca⁺⁺):** 9.0 to 10.5 mg/dL
D. **Magnesium (Mg⁺⁺):** 1.3 to 2.1 mEq/L
E. **Phosphorus (PO₄):** 3.0 to 4.5 mg/dL
F. **Chloride (Cl):** 98 to 106 mEq/L

II Arterial Blood Gases (ABGs)

A. **pH:** 7.35 to 7.45
B. **PaCO₂:** 35 to 45 mm Hg
C. **PaO₂:** 80 to 100 mm Hg
D. **HCO₃ (bicarbonate):** 21 to 28 mEq/L

III CBC

A. **RBCs:** Males 4.7 to 6.1 million/uL; females 4.2 to 5.4 million/uL
B. **Hgb:** Males 14 to 18 g/dL; females: 12 to 16 g/dL
C. **Hct:** Males: 42% to 52%; females 37% to 47%
D. **WBCs:** 5,000 to 10,000 mm³
E. **Erythrocyte sedimentation rate (ESR):** less than 20 mm/hr

IV Blood Lipid Levels

A. **Total serum cholesterol:** Desirable less than 200 mg/dL; risk for cardiac or stroke event with levels greater than 150 mg/dL is the target range for therapy and has been shown to be the cut point to decrease cerebrovascular or arterial incidences.
B. **LDL (low-density lipids):** Desirable less than 130 mg/dL
C. **HDL (high-density lipids):** Males greater than 45 mg/dL; females greater than 5 mg/dL
D. **Triglycerides:** Desirable less than 150 mg/dL; males 40 to 160 mg/dL; females 35 to 135 mg/dL

V Anticoagulant Therapy Coagulation Times

A. **PT:** 11 to 12.5 seconds. Therapeutic range for anticoagulant therapy is 1.5 to 2 times the normal or control value. Critical value greater than 20 seconds.
B. **Activated Partial Thromboplastin Time (aPTT):** 30 to 40 seconds. Critical value greater than 70 seconds.
C. **Partial Thromboplastin Time (PTT):** 60 to 70 seconds, greater than 100 seconds.
D. Therapeutic range for anticoagulant therapy is 1.5 to 2 times the normal or **control value.**

E. **INR**
1. Normal INR is 0.8 to 1.1.
2. If the client requires anticoagulation, the desired value is increased to approximately 2 to 3. Critical value greater than 5.
3. The INR is a corrected ratio of a client's prothrombin time to normal.
4. Universal test is not affected by variations in laboratory norms.
F. **Platelets:** 150,000 to 400,000/mm³. Critical value less than 20,000 or greater than 1 million/mm³.

VI Liver Function Tests

A. **Albumin:** 3.5 to 5 g/dL
B. **Ammonia:** 10 to 80 mcg/dL
C. **Total bilirubin:** 0.1 to 1.0 mg/dL
D. **Total protein:** 6 to 8 g/dL

VII Urinalysis

A. **Specific gravity:** 1.005 to 1.030
B. **Protein:** 0 to 8 mg/dL
C. **Glucose:** less than 0.5 g/day
D. **Ketones:** none
E. **pH:** 4.6 to 8
F. **WBC:** males 0 to 3 per high-power field; females 0 to 5 per high-power field

VIII Renal Function

A. **Serum creatinine:** Males 0.6 to 1.2 mg/dL; females 0.5 to 1.1 mg/dL
B. **BUN:** 10 to 20 mg/dL
C. **Creatinine clearance test:** Males 90 to 139 mL/min; females 80 to 125 mL/min. This is a calculation of GFR and is the best indicator of overall renal function.

IX Therapeutic Medication Monitoring

A. **Digoxin level:** 0.8 to 2.0 ng/mL
B. **Lithium level:** 0.4 to 1.4 mEq/L
C. **Phenobarbital:** 10 to 40 mcg/mL
D. **Theophylline:** 10 to 20 mcg/mL
E. **Dilantin:** 10 to 20 mcg/mL

X Blood Glucose Levels

A. **Glucose (fasting):** 70 to 105 mg/dL
B. **Glycosylated hemoglobin (HbA1c):** 4% to 6% is within the expected reference range. Greater than 8% indicates poor diabetes mellitus control.

NOTE: Normal laboratory value reference ranges can have slight variations depending on the facility or organization. To recognize deviations, candidates should know the laboratory value ranges. It is important to recognize values that are elevated or low.

Mental Health Nursing

Overview

I Mental Health

A state of well-being in which each individual is able to realize their own potential, cope with the normal stresses of life, work productively and fruitfully, and contribute to the community.

II Mental Illness

Refers to all mental disorders with definable diagnoses and includes developmental, biological, and psychological disturbances in mental functioning.

III Mental Health Nursing

This type of nursing employs a purposeful use of self as its art and a wide range of nursing, psychosocial, and neurobiological theories and research evidence as its science.

MENTAL HEALTH-ILLNESS CONTINUUM

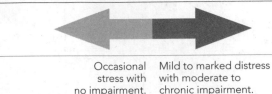

Occasional stress with no impairment.	Mild to marked distress with moderate to chronic impairment.

A. **Theoretical Models**
  1. Psychoanalytic
    a. **Sigmund Freud**
      1) Id, ego, superego
      2) Five Stages of Development
        a) Oral: Birth to 1 year
        b) Anal: 1 to 3 years
        c) Phallic: 3 to 6 years
        d) Latency: 6 to 12 years
        e) Genital: 12 years to young adult
      3) Transference
      4) Countertransference

  b. **Erik Erikson**
    1) Eight Stages of Growth and Development
      a) Infancy: Birth to 1 year
        Trust vs. Mistrust
      b) Early Childhood: 1 to 3 years
        Autonomy vs. Shame and Doubt
      c) Preschooler: 3 to 6 years
        Initiative vs. Guilt
      d) School Age: 6 to 12 years
        Industry vs. Inferiority
      e) Adolescence: 12 to 20 years
        Identity vs. Role Confusion
      f) Young Adult: 20 to 35 years
        Intimacy vs. Isolation
      g) Middle Adult: 35 to 65 years
        Generativity vs. Stagnation
      h) Older Adult: 65 years and older
        Integrity vs. Despair
  2. Behavioral
    a. **Ivan Pavlov:** Classical Conditioning
    b. **B. F. Skinner:** Operant Conditioning
  3. Humanistic
    a. **Abraham Maslow:** Hierarchy of Needs

Self-actualization
Self-esteem
Love and belonging
Safety and security
Physiological

MAJOR THEORETICAL CONTRIBUTIONS	MAJOR CONTRIBUTIONS USED IN NURSING

Psychoanalyst: Sigmund Freud

Interactive systems of the personality: Id, ego, and superego **Five Stages of Development**: Oral, anal, phallic, latency, and genital Erik Erikson later expanded upon these stages.	**Transference** develops when the client experiences feelings toward the nurse or therapist that were originally held toward significant others. **Countertransference** is the health care worker's unconscious, personal response to the client.

Psychoanalyst: Erik Erickson

Eight Stages of Growth and Development	Erikson's developmental framework helps the nurse identify age-appropriate behaviors during data collection.
Infancy (Birth to 1 year): Trust vs. Mistrust Behavior: Hopefulness, trusting vs. withdrawn, alienated	Success: Trust should be seen with the primary caregiver. Crisis: Infant is withdrawn and unresponsive.
Early Childhood (1 to 3 years): Autonomy vs. Shame and Doubt Behavior: Self-control and using willpower vs. uncertainty of doing anything at all	Success: A toddler shows signs of self-control in toilet training. Crisis: A toddler shows signs of doubt in being able to toilet train.
Preschooler (3 to 6 years): Initiative vs. Guilt Behavior: Ability to initiate activities vs. feeling conflicted about what was initiated	Success: A preschooler may initiate helping set the table for dinner. Crisis: A preschooler took candy without paying for it and knew it was wrong.
School Age (6 to 12 years): Industry vs. Inferiority Behavior: Feeling competent in activities and work vs. feelings of low self-esteem	Success: "I'm getting really good at piano since I started taking lessons." Crisis: "I'm dumb because I can't read as fast as everyone else."
Adolescence (12 to 20 years): Identity vs. Role Confusion Behavior: A sense of self vs. becoming confused about self	Success: "I am fine with who I am." Crisis: "I belong to a gang because I am nothing without them."
Young Adult (20 to 35 years): Intimacy vs. Isolation Behavior: Ability to love deeply and commit oneself in relationships vs. remaining uncommitted and alone	Success: "My partner has been my best friend for 10 years." Crisis: "No one is worthy of being in a relationship with me."
Middle Adult (35 to 65 years): Generativity vs. Stagnation Behavior: Ability to give and care for others vs. self-absorption and inability to grow as a person	Success: "I will be taking a leave of absence for 3 months to stay with my mother who is terminally ill." Crisis: "I just want to be by myself and watch television all night."
Older Adult (65 years and older): Integrity vs. Despair Behavior: Sense of accomplishment in life vs. feeling dissatisfied with life	Success: "I have led a happy and productive life." Crisis: "My life has been a waste."

Behaviorist: Ivan Pavlov

Classical conditioning: Pavlov discovered when a neutral stimulus (bell) was repeatedly paired with another stimulus (food that triggered salivation), eventually the sound of the bell alone could elicit salivation in dogs.	Humans can also experience classically conditioned responses that are involuntary and not spontaneous choices.

Behaviorist: B.F. Skinner

Operant conditioning: Voluntary behaviors are learned through consequences and behavioral responses are elicited through reinforcement, which causes a behavior to occur more frequently.	Positive behavior can be encouraged to continue through positive reinforcement, such as offering a reward or returning a privilege.

Humanistic: Abraham Maslow

The Hierarchy of Needs Pyramid

	Self-actualization	People strive to become everything they are capable of.
	Self-esteem	People need to have a high self-regard, and have it reflected to them from others.
	Love and belonging	This involves the need for intimate relationships and experiencing love and affection from others.
	Safety and security	Once physiological needs are met, the safety needs emerge. These needs include security; protection; freedom from fear; and the need for structure, order, and limits.
	Physiological	The most basic needs are food, oxygen, water, sleep, sex, and a constant body temperature. If all needs were deprived, this level would take priority.

THEORY REVIEW

List Erikson's (E) stage of growth and development and Maslow's (M) priority need for the following scenarios.

1. A teenager has been admitted to the emergency department for a drug overdose.

E:

M:

2. An elderly client who lives alone is being discharged following a total hip replacement.

E:

M:

3. An infant is born weighing 1 lb 4 oz (635 g).

E:

M:

4. A young college graduate who was recently engaged receives a diagnosis of tinea corporis.

E:

M:

5. A student who is in the fourth grade has been admitted to a psychiatric hospital for depression and suicidal ideation.

E:

M:

Answer Key: 1. Identity vs. Role Confusion, Physiological (The basic needs to sustain life are priority due to the drug overdose); 2. Integrity vs. Despair, Physiological (The basic needs to maintain life is priority because the client lives alone and is physically compromised); 3. Trust vs. Mistrust, Physiological (The basic needs to maintain life are priority); 4. Intimacy vs. Isolation, Love and Belonging (Physiological and Safety are not priority with tinea corporis because neither are threatened with this diagnosis. However, intimacy and love and belonging are priority needs); 5. Industry vs. Inferiority, Safety (This pediatric client must have protective/safe measures taken to maintain life).

B. **Nursing Process**

1. **Monitor** using the Mental Status Examination (MSE).

    a. Appearance: Grooming, dress, hygiene, facial expression

    b. Behavior: Excessive or reduced body movements, level of eye contact

    c. Speech: Slow, rapid, normal, loud, soft, disorganized, slurred

    d. Mood: Sad, labile, euphoric, flat, bland affect

    e. Thoughts: Disorganized, flight of ideas, obsessions

    f. Perceptual disturbances: Hallucinations, delusions

    g. Cognition: Orientation to time, place, and person; level of consciousness; remote and recent memory; judgment

    h. Ideas of harming self or others: Presence of a plan, means, and opportunity to carry out the plan

2. **Diagnose** with input from the treatment team.

    a. The problem should include related factors and defining characteristics with the probable cause and supporting data.

    b. Example: Hopelessness (problem) related to abandonment (related factor) as evidenced by client statement "Nothing will change" (defining characteristic).

3. **Plan** interventions based on the following criteria.

    a. Safe for client, other clients, staff, and family

    b. Compatible with other therapies, client's personal goals, and cultural values

    c. Realistic and individualized with consideration given to the client's age, physical condition, willingness to change, and community resources

    d. Evidence-based, when available

4. **Implementation** should include the following.

    a. Coordination of care with all members of the treatment team

    b. Reinforcing health teaching and promotion

    c. Milieu therapy

    d. Pharmacological and integrative therapies

5. **Evaluation** should be based on the following.

    a. Ongoing review of data for consideration of revisions in the treatment plan

    b. Realistic outcomes for each client

C. **Nurse-Client Relationship**

1. Orientation phase: This phase can last for a few meetings or longer.

    a. Rapport and trust is established.

    b. The nurse's role is clarified, and all roles are defined.

    c. Confidentiality is established.

    d. The terms of termination are introduced.

    e. The nurse becomes aware of transference and countertransference issues.

    f. Client problems are articulated, and mutually agreed-upon goals are established.

2. Working phase: This allows for a strong working relationship.

    a. Maintain the client relationship.

    b. Share information and gather further data.

    c. Promote the client's problem-solving skills.

    d. Facilitate behavioral change.

    e. Overcome resistance behaviors.

    f. Evaluate problems and goals.

    g. Promote practice and expression of alternative adaptive behaviors.

3. Termination phase: This is the final phase of the nurse–client relationship.

   a. Summarize the goals achieved.

   b. Discuss new coping strategies.

   c. Review situations that occurred during the relationship.

   d. Exchange memories and validate experiences of the relationship to promote closure.

4. Factors that Promote Client Growth

   a. Communicating genuineness

   b. Expressing empathy

   c. Having positive regard for client

D. **Communication Techniques**

1. Therapeutic

   a. Active listening includes the following.

      1) Observing the client's nonverbal behaviors

      2) Understanding and reflecting on the client's verbal message

   b. **Clarifying techniques**

      1) **Restating** allows the nurse to mirror overt and covert messages.
         Client: "I can't focus."
         Nurse: "You are having problems focusing?"

      2) **Reflecting** provides a means to assist clients to better understand their thoughts and feelings.
         Client: "What should I do about my son's addiction?"
         Nurse: "What do you think you should do?"

      3) **Exploring** allows the nurse to examine ideas and experiences in more depth.
         "Tell me more about…"

   c. Ask open-ended questions to elicit client responses.
      "What do you perceive as your biggest stressor right now?"

   d. Offer self.
      "I would like to spend time talking with you."

   e. Offer general leads.
      "And then?"

   f. Focus.
      "You've mentioned many events. Let's talk about your wanting to end it all again."

2. Nontherapeutic

   a. Giving premature advice
      "You should leave your home immediately."

   b. Minimizing feelings
      "Things often get worse before they get better."

   c. False reassurance
      "Everything is going to be fine."

   d. Disapproval
      "I disagree with that."

   e. Making value judgments
      "You wife is dying of lung cancer, and you smoke?"

3. **Group Therapy:** A group of individuals interacting together with a shared purpose

   a. Phases of Group Development

      1) Orientation phase defines the purpose of the group.

      2) Working phase allows for a focus on problem-solving.

      3) Termination phase promotes reflection on the progress that has been made, and identifies post termination goals.

   b. Therapeutic Factors of Groups

      1) Instill hope: The leader promotes optimism about success of group treatment.

      2) Altruism: Members gain from giving support to others, allowing for an improvement of self-worth.

      3) Universality: Members realize that they are not alone with the problems they face.

COMMUNICATION REVIEW

Analyze the following communication scenarios and determine whether the nurse's responses are therapeutic or nontherapeutic and which communication technique is used.

1. Client: "I wish I were dead."
   Nurse: "I know what you mean."
   ☐ THERAPEUTIC
   ☐ NONTHERAPEUTIC
   COMMUNICATION TECHNIQUE:

2. Client: "I am so worried."
   Nurse: "What specifically are you worried about?"
   ☐ THERAPEUTIC
   ☐ NONTHERAPEUTIC
   COMMUNICATION TECHNIQUE:

3. Client: "I haven't taken my medicine in 4 days."
   Nurse: "Why would you stop taking your medications?"
   ☐ THERAPEUTIC
   ☐ NONTHERAPEUTIC
   COMMUNICATION TECHNIQUE:

4. Client: "I wish everyone would leave me alone."
   Nurse: "You are going to do fine, you'll see."
   ☐ THERAPEUTIC
   ☐ NONTHERAPEUTIC
   COMMUNICATION TECHNIQUE:

Answer Key: 1. Nontherapeutic/minimizing feelings; 2. Therapeutic/clarifying with reflection; 3. Nontherapeutic/confrontational, asking "why."; 4. Nontherapeutic/false reassurance

Anxiety and Anxiety Disorders

A. Anxiety

1. Definition: A universal human experience that is considered the most basic of human emotions

2. Levels of Anxiety

   a. Mild: Occurs in normal experience of everyday life, and promotes a sharp focus of reality

   b. Moderate: Narrows the perceptual field, and some details become excluded

   c. Severe: Severely narrows the perceptual field, and the right amount of focus on detail is lost

   d. Panic: Extreme level of anxiety; leaves a person unable to process the environment

LEVELS OF ANXIETY

	MANIFESTATIONS	NURSING INTERVENTIONS
Mild	Heightened perceptual field, alert and can grasp what is going on, restless, irritable or impatient, foot or finger tapping	Help the client identify the anxiety. Anticipate anxiety-provoking situations. Demonstrate interest in the client by leaning forward and maintaining eye contact. Ask questions to clarify what is said. Encourage problem-solving.
Moderate	Narrow perceptual field, voice tremors, difficulty concentrating, increased respiratory and heart rate, pacing, banging hands on table	
Severe	Greatly reduced perceptual field, problem-solving feels impossible, feelings of dread, confusion, chest discomfort, diaphoresis, loud and rapid speech, threats and demands	Maintain calm manner. Remain with the client. Minimize environmental stimuli. Use clear, simple statements. Use low-pitched voice. Listen for themes in communication. Attend to physical and safety needs.
Panic	Inability to focus on the environment, can feel unreal, cannot process what is happening, hallucinations or delusions can occur, somatic reports increase	

B. Defense Mechanisms

1. Definition: Automatic coping styles that protect individuals from anxiety and maintain self-image

2. Adaptive use: Allows anxiety to be lowered and goals to be achieved

3. Maladaptive use: Occurs when one or several are used in excess, disallowing goals to be achieved

4. Defense Mechanisms

   a. Denial: Attempt to escape unpleasant realities

      1) Adaptive use: Client states, "I don't believe you" when hearing news that a loved one died.

      2) Maladaptive use: A client who lost her partner 3 years ago keeps his clothes hanging in the closet and talks about him in the present tense.

   b. Projection: Unconscious rejection of emotionally unacceptable features and attributing them to others. This is an immature defense mechanism. There is no adaptive example.

      1) Example: A woman who has repressed an attraction toward other women refuses to socialize, fearing other women will make homosexual advances.

   c. Regression: Reverting to an earlier developmental level

      1) Adaptive use: A 5-year-old begins sucking his thumb when a new sibling is born.

      2) Maladaptive use: An employee who is not promoted begins missing appointments and showing up late for meetings.

   d. Sublimation: Directing unacceptable behaviors into a socially acceptable area. This is always adaptive.

      1) Example: A student who is angry with a faculty member writes a short story of a hero.

C. Anxiety/Obsessive Compulsive Disorders

1. Clients who have anxiety disorders can use ineffective behaviors to try to control their anxiety.

2. Types of Anxiety Disorders

   a. Phobias

      1) Definition: Persistent, irrational fear of a specific object, activity, or situation that leads to avoidance

      2) Examples

         a) Acrophobia: Fear of heights

         b) Social anxiety disorder: Social phobia characterized by severe anxiety or fear provoked by exposure to social or performance situations

         c) Claustrophobia: Fear of closed spaces

   b. Panic

      1) Definition: Panic attacks are the most commonly seen feature of this disorder. Panic attacks are characterized as a sudden onset of extreme apprehension or fear usually associated with impending doom.

c. Obsessive-Compulsive Disorder (OCD)

   1) Definition: Obsessions are thoughts, impulses, or images that persist and cannot be dismissed from the mind even though the individual makes attempts to do so. Compulsions are ritualistic behaviors an individual feels driven to perform to attempt a reduction of anxiety. Obsessions and compulsions often occur together, and the rituals become time-consuming, interfering with normal routines and relationships.

d. Generalized Anxiety Disorder (GAD)

   1) Definition: Characterized by excessive anxiety or worry about numerous situations, and the anxiety is out of proportion to the true effect of the event.

e. Separation Anxiety Disorder

   1) Definition: This is a normal part of early development, but it can continue into adulthood, and inappropriate levels of concern over being away from a significant other can be exhibited.

ANXIETY/OBSESSIVE COMPULSIVE DISORDERS

	SIGNS AND SYMPTOMS
Phobias	Irrational fear of an object or situation that persists
Panic disorder	Recurrent episodes of panic attacks that can include palpitations, chest pain, breathing difficulties, nausea, and feelings of choking
Obsessive-compulsive disorder (OCD)	Obsessions: persistent intrusive thoughts Compulsions: repetitive behaviors that a client feels driven to perform (such as hand washing)
Generalized anxiety disorder (GAD)	Excessive anxiety/worry more days than not over 6 months associated with restlessness, fatigue, difficulty concentrating, sleep disturbances, and irritability
Separation anxiety disorder	Adults exhibit worry, shyness, uncertainty, and lack of self-direction.

3. Medications for Anxiety Disorders

  a. Antidepressants

    1) Selective Serotonin Reuptake Inhibitors (SSRIs)

      a) Citalopram

      b) Fluoxetine

      c) Sertraline

    2) Serotonin Norepinephrine Reuptake Inhibitors (SNRIs)

      a) Venlafaxine

      b) Duloxetine

    3) Tricyclics

      a) Imipramine

      b) Amitriptyline

  b. Antianxiety Agents

    1) Benzodiazepines

      a) Alprazolam

      b) Clonazepam

      c) Diazepam

    2) Nonbenzodiazepines

      a) Buspirone

  c. Anticonvulsants

    1) Gabapentin

ANXIETY DISORDER REVIEW

Match the disorder with the correct nursing communication.

_____ 1. Phobias

_____ 2. Panic disorder

_____ 3. Generalized anxiety disorder

_____ 4. Obsessive-compulsive disorder

_____ 5. Separation Anxiety Disorder

a. "Tell me more about how you feel since your mom has been away."

b. "Tell me more about how your partner responds to your returning home each day to check the coffee pot."

c. "Where would you like to begin our discussion regarding your fear of flying?"

d. "What do you believe brings on your episodes of chest pain and difficulty breathing?"

e. "You have mentioned a lot of stressors that have been occurring for several months. Which situation is causing the greatest stress for you?"

Answer Key: 1. C; 2. D; 3. E; 4. B; 5. A

SECTION 3

Schizophrenia

A. **Schizophrenia**

1. Definition: A complex brain disorder that affects thinking, language, emotions, social behavior, and the ability to perceive reality correctly

2. Phases

  a. Acute: Onset or exacerbation of symptoms with loss of functional abilities.

  b. Stabilization: Symptoms diminish and the client progresses toward previous level of functioning.

  c. Maintenance: The client is at or near baseline functioning.

3. Data Collection

  a. Positive symptoms are the presence of something that is not normally present, such as the following.

    1) Alterations in thought include delusions which are false, fixed beliefs that cannot be corrected with reasoning.

    2) Alterations in speech can include word salad (meaningless jumble of words) or echolalia (pathological repeating of another's words).

    3) Alterations in perception include hallucinations that involve a sensory experience for which no external stimulus exists (hearing voices, seeing things, experiencing tastes).

  b. Negative symptoms refer to the absence of something that should be present. Examples include flat or blunted affect and inappropriate emotional response.

  c. Cognitive symptoms are subtle changes in memory or thinking leading to an inability to cope and effectively make decisions.

4. **Nursing Interventions**

   a. Provide a structured, safe environment (milieu) for the client in order to decrease anxiety and to distract the client from constant thinking about hallucinations.

   b. Promote therapeutic communication to lower anxiety, decrease defensive patterns, and encourage participation in the milieu.

   c. Establish a trusting relationship with the client.

   d. Use appropriate communication to address hallucinations and delusions.

      1) Ask the client directly about hallucinations. Do not argue or agree with the client's view of the situation.

      2) Do not argue with a client's delusions, but focus on the client's feelings and possibly offer reasonable explanations.

      3) Monitor for paranoid delusions, which can increase the risk for violence against others.

      4) Attempt to focus conversations on reality-based subjects.

   e. First-Generation Antipsychotics (treat positive symptoms)

      1) Thioridazine

      2) Haloperidol

      3) Loxapine

   f. Second-Generation Antipsychotics (treat positive and negative symptoms)

      1) Clozapine

      2) Olanzapine

      3) Quetiapine

      4) Risperidone

   g. Therapy

      1) Cognitive behavioral therapy can assist in controlling symptoms.

SCHIZOPHRENIA REVIEW

Determine whether the following symptoms are positive or negative.

1. The client shows a flattened affect.	☐ POSITIVE	☐ NEGATIVE
2. The client states the CIA is spying on his every move.	☐ POSITIVE	☐ NEGATIVE
3. The client stops speaking to everyone.	☐ POSITIVE	☐ NEGATIVE
4. The client does not complete a task.	☐ POSITIVE	☐ NEGATIVE
5. The client states she feels spiders crawling all over her body.	☐ POSITIVE	☐ NEGATIVE

Answer Key: 1. Negative; 2. Positive; 3. Negative; 4. Negative; 5. Positive

---

Childhood Disorders

A. **Motor Disorders**

   1. Stereotypic Movement Disorder

      a. Definition: A complex neurobiological and developmental disability that typically appears before 3 years of age

   2. Tourette Syndrome

      a. Definition: Motor and verbal tics appearing between 2 and 7 years of age. These symptoms cause marked distress and impairment in social and occupational functioning. This disorder is usually permanent.

      b. Interventions include antipsychotics and behavioral techniques.

   3. **Nursing Interventions**

      a. Motor Disorders

         1) Maintain safe environment. (For example, a helmet can be required for head banging.)

         2) Use positive reinforcement for correct behavior response.

         3) Determine the parents' understanding of the motor disorder.

         4) Encourage participation in behavioral therapy and support groups.

B. **Intellectual Development Disorder (IDD)**

   1. Characterized by deficits in intellectual functioning, social functioning, and managing activities of daily living. Impairments can range from mild to severe.

   2. Interventions

      a. Monitor cognitive and physical development and functioning.

      b. Care and teaching should be individualized to the client's needs.

      c. Make appropriate referrals (early intervention program, social work, speech therapy, physical therapy, occupational therapy).

      d. Add visual cues with verbal instruction.

      e. Give one-step instructions.

C. **Attention Deficit Disorder (ADD) Attention Deficit Hyperactivity Disorder (ADHD)**

   1. Definition: Children with ADD show an inappropriate degree of inattention and impulsiveness. These symptoms are present with the addition of hyperactivity for children who have ADHD.

   2. **Nursing Interventions**

      a. Observe for level of physical activity, attention span, talkativeness, frustration tolerance, and the ability to follow directions.

      b. Monitor social skills, problem-solving skills, and school performance.

      c. Monitor for comorbidities (anxiety, depression).

   3. Medications

      a. Stimulants

         1) Methylphenidate

         2) Amphetamine and dextroamphetamine

D. **Autism Spectrum Disorders (ASDs)**

1. Definition: Complex neurobiological and developmental disabilities that typically appear during the first 3 years of life.

2. Symptoms include deficits in social relatedness, including communication, nonverbal behavior, and interactions.

3. Interventions should begin early within the second or third year of life through specialized treatment programs.

   a. Assist with behavior modification program.

   b. Promote positive reinforcement.

   c. Structure opportunities for small successes.

   d. Set clear rules.

   e. Decrease environmental stimulation.

   f. Introduce the child to new situations slowly.

CHILDHOOD DISORDERS REVIEW

Match the following disorder with the correct expected findings.

_____ 1. Tourette syndrome

_____ 2. Intellectual development disorder

_____ 3. Attention deficit hyperactivity disorder

_____ 4. Autism spectrum disorder

a. A child has delays in both cognitive and physical functioning and an inability to do age-appropriate activities.

b. A child lacks speech.

c. A child fidgets and does not pay attention during an interview.

d. A 4-year-old child consistently protrudes their tongue.

Answer Key: 1. D; 2. A; 3. C; 4. B

SECTION 5

Depressive/Bipolar Disorders

A. **Major Depressive Disorder (MDD)**

1. Definition: Persistently depressed mood lasting for a minimum of 2 weeks

2. Symptoms

   a. Fatigue

   b. Anhedonia

   c. Changes in appetite

   d. Insomnia or hypersomnia

   e. Anergia

   f. Feelings of worthlessness

   g. Persistent thoughts of suicide

3. Primary Risk Factors

   a. Female gender

   b. Unmarried status

   c. Low socioeconomic class

   d. Early childhood trauma

   e. Family history of depression

   f. Postpartum period

   g. Medical illness

4. Three Phases of Treatment and Recovery

   a. Acute is focused on reducing depressive symptoms and lasts 6 to 12 weeks.

   b. Continuation is focused on prevention of a relapse through pharmacotherapy, education, and psychotherapy. It lasts 4 to 9 months.

   c. Maintenance is focused on prevention of further episodes and lasts 1 year or more.

5. **Nursing Interventions**

   a. Evaluate the client's risk of harm to self or others.

   b. Evaluate the client's use of drugs and alcohol.

   c. Determine the client's history of depression.

   d. Determine the client's support systems.

6. Medications

   a. SSRIs

      1) Citalopram

      2) Escitalopram

   b. Selective Serotonin Reuptake Inhibitor and Serotonin Receptor Agonist

      1) Vilazodone

   c. SNRIs

      1) Venlafaxine

      2) Duloxetine

   d. Norepinephrine Dopamine Reuptake Inhibitor (NDRI)

      1) Bupropion

   e. Tricyclic Antidepressants (TCAs)

      1) Imipramine

   f. Monoamine Oxidase Inhibitors (MAOIs)

      1) Phenelzine

      2) Tranylcypromine

7. Electroconvulsive Therapy (ECT)

   a. Induced seizure activity that is found to be helpful in treating clients who have MDD. Clients can experience temporary short-term memory loss after several ECT treatments.

8. Transcranial Magnetic Stimulation (TMS)

   a. Noninvasive treatment that uses magnetic pulses to stimulate the cerebral cortex. There have been no neurological deficits or memory problems noted.

B. **Suicide**

   1. Definition: The intentional act of killing oneself by any means

   2. **Nursing Interventions**

     a. Monitor for suicidal ideation with intent.

     b. Monitor for a lethal suicide plan.

     c. Identify coexisting psychiatric or medical illness.

     d. Identify family history of suicide.

     e. Identify recent lack of support.

     f. Monitor for feelings of hopelessness and helplessness.

     g. Monitor for covert statements such as, "Things will never work out."

     h. Monitor for overt statements such as, "I can't take it anymore."

   3. Environmental Guidelines for Suicide Prevention

     a. Meal trays should not contain glass or metal silverware.

     b. Hands should be in full view while the client is sleeping.

     c. Carefully observe clients swallow medication.

     d. Screen all potentially harmful gifts (such as flowers in a glass vase).

     e. Injury-proof rooms and bathrooms.

     f. Remove all possessions from client that could lead to injury.

     g. One-on-one constant supervision.

C. **Bipolar Disorder**

   1. Definitions

     a. Bipolar I: Mood disorder characterized by at least one week-long manic episode. Manic episodes can alternate with depression.

     b. Bipolar II: Low-level mania alternates with profound depression.

   2. Mania Characteristics

     a. Inflated sense of self-importance

     b. Extreme energy

     c. Excessive talking with pressured speech

     d. Indiscriminate spending, reckless sexual encounters, risky investments

   3. **Nursing Interventions**

     a. Identify whether the client is a danger to self or others.

     b. Identify the need to protect client from uninhibited behaviors.

     c. Monitor for coexisting medical conditions, such as substance use disorder.

   4. Medications

     a. Mood Stabilizers: Lithium

     b. Anticonvulsants: Valproic acid

     c. Atypical Antipsychotics

       1) Aripiprazole

       2) Risperidone

     d. Antianxiety Agents: Clonazepam

DEPRESSIVE/BIPOLAR DISORDERS REVIEW

Place a check by the nursing interventions that are therapeutic for a client experiencing the following.

Depression

☐ 1. Encourage exercise.

☐ 2. Encourage overgeneralizations.

☐ 3. Encourage problem-solving.

☐ 4. Encourage formation of supportive relationships.

Mania

☐ 1. Provide long explanations.

☐ 2. Use firm, calm approach.

☐ 3. Provide frequent high-calorie fluids.

☐ 4. Maintain low-level stimuli.

Answer Key:

Depression/Therapeutic: 1, 3, & 4. Overgeneralizations, such as "She always" or "He never," lead to negative appraisals, making 2 incorrect.

Mania/Therapeutic: 2, 3, & 4. Long explanations could be poorly understood by a client experiencing mania; short statements are preferred, making 1 incorrect.

SECTION 6

Personality Disorders

A. **Personality Disorders**

   1. All personality disorders share characteristics of inflexibility and difficulties in interpersonal relationships that impair social or occupational functioning.

   2. Cluster A

     a. Paranoid

     b. Schizoid

     c. Schizotypal

   3. Cluster B

     a. Antisocial

     b. Borderline

     c. Narcissistic

     d. Histrionic

   4. Cluster C

     a. Dependent

     b. Obsessive-compulsive

     c. Avoidant

B. **Medications**
1. Depend on the disorder
   a. Antidepressants
   b. Antianxiety agents
   c. Antipsychotics

PERSONALITY DISORDERS

DISORDER	🩺 NURSING INTERVENTIONS

Cluster A (Odd/Eccentric)

DISORDER	NURSING INTERVENTIONS
Paranoid Distrust, suspiciousness of others, and hypervigilance	Avoid being too nice or too friendly. Give clear explanations. Warn about changes in treatment plan and explain reasons for delays.
Schizoid Emotional detachment, isolates self, few close relationships Content being an observer	Not affected by approval or rejection of others. Do not try to increase socialization.
Schizotypal Can exhibit extreme anxiety in social situations related to severe social and interpersonal deficits	Respect the client's need for social isolation. Be aware of the client's suspicious behavior. Be aware that superstition and magical thinking are common.

Cluster B (Dramatic/Emotional)

DISORDER	NURSING INTERVENTIONS
Antisocial Disregard for the rights of others, impulsive risk-taking behaviors common, lacks empathy	Be aware of and monitor for substance use disorder. Set clear limits on specific behavior. Be cautious of manipulation through guilt when clients don't get what they want.
Borderline Extreme emotional lability, impulsivity, and self-image distortions that severely impair functioning	Provide clear and consistent boundaries. Use clear communication. Review therapeutic goals and boundaries when behavior issues are evident. Monitor for self-mutilating behaviors.
Narcissistic Lack of empathy impairs relationships, can appear arrogant due to over-inflated sense of self, difficulty with criticism	Remain neutral and avoid power struggles. Convey unassuming self-confidence.
Histrionic Attention-seeking, frustrates easily, often melodramatic and seductive	Understand seductive behavior as a response to distress. Monitor for suicidal behavior if admiration is withdrawn. Model concrete, descriptive (not vague) language.

PERSONALITY DISORDERS (CONTINUED)

DISORDER	🩺 NURSING INTERVENTIONS

Cluster C (Anxious/Fearful)

DISORDER	NURSING INTERVENTIONS
Dependent Excessive clinging and need to be taken care of, submissive	Be aware of countertransference that can occur due to client's clinging behavior. Identify current stresses. Satisfy the client's needs when setting limits.
Obsessive-Compulsive Preoccupied with orderliness, perfectionism, and control; rigid and inflexible; fears failure	Guard against power struggles with the client, as the need to control is high. Monitor for the use of intellectualization, rationalization, and reaction formation as defense mechanisms. Be aware of the client's critical nature toward self and others.
Avoidant Social inhibition, feelings of inadequacy, hypersensitivity to negative evaluation	Maintain a friendly, accepting, reassuring approach. Do not push the client into social situations.

PERSONALITY DISORDERS REVIEW

Select whether the following nursing interventions are therapeutic or nontherapeutic.

1. Communicate behavioral expectations that are easily understood and nonpunitive.	☐ THERAPEUTIC ☐ NONTHERAPEUTIC
2. Discuss concerns about behavior with the client.	☐ THERAPEUTIC ☐ NONTHERAPEUTIC
3. Assist the client to identify consequences and benefits of her behavior.	☐ THERAPEUTIC ☐ NONTHERAPEUTIC
4. Bargain with the client to establish behavioral expectations.	☐ THERAPEUTIC ☐ NONTHERAPEUTIC
5. Encourage the client to participate in problem-solving.	☐ THERAPEUTIC ☐ NONTHERAPEUTIC

Answer Key: 1. T/Helps establish trust and a positive rapport with client; 2. T/Allows the client to reflect on behavior; 3. T/Allows the client to reflect on behavior; 4. NT/Client behavioral expectations should be achievable and mutually agreed upon. A manipulative personality will seek to bargain, and the nurse must not participate; 5. T/The client should consistently participate in problem-solving with professional guidance.

Addictive Disorders

A. **Definitions**

1. Substance use disorder: Pathologic and disordered use of a substance that can lead to intoxication and withdrawal if the substance is removed.

2. Codependency: Over-responsibility for the behaviors of others, often ignoring own needs and desires. Self-worth is defined in terms of caring for others.

    a. Behaviors can include finding excuses for the person's substance use or destroying the person's drug or alcohol supply.

CENTRAL NERVOUS SYSTEM DEPRESSANTS

DRUG	Barbiturates Benzodiazepines Alcohol
INTOXICATION	Slurred speech, unsteady gait, drowsiness, impaired judgment
WITHDRAWAL	Nausea, vomiting, tachycardia, diaphoresis, tremors, tonic-clonic seizures, restlessness, irritability

CENTRAL NERVOUS SYSTEM STIMULANTS

DRUG	Cocaine Amphetamines Methamphetamines
INTOXICATION	Tachycardia, dilated pupils, elevated blood pressure, grandiosity, impaired judgment, paranoia with delusions
WITHDRAWAL	Fatigue, depression, agitation, apathy, anxiety, craving, increased appetite

OPIATES

DRUG	Heroin Meperidine Fentanyl Hydromorphone
INTOXICATION	Constricted pupils, decreased respirations, decreased heart rate, decreased blood pressure, initial euphoria followed by dysphoria
WITHDRAWAL	Yawning, insomnia, panic, diaphoresis, cramps, nausea, vomiting, chills, fever, diarrhea

B. **Nursing Interventions**

1. Monitor vital signs.
2. Monitor for dehydration.
3. Monitor for low self-worth.
4. Provide for client safety.
5. Monitor toxicology screen/blood alcohol level.
6. Monitor for severe withdrawal syndrome.
7. Monitor for an overdose that warrants immediate medical attention.
8. Monitor for suicidal thoughts and behaviors.
9. Monitor family members for codependency.
10. Explore the client's interest in participating in a 12-step program (Alcoholics Anonymous, Narcotics Anonymous).
11. Explore the family's interest in participating in self-help groups (Al-Anon, Alateen).

ADDICTIVE DISORDERS REVIEW

Which of the following nursing diagnoses could apply to a client who has a new diagnosis of substance use disorder?

1. Disturbed sleep pattern	☐ YES ☐ NO
2. Fluid volume overload	☐ YES ☐ NO
3. Interrupted family processes	☐ YES ☐ NO
4. Ineffective coping	☐ YES ☐ NO
5. Disturbed sensory perception	☐ YES ☐ NO

Answer Key: 1. Yes; 2. No (Clients who have substance use disorder typically have imbalanced nutrition: less than body requirements and deficient volume); 3. Yes; 4. Yes; 5. Yes

Neurocognitive Disorders

A. **Delirium and Dementia**

1. **Delirium** is characterized by a disturbance of consciousness and a change in cognition that develop over a short period of time.

2. **Dementia** is a progressive deterioration of cognitive functioning and global impairment of intellect with no change in consciousness.

COGNITIVE DISORDERS

	Delirium	Dementia
ONSET	Sudden, over hours to days	Slowly, over months to years
CONTRIBUTING FACTORS	Fever, hypotension, infection, hypoglycemia, adverse medication reaction, head injury, emotional stress, seizures	Alzheimer's disease, neurological disease, vascular disease, alcohol use disorder, head trauma
COGNITION	Impaired memory, judgment, and attention span that can fluctuate	Impaired memory, judgment, and attention span; abstract thinking
SPEECH	Rapid, inappropriate, incoherent	Slow, inappropriate, incoherent
PROGNOSIS	Reversible with treatment	Not reversible

3. **Alzheimer's disease** is the most common cause of dementia in older adult clients. It is marked by impaired memory and thinking skills. This disease is classified into three stages.

   a. Stage 1: Mild

      1) Memory lapses

         a) Losing or misplacing items

         b) Difficulty concentrating and organizing

         c) Unable to remember material just read

         d) Still able to perform ADLs

         e) Short-term memory loss noticeable to close relations

   b. Stage 2: Moderate

      1) Forgetting events of one's own history

         a) Difficulty performing tasks that require planning and organizing (paying bills, managing money)

         b) Difficulty with complex mental arithmetic

         c) Personality and behavioral changes (appearing withdrawn or subdued, especially in social or mentally challenging situations; compulsive, repetitive actions)

         d) Changes in sleep patterns

         e) Can wander and get lost

         f) Can be incontinent

         g) Clinical findings that are noticeable to others

   c. Stage 3: Severe

      1) Losing ability to converse with others

         a) Assistance required for ADLs

         b) Incontinence

         c) Losing awareness of one's environment

         d) Progressing difficulty with physical abilities (walking, sitting, and eventually swallowing)

         e) Eventually losses all ability to move; can develop stupor and coma

         f) Death frequently related to choking or infection

4. Medications for Clients who have Alzheimer's Disease

   a. Cholinesterase Inhibitors

      1) Donepezil

      2) Galantamine

   b. NMDA Antagonist

      1) Memantine

   c. SSRIs

      1) Citalopram

      2) Paroxetine

   d. Antianxiety Agents

      1) Lorazepam

      2) Oxazepam

5. **Nursing Interventions** for Dementia

   a. Evaluate the client's level of cognitive and daily functioning.

   b. Identify threats to client's safety.

   c. Review all medications the client is taking.

   d. Interview family members to obtain a full history.

   e. Use short, simple words and phrases.

   f. Speak slowly.

   g. Have clocks, calendars, and personal items in clear view.

   h. Explore how well the family understands the disease progression.

   i. Review resources available to the family.

   j. Maintain consistent routine.

6. **Nursing Interventions** for Delirium

   a. Establish the client's baseline level of consciousness by interviewing family members.

   b. Monitor vital signs and perform neurological checks.

   c. Monitor for acute onset and fluctuating levels of consciousness.

   d. Monitor the client's ability to function in the immediate environment.

   e. Determine the physiologic reason delirium is occurring.

   f. Maintain safety.

NEUROCOGNITIVE DISORDERS REVIEW

Place a check by the nursing interventions that could apply to a client who has Alzheimer's disease.

☐	1. Keep the client in a locked setting.
☐	2. Monitor for a physiological reason for confusion.
☐	3. Give step-by-step instructions.
☐	4. Perform neurological checks.
☐	5. Administer donepezil as prescribed.

Answer Key

Correct: 1. Wandering begins to occur in stage 2, and a locked setting is needed; 3. Clear, simple instructions can be needed as early as stage 1; 5. This is a commonly prescribed medication for a client who has Alzheimer's.

Incorrect: 2. This intervention is best for a client who has delirium.; 4. Neurological checks are used for clients who have delirium, rather than dementia.

Eating Disorders

A. **Anorexia Nervosa**

1. Definition: An eating disorder characterized by an extreme fear of gaining weight and altered perception of one's own body weight

2. Manifestations

   a. Describes self as "fat"

   b. Preoccupation with thoughts of food

   c. Judges self-worth by body weight

   d. Low body weight

   e. Amenorrhea

   f. Cold extremities

   g. Constipation

   h. Hypotension, bradycardia

   i. Impaired renal function

   j. Hypokalemia

3. **Nursing Interventions**

   a. Develop a supportive relationship with the client.

   b. Monitor electrolytes and vital signs.

   c. Monitor food and fluid intake.

   d. Set achievable weight goals.

   e. Limit exercise regimen to promote weight gain.

   f. Explore the client's feelings of self-worth.

   g. Assist in development of effective coping strategies.

   h. Encourage client attendance in behavior modification therapy.

   i. Encourage family support groups.

   j. Administer antidepressants as prescribed.

   k. Provide positive reinforcement for weight gain.

B. **Bulimia Nervosa**

1. Definition: An uncontrollable compulsion to consume large amounts of food in a short period (binge eating), followed by a compensatory need to rid the body of the calories consumed

   a. Purging: Client uses self-induced vomiting, laxatives, diuretics, and enemas to lose or maintain weight.

   b. Nonpurging: Client compensates for binge eating through other means, such as excessive exercise.

2. Manifestations

   a. Bradycardia, hypotension

   b. Electrolyte imbalances

   c. Erosion of teeth

   d. Esophageal tears from vomiting

   e. Normal to slightly low body weight

   f. Muscle weakening

   g. Calluses/scars on hand from self-induced vomiting

3. **Nursing Interventions**

   a. Develop a supportive relationship with the client.

   b. Monitor electrolytes and vital signs.

   c. Monitor food and fluid intake.

   d. Monitor the client 30 to 60 min after a meal.

   e. Monitor exercise regimen.

   f. Explore the client's feelings of self-worth.

   g. Observe teeth for erosion and caries.

   h. Observe the room for food hoarding.

   i. Encourage client attendance in behavior modification therapy.

   j. Encourage family support groups.

   k. Administer antidepressants as prescribed.

EATING DISORDERS REVIEW

Determine whether the following nursing interventions support restricting anorexia, purging bulimia, or both.

1. Monitor dental erosion.	☐ ANOREXIA	☐ BULIMIA
2. Monitor ECG for arrhythmias.	☐ ANOREXIA	☐ BULIMIA
3. Monitor exercise regimen.	☐ ANOREXIA	☐ BULIMIA
4. Check for calluses on hands.	☐ ANOREXIA	☐ BULIMIA
5. Identify significant weight loss.	☐ ANOREXIA	☐ BULIMIA

Answer Key: 1. Bulimia due to self-induced vomiting; 2. Both have electrolyte imbalances that can lead to arrhythmias; 3. Both. Clients who have anorexia have a weight gain goal and exercise should be monitored. Clients who have bulimia use exercise as a way to purge calories; 4. Bulimia due to self-induced vomiting; 5. Anorexia. Clients who have bulimia have normal to slightly low body weight.

Anger/Violence, Abuse, and Assault

A. **Anger and Violence**

1. Feelings that can precipitate anger: Discounted, embarrassed, guilty, humiliated, hurt, ignored, unheard, rejected, threatened, tired, vulnerable

2. Definitions

   a. Anger is an emotional response to frustration of desires and can be expressed in a healthy way. Problems begin to occur when anger is expressed through violence.

   b. Violence is always an objectionable act that involves intentional use of force that can result in injury or death.

3. Predictors of Violence

   a. Loud voice

   b. Intense avoidance of eye contact

   c. Verbal abuse

   d. Pacing and restless

   e. Jaw clenching, rigid posture

   f. Stone silence

   g. Alcohol or drug intoxication

4. **Cycle of Violence**

a. **Tension-Building Stage** is characterized by minor incidents by the abuser, such as pushing and verbal abuse. The victim often accepts blame.

b. **Battering Stage** is characterized by the abuser releasing built-up tension by beating the victim brutally. The victim might try to cover the injury or look for help.

c. **Honeymoon Stage** is characterized by kindness and loving behaviors such as flowers given by the abuser. The victim is hopeful and wants to believe the abuser will change.

CYCLE OF VIOLENCE

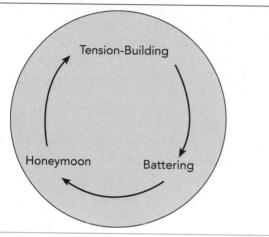

5. **Nursing Interventions**

a. De-escalation

   1) Maintain a calm approach.
   2) Use short, simple sentences.
   3) Avoid verbal struggles/conflict.
   4) Identify the client's perceived need.
   5) Monitor for stressors.
   6) Use a nonaggressive posture.
   7) Maintain client's self-esteem/dignity.
   8) Maintain a large personal space.

b. Medications

   1) Antianxiety Agents
      a) Lorazepam
      b) Alprazolam
      c) Diazepam
   2) Antipsychotics
      a) Haloperidol
      b) Chlorpromazine

c. Restraints and Seclusion

   1) Restraints are a manual method to prevent client movement with the intention to protect the client from self-harm or assaulting others.
   2) Seclusion is the involuntary confinement of a client alone in a room. The goal is always centered around the safety of the client and others and is never punitive.

B. **Abuse**

1. **Physical abuse** is the infliction of physical pain or bodily harm (hitting, choking).

2. **Sexual abuse** is any form of sexual contact or exposure without consent. This is often referred to as assault when referring to adults.

3. **Emotional abuse** is the infliction of mental anguish, such as threatening or intimidating.

4. **Neglect** can be physical or emotional and includes failure to meet the needs of education and appropriate medical care.

5. **Economic abuse** is the withholding of financial support or illegal use of funds for one's personal gain.

THE VICTIM INTERVIEW

DO	DO NOT
Conduct the interview in private.	Try to prove abuse.
Be direct, honest, and professional.	Display horror, anger, or shock.
Be understanding and attentive.	Place blame or make judgments.
Monitor client safety.	Force anyone to remove clothing.

C. **Sexual Assault**

1. Any type of sexual activity to which the victim does not consent, ranging from inappropriate touching to penetration.

2. Rape is nonconsensual vaginal, anal, or oral penetration obtained by force or by threat of bodily harm, or when consent is unobtainable.

   a. Drugs associated with date rape
      1) Gamma-hydroxybutyrate (GHB) produces relaxation, euphoria, and disinhibition.
      2) Flunitrazepam causes sedation, muscle relaxation, and amnesia.
      3) Ketamine causes a dreamlike state and compliance of the victim.

3. Rape Trauma Syndrome

   a. This is a variant of posttraumatic stress disorder that can last for weeks following rape. Symptoms can include feelings of numbness, disbelief, fear, denial, flashbacks, and emotional lability.

4. **Nursing Interventions**

   a. Use a nonjudgmental and empathic approach.
   b. Monitor, treat, and document all injuries.
   c. Provide a private environment and limit personnel who examine the client.
   d. Monitor client emotions, and provide support.

ANGER/VIOLENCE, ABUSE, AND ASSAULT REVIEW

Match the following.

_____ 1. A nonpunitive intervention used to protect the client from harming self or others

_____ 2. A stage of violence in which gifts and apologies are given

_____ 3. Antianxiety agent

_____ 4. Failure to make educational provisions for a child

_____ 5. Intense eye contact

_____ 6. Antipsychotic

a. Lorazepam

b. Seclusion

c. Predictor of violence

d. Honeymoon

e. Haloperidol

f. Neglect

Answer Key: 1. B; 2. D; 3. A; 4. F; 5. C; 6. E

Trauma- and Stressor-Related Disorders

A. **Acute Stress Disorder (ASD)**

1. Definition: Diagnosed 3 days to 1 month after exposure to a highly traumatic event. Can cause change in mood, sleep patterns, and physiologic reactivity.

B. **Posttraumatic Stress Disorder (PTSD)**

1. Definition: Diagnosed after 1 month to years after a traumatic event. Persistent re-experiencing of a highly traumatic event that involved actual or threatened death or serious injury to self or others to which the individual responded with intense fear, helplessness, or horror.

2. **Nursing Interventions** (ASD, PTSD)

   a. Establish a therapeutic relationship.

   b. Monitor for persistent re-experiencing of a highly traumatic event through dreams, flashbacks, thoughts, or images.

   c. Monitor for suicidal ideation or violence.

   d. Identify family and social support.

   e. Monitor for current life stressors and social withdrawal.

   f. Monitor for insomnia.

   g. Monitor for agitation and restlessness.

   h. Maintain stable, nonthreatening environment.

3. Medications (ASD, PTSD)

   a. SSRIs: fluoxetine, paroxetine

   b. SNRIs: venlafaxine

   c. Tricyclic antidepressants: amitriptyline

   d. Alpha agonists: clonidine, prazosin

   e. Beta blocker: propranolol

Legal Aspects of Mental Health Nursing

A nurse who works in a mental health setting is responsible for providing ethical, competent, and safe care consistent with local, state, and federal laws.

A. **Types of Admissions**

1. Voluntary

   a. Admits self

   b. Consents to all treatment

   c. Can refuse treatment, including medications, unless a danger to self or others

   d. Can demand and receive discharge

2. Involuntary

   a. The client is deemed by lawful authority to be a danger to self or others.

   b. At the end of a specified time, the client must have a hearing or be released.

B. **Informed consent required for**

1. Electroconvulsive therapy

2. Medications

3. Seclusion

4. Restraints

C. **Client Rights**

1. Clients who have a diagnosis of or are hospitalized with a mental health disorder are guaranteed the same civil rights as any other citizens.

   a. Right to plan of care

   b. Right to receive or refuse treatment

   c. Access to stationery and postage

   d. Receipt of unopened mail

   e. Visits by health care provider, attorney, or clergy

   f. Daily interaction with visitors or phone access

   g. Right to have and/or spend money

   h. Storage space for personal items

   i. Right to own property, vote, and marry

   j. Right to make wills and contracts

   k. Access to educational resources

   l. Right to sue, or be sued, including challenging one's hospitalization

Point to Remember

A nurse's priority is to promote and provide care to a client in the least restrictive environment possible.

Maternal and Newborn Nursing

Female Reproductive System

ı Reproduction

A. **Reproductive Organs**

1. Ovaries
2. Fallopian tubes
3. Uterus
4. Cervix
5. Vagina

B. **Fertilization and Fetal Development**

1. Conception (i.e., fertilization): Union of sperm and ovum
2. Conditions necessary for fertilization
   a. Mature egg and sperm
   b. Timing
      1) Lifetime of ovum is 24 hr.
      2) Lifetime of sperm in female genital tract is 72 hr.
      3) Menstruation begins approximately 14 days after ovulation if conception has not occurred.
   c. Vaginal and cervical secretions
      1) Less acidic during ovulation (sperm cannot survive in a highly acidic environment)
      2) Thinner during ovulation (sperm can penetrate more easily)
   d. Process of fertilization (7 to 10 days)
      1) Ovulation occurs.
      2) Ovum travels to fallopian tube.
      3) Sperm travels to fallopian tube.
      4) One sperm penetrates the ovum.
      5) Zygote forms (i.e., fertilized egg).
      6) Zygote migrates to uterus.
      7) Zygote implants in uterine wall.
      8) Progesterone and estrogen are secreted by the corpus luteum to maintain the lining of the uterus and prevent menstruation until the placenta starts producing these hormones. (Progesterone is a thermogenic hormone that raises body temperature, an objective sign that ovulation has occurred.)
3. Placental development
   a. Chorionic villi
      1) Secrete human chorionic gonadotropin (hCG), which stimulates production of estrogen and progesterone from the corpus luteum.
         a) Production of hCG begins on the day of implantation and can be detected by day 6.
      2) Burrow into the endometrium, forming the placenta.
   b. Placental hormones
      1) hCG
      2) Human chorionic somatomammotropin (hCS): Acts as growth hormone and insulin antagonist
      3) Estrogen and progesterone

4. Fetal membranes develop and surround the fetus.
   a. Amnion: Inner membrane
   b. Chorion: Outer membrane
5. Umbilical cord
   a. Two arteries carry deoxygenated blood to the placenta.
   b. One vein carries oxygenated blood to the fetus.
   c. No pain receptors
   d. Encased in Wharton's jelly (thick substance that surrounds the umbilical cord and acts as a buffer, preventing pressure on the vein and arteries in the umbilical cord)
   e. Covered by chorionic membrane
6. Amniotic fluid
   a. Replaced every 3 hr
   b. 800 to 1,200 mL at end of pregnancy
   c. Functions: Temperature regulation, protection, and promoting musculoskeletal development of the fetus

Pregnancy

ı Prenatal Period

Begins with conception and ends before birth.

A. **Anatomy and Physiology**

1. **Female Anatomy**: Hormones, ovulation, organs
2. **Male Anatomy**: Sperm, vas deferens, seminal fluid
3. **Fetal/Maternal Circulation:** Fetal and maternal blood do not mix

PSYCHOLOGICAL AND PHYSIOLOGICAL ADAPTATIONS OF PREGNANCY

TRIMESTER	NURSING INTERVENTIONS
Ambivalence	
1st	Collect data to determine meaning of pregnancy to the client/partner and socioeconomic supports. Refer if needed.
Accepting	
2nd	Collect data to determine if ambivalence is increased and how the client views the fetus.
Preparing for birth	
3rd	Reinforce manifestations of onset of labor, newborn care, feeding methods, birth control, and home preparations for the baby. Review birthing plan.
Skin: Striae, linea nigra, chloasma	
2nd, 3rd	Commercial treatments are not useful. Pigmentation usually disappears after pregnancy. Striae can fade.
Breasts: Size, striae, tenderness	
1st	Fullness and sensitivity is hormone-related. Wear a supportive bra. Over-the-counter products do not reduce stretch marks.

PSYCHOLOGICAL AND PHYSIOLOGICAL ADAPTATIONS OF PREGNANCY (CONTINUED)

TRIMESTER	🩺 NURSING INTERVENTIONS

Breasts: Colostrum

2nd, 3rd	Colostrum may be expressed as early as 16 weeks. Discuss breast care (pads), nipple care (keep dry).

Respiratory: Dyspnea

2nd, 3rd	Sleep propped or sitting up. Lightening (fetus begins descent into pelvis) between 38 to 40 weeks—can breathe easier.

Cardiovascular: Faintness and syncope

2nd	Encourage moderate exercise, deep breathing, and side-lying position. Avoid sudden changes in position.

Cardiovascular: Varicose veins

2nd, 3rd	Monitor activity (sitting/standing, constrictive clothing, crossing legs). Reinforce teaching about leg elevation, position changes, support hose, and exercise.

GI: Nausea/vomiting

1st	Reinforce teaching about diet (dry crackers, five to six small meals, ginger, raspberry). Avoid fried, odorous, spicy foods and foods with strong smells. Monitor weight, urine output (UO), and signs of hyperemesis. Call the provider if cannot eat/drink for more than 24 hr, urine becomes scant and dark, heart pounds, or client becomes dizzy.

GI: Constipation

2nd, 3rd	Reinforce teaching about activity, fluids, and fiber.

GI: Heartburn

2nd, 3rd	Encourage small meals. Sit upright for 30 min or longer after eating. Avoid spicy, fatty foods. Drink hot herbal tea.

GU: Frequency

1st, 3rd	Monitor for urinary tract infection (UTI). Reinforce teaching of frequent voiding. Do not decrease fluids. Urinate after intercourse. Call provider for dysuria, cloudy or foul-smelling urine, or flank pain. Perform Kegel exercises.

GU: Leukorrhea

2nd, 3rd	This is normal. Do not douche. Maintain good hygiene. Wear perineal pads. Report if accompanied by pruritus, foul odor, or change in character.

GU: Braxton Hicks

2nd, 3rd	Reinforce teaching about the difference between Braxton Hicks and true labor. (See table on false vs. true labor in this unit.)

Nutrition

1st, 2nd, 3rd	Monitor and reinforce teaching about weight gain patterns; average weight gain is 25 to 35 lb. Caloric increase 300 to 400 kcal/day; protein increase by 25 g/day; iron intake 30 mg/day; folate intake 600 mcg/day. Take prenatal vitamins. Limit caffeine intake.

SIGNS/SYMPTOMS OF PREGNANCY

Presumptive: Subjective signs/symptoms

Amenorrhea

Fatigue

Nausea and vomiting

Urinary frequency

Breast changes: Darkened areola, enlarged Montgomery's tubules

Quickening: Slight fluttering movements of the fetus felt by the client, usually between 16 to 20 weeks of gestation

Probable: Objective signs

Cervical changes

Hegar's sign: Softening and compressibility of lower uterus

Chadwick's sign: Deepened violet-bluish color of vaginal mucosa secondary to increased vascularity of the area

Goodell's sign: Softening of cervical tip

Ballottement: Rebound of unengaged fetus

Braxton Hicks contractions: False contractions, painless, irregular, and usually relieved by walking

Positive pregnancy test

Positive: Signs related to presence of fetus

Fetal heart tones

Visualization of fetus by ultrasound

Fetal movement palpated by an experienced examiner

B. **Verifying Pregnancy**

1. Serum and urine tests provide an accurate measure for the presence of hCG.

2. hCG can be detected 6 to 11 days in serum and 26 days in urine after conception following implantation.

   a. Production begins with implantation, peaks at about 60 to 70 days of gestation, and then declines until around 80 days of pregnancy, when it begins to gradually increase until term.

   b. Higher levels can indicate multifetal pregnancy, ectopic pregnancy, hydatidiform mole (gestational trophoblastic disease), or a genetic abnormality such as Down syndrome.

   c. Lower blood levels of hCG can suggest a miscarriage or ectopic pregnancy. Some medications (anticonvulsants, diuretics, tranquilizers) can cause false-positive or false-negative pregnancy results.

C. **Calculating Delivery Date**

1. Nägele's rule: Formula for calculating estimated date of confinement (EDC) or estimated date of birth (EDB). To calculate EDB, subtract 3 months and add 7 days to the first day of the last menstrual period.

2. McDonald's rule: Measure uterine fundal height in centimeters from the symphysis pubis to the top of the uterine fundus. Between 18 and 32 weeks of gestation, the fundal height measurement should approximate gestational age.

D. **Antepartum Fetal Data Collection**

1. Ultrasound

   a. Indications for use

      1) Confirm pregnancy and location (uterine vs. ectopic).

      2) Evaluate fetus: Number, heartbeat, gestational age, abnormalities, growth and development, activity (biophysical profile [BPP]).

      3) Evaluate placenta: Location (previa, abruption), grading.

      4) Evaluate amniotic fluid volume.

   b. **Nursing Interventions**

      1) Preparation of a client

         a) Explain the procedure.

         b) Ensure client has a full bladder.

2. Non-stress test (NST)

   a. Most widely used test for evaluating fetal well-being

   b. Noninvasive

   c. Monitors response of the fetal heart rate (FHR) to fetal movement

   d. Indications for use

      1) Monitor for fetal well-being and an intact CNS during the third trimester.

      2) Monitor fetus of clients who have high-risk pregnancies (maternal diabetes mellitus, hypertension, heart disease, IUGR, postdates, history of stillbirth, decreased fetal movement).

   e. Interpretation of findings

      1) Reactive NST (normal)

         a) Two or more fetal heart rate accelerations (increase in FHR of at least 15/min above the baseline and last 15 seconds) within a 20-min period.

         b) Before 32 weeks gestation, acceleration is defined as increase of at least 10/min lasting at least 10 seconds in FHR.

      2) Non-reactive NST (abnormal)

         a) Does not produce two or more qualifying accelerations in 20 min.

         b) If does not meet criteria in 40 min, additional testing is indicated: contraction stress test (CST) or BPP.

   f. **Nursing Interventions**

      1) Seat the client in a reclining chair or place in a semi-Fowler's or left-lateral position.

      2) Apply two belts and transducers to the client's abdomen.

REACTIVE NST

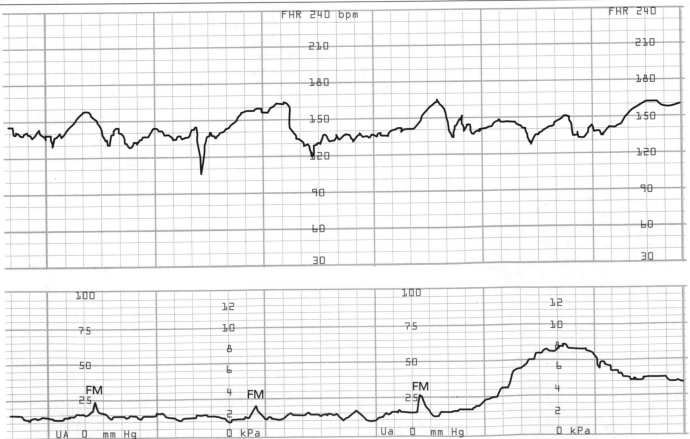

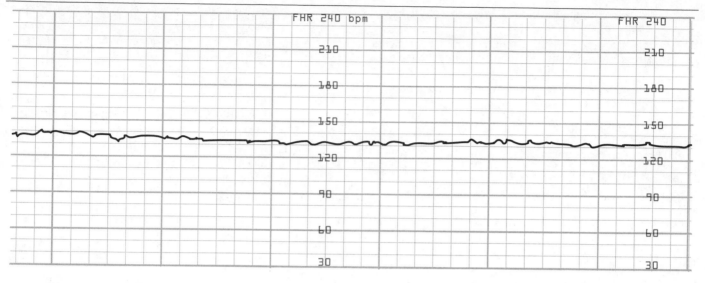

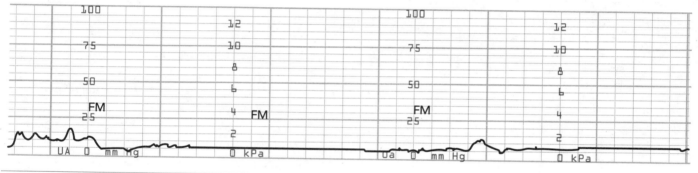

3. Contraction stress test (CST)

  a. Method

    1) Nipple stimulation

    2) Oxytocin IV

  b. Indications for use

    1) Non-reactive NST

    2) High-risk pregnancies; same as indications for NST

  c. **Nursing Interventions**

    1) Explain procedure and obtain informed consent.

    2) Obtain baseline FHR, fetal movement, and contraction pattern 10 to 20 min before and 30 min afterward.

    3) Initiate method and observe for uterine tachysystole (hyperstimulation).

    4) Obtain at least three contractions in a 10-min period, each lasting 40 to 60 seconds.

    5) Maintain bed rest during the procedure.

  d. Interpretation of findings

    1) Test results are negative, positive, equivocal, suspicious, or unsatisfactory.

    2) Negative CST (normal)

      a) At least three uterine contractions in 10 min, with no late decelerations

      b) Reassuring finding

    3) Positive CST (abnormal)

      a) Late decelerations occur with 50% or more of contractions

      b) Nonreassuring finding

      c) Suggestive of uteroplacental insufficiency

4. Biophysical profile

   a. Uses real-time ultrasound to visualize physiological characteristics of the fetus

   b. Monitors five variables: Fetal breathing movements, gross body movements, fetal heart rate, reactive FHR (NST), amniotic fluid volume

   c. Award score of 0 (abnormal finding) or 2 (normal finding) to each variable

BIOPHYSICAL PROFILE

Fetal breathing movements

NORMAL SCORE:	2	At least one episode of 30 seconds in 30 min
ABNORMAL SCORE:	0	Absent or less than 30 seconds duration

Gross body movements

NORMAL SCORE:	2	At least three body or limb extensions with return to flexion in 30 min
ABNORMAL SCORE:	0	Less than three episodes

Fetal tone

NORMAL SCORE:	2	At least one episode of extension with return to flexion
ABNORMAL SCORE:	0	Slow extension and flexion, lack of flexion, or absence of movement

Reactive FHR

NORMAL SCORE:	2	Reactive NST
ABNORMAL SCORE:	0	Nonreactive NST

Amniotic fluid volume

NORMAL SCORE:	2	At least one pocket of fluid equal to or greater than 2 cm, or more than 5 cm total fluid
ABNORMAL SCORE:	0	Pockets absent or less than 5 cm total

Total Score

The score will be even numbers only, ranging from 0 to 10.
Normal = 8 to 10
Equivocal/borderline = 6
Abnormal = 0 to 4

5. Amniocentesis

   a. Early pregnancy

      1) Genetic work-up for fetal anomalies (Down syndrome, Trisomy 18, Trisomy 13)

      2) Detect presence of AChE in neural tube defects (NTDs)

      3) Performed at 14 to 16 weeks

   b. Late in pregnancy

      1) Monitor fetal lung maturity and fetal well-being.

      2) L:S ratio of 2:1 indicates fetal lung maturity.

   c. **Nursing Interventions** for amniocentesis

      1) Preprocedure: Explain the procedure and risks to the client, and obtain informed consent.

      2) Ensure the client has a patent IV.

      3) Postprocedure

         a) Monitor FHR and fetal activity.

         b) Monitor for signs of labor.

         c) Monitor for vaginal bleeding or hemorrhage.

         d) Administer Rho(D) immune globulin if client is Rh-negative.

      4) Education on complications to report

         a) Bleeding

         b) Contractions

         c) Signs and symptoms of infection

NOTE: According to the NCLEX® scope of practice, only RNs may administer Rho(D) immune globulin IM. It is a blood product!

6. Percutaneous umbilical blood sampling (PUBS)

   a. Also referred to as cordocentesis

   b. Direct access to fetal circulation

   c. Used for fetal blood sampling and transfusion

   d. Performed in high-risk centers

   e. In many centers replaced by placental biopsy

7. Chorionic villi sampling

   a. Obtain sample of chorionic villi (placental) tissue.

   b. Identify fetal genetic abnormalities.

   c. Performed transcervical or transabdominal.

   d. Performed during the first trimester.

   e. Similar risk and nursing interventions as amniocentesis.

8. Maternal serum alpha-fetoprotein screening (MSAFP)

   a. Screening tool for NTDs

   b. Ideally performed at 16 to 18 weeks

   c. Lower than normal levels: Follow up for Down syndrome

   d. Higher than normal levels: Follow up for neural tube defects

E. **Fetal Data Collection**

   1. FHR expected reference range is 110 to 160/min.

   2. Fundal height used to evaluate gestational age and growth of fetus.

   3. Fetal activity: Kick counts or daily fetal movement counts.

      a. Contact provider if fetal movement decreases or ceases entirely for 12 hr.

      b. Contact if less than 10 kicks/2 hr.

      c. Try to do at the same time each day.

      d. Most active after meals and in the evening.

      e. Fetal movement can be decreased by illicit drugs, prescribed medications, alcohol, and cigarette smoke.

      f. Obesity can hinder the sensation of fetal activity.

II Obstetrical Terminology

A. Pregnancy Outcome

1. Gravidity: Number of pregnancies
2. Parity: Number of pregnancies that reach viability (20 weeks)
3. Five-digit system (GTPAL)
   a. **G** – Gravidity (number of pregnancies, including this pregnancy)
   b. **T** – Term births (38 weeks or more)
   c. **P** – Preterm births (from 20 weeks up to 37 completed weeks)
   d. **A** – Abortions/miscarriages (prior to viability)
   e. **L** – Living children

III Collaborative Care

A. Prenatal Care

1. Initial exam
   a. Psychosocial data collection
   b. Complete history including medications, pertinent history from partner, and family history of genetic concerns
   c. Complete physical
   d. Baseline laboratory values
      1) CBC
      2) Blood type and Rh
      3) Urinalysis
      4) STI screen, including the following
         a) HIV
         b) Rubella titer
         c) Hepatitis B
   e. Nutritional counseling (See the table on psychological and physiological adaptations of pregnancy in this unit.)
   f. Teratogens: Fetus especially vulnerable during first trimester
      1) Drugs
         a) Category C and D medications (warfarin, lithium, methimazole, phenytoin, tetracycline, antipsychotics)
         b) Illicit drugs
      2) Cigarettes and alcohol
         a) Smoking increases incidence of abortion, prematurity, SGA, and SIDS.
         b) Quantity of alcohol to produce fetal effects (IUGR, CNS malformation, neurologic problems) is unclear.
      3) Thermal risks and radiation
         a) Avoid hot tubs, long baths, or excessively hot showers.

4) Infections
   a) Group B Strep
      (1) Culture obtained at 35 to 36 weeks.
      (2) Treat positive culture with PCN IVPB every 4 hr during labor.
      (3) Monitor newborn for infection.
   b) TORCH
      (1) **T** – Toxoplasmosis
      (2) **O** – Other (syphilis, varicella, parvovirus)
      (3) **R** – Rubella
      (4) **C** – Cytomegalovirus
      (5) **H** – Herpes infections
   c) See the table on sexually transmitted Infections table in this unit.

2. Initial and subsequent exams
   a. Weight
   b. Fundal height
   c. FHR
   d. Fetal activity (include date of quickening)
   e. Urine check for glucose and protein
   f. Anticipatory guidance. (See the table on psychological and physiological adaptations of pregnancy in this unit.) Review when to contact provider.
      1) Rupture of membranes prior to 37 weeks
      2) Abdominal or back pain (contractions) before 37 weeks
      3) Vaginal bleeding
      4) Elevated temperature
      5) Dysuria, oliguria
      6) Severe headache with vision changes

3. 16 to 22 weeks
   a. Screen for NTDs with maternal serum alpha fetoprotein.

4. 28 weeks
   a. Screen for diabetes mellitus.
   b. Administer Rho(D) immune globulin if Rh-negative.
   c. Begin NST testing twice a week for any pregnancy at risk for intrauterine fetal death.

5. 35 weeks
   a. Test for group B strep.

B. **Anticipatory Care:** Do not assume manifestations are normal adaptations of pregnancy.

   1. Physiological changes

      a. Physiological changes in pregnancy are the result of hormone production and the enlarging uterus.

PHYSIOLOGICAL CHANGES

SYSTEM	CHANGES
Reproductive	Uterus increases in size, shape, position Ovulation and menses cease
Cardiovascular	Increased cardiac output and blood volume Increased heart rate Increased coagulation
Respiratory	Increased maternal oxygen needs Uterine enlargement displaces diaphragm causing increased respiratory rate and decreased total lung capacity
Musculoskeletal	Pelvic joint relaxation Body alterations require adjustment in posture Separation of rectus abdominis muscles
Gastrointestinal	Nausea, vomiting, slowed digestive processes, constipation
Renal	Increased glomerular filtration, urinary frequency
Endocrine/ Metabolic	Increased hormone production (hCG, progesterone, estrogen, HCS, and prostaglandins) Increased thyroid and parathyroid activity Insulin resistance
Integument	Hyperpigmentation causing chloasma, linea nigra, striae gravidarum, and palmar erythema

   b. Changes in physical appearance can lead to a negative body image. The client can make statements of resentment toward the pregnancy and express anxiousness for it to be over soon.

   2. Expected vital signs

      a. Blood pressure

         1) Within the prepregnancy range during the first trimester

         2) Decreases 5 to 10 mm Hg during the second trimester

         3) Position affects blood pressure; supine position can cause supine hypotensive syndrome or vena cava syndrome. Manifestations include dizziness, lightheadedness, and pale, clammy skin. Interventions include left–lateral side, semi–Fowler's position, or wedge under one hip if supine.

      b. Pulse

         1) Increases by 10 to 15/min around 20 weeks

      c. Respirations

         1) Increases by 1 to 2/min due to elevation of the diaphragm

   3. Fetal heart tones

      a. Normal baseline rate 110 to 160/min

      b. Accelerations are reassuring, indicate intact fetal CNS

SECTION 3

Complications of Pregnancy

Medical Problems

Preexisting conditions can complicate pregnancy. Some medical conditions develop during pregnancy and cause complications.

NOTE: Remember that only the RN may care for or assess high-risk or unstable clients, according to the NCLEX® scope of practice.

A. **Cardiac Disease**

   1. Contributing Factors

      a. Preexisting heart condition

      b. Increased maternal plasma volume

   2. Greatest risks for heart failure

      a. End of second trimester (28 to 32 weeks)

      b. During labor

      c. After delivery (first 48 hr)

   3. Manifestations

      a. Subjective data

         1) Dizziness

         2) Shortness of breath

         3) Weakness

         4) Fatigue

         5) Chest pain on exertion

         6) Anxiety

      b. Objective data: Physical findings

         1) Arrhythmias

         2) Irregular heart rate

         3) Tachycardia

         4) Heart murmur

         5) Distended jugular veins

         6) Cyanosis of nails or lips

         7) Pallor

         8) Generalized edema

         9) Diaphoresis

         10) Increased respirations

         11) Moist, frequent cough

         12) Hemoptysis

         13) Crackles at base of lungs

         14) Intrauterine growth restriction

         15) Decreased amniotic fluid

         16) FHR with decreased variability

   4. Laboratory and Diagnostic Testing

      a. Laboratory tests

         1) Hgb

         2) Hct

         3) WBC

         4) Chemistry profile

5) Sedimentation rate
6) Maternal ABGs
7) Clotting studies
    b. Other diagnostic procedures
        1) Echocardiogram
        2) Holter monitoring
        3) Chest x-ray
        4) Ultrasound
        5) Pulse oximetry
        6) NST
        7) Biophysical profile
5. Collaborative Care
    a. **Nursing Interventions**
        1) Monitor for manifestations of fatigue, anemia, weight gain more than 2 lb/week, pulmonary edema, peripheral edema, palpitations, tachycardia, angina.
        2) Prevent infection.
        3) Reinforce teaching (well-balanced diet with iron and folic acid).
    b. **Medications:** Pharmacological management is determined by the client's cardiac diagnoses and clinical presentation.
        1) Propranolol: beta blocker; used to treat tachyarrhythmias and to lower maternal blood pressure
        2) Ampicillin antibiotic; prophylaxis given to prevent endocarditis
        3) Heparin sodium: Anticoagulant used in treating clients who have pulmonary embolus, deep-vein thrombosis, prosthetic valves, cyanotic heart defects, and rheumatic heart disease
        4) Digoxin: Cardiac glycoside; used to increase cardiac output during pregnancy; may be prescribed if fetal tachycardia is present
        5) Anticoagulant therapy (heparin)
            a) Reinforce bleeding precautions.
            b) Report any bleeding.

B. **Hypertension in Pregnancy:** Hypertensive disease in pregnancy is divided into clinical subsets: gestational hypertension; mild and severe preeclampsia; eclampsia; hemolysis, elevated liver enzymes, and low platelets (HELLP) syndrome.

1. **Vasospasm** contributing to poor tissue perfusion is the underlying mechanism for the manifestations of pregnancy hypertensive disorders.

2. **Gestational hypertension (GH)**
    a. Begins after the 20th week of pregnancy.
    b. Presents with elevated blood pressure of 140/90 mm Hg or greater on two occasions, at least 4 hr apart, within 1 week.
    c. There is no proteinuria.
    d. Blood pressure returns to baseline by 6 weeks postpartum.

3. **Mild preeclampsia is GH** with the addition of proteinuria of 1 to 2+.

4. **Severe preeclampsia**
    a. Blood pressure 160/110 mm Hg or greater on two separate occasions 6 hr apart on bed rest
    b. Proteinuria greater than 3+ (dipstick)
    c. Oliguria
    d. Serum creatinine greater than 1.1 mg/dL
    e. Cerebral or visual disturbances (headache, blurred vision)
    f. Hyperreflexia with possible ankle clonus
    g. Pulmonary or cardiac involvement
    h. Extensive peripheral edema
    i. Hepatic dysfunction (elevated liver function tests)
    j. Epigastric and right upper-quadrant pain
    k. Thrombocytopenia

5. **Eclampsia**
    a. Severe preeclampsia plus seizure activity
    b. Usually preceded by persistent headache, blurred vision, severe epigastric or right upper quadrant abdominal pain, and altered mental status

6. **HELLP** syndrome is a variant of GH in which hematologic conditions coexist with severe preeclampsia involving hepatic dysfunction. HELLP syndrome is diagnosed by laboratory tests, not clinically.
    a. **H** – hemolysis resulting in anemia and jaundice
    b. **EL** – elevated liver enzymes resulting in elevated ALT and AST, epigastric pain, nausea, and vomiting
    c. **LP** – low platelets (less than 100,000/mm³), resulting in thrombocytopenia, abnormal bleeding and clotting time, bleeding gums, petechiae, and possible DIC

NOTE: Gestational hypertensive disease and chronic hypertension can occur simultaneously. Gestational hypertensive diseases are associated with placental abruption, acute kidney failure, hepatic rupture, preterm birth, and fetal and maternal death.

7. Contributing Factors
    a. No single profile identifies risks for gestational hypertensive disorders, but some high risks include the following.
        1) Maternal age younger than 20 or older than 40
        2) First pregnancy
        3) Obesity
        4) Multifetal gestation
        5) Chronic kidney disease
        6) Chronic hypertension
        7) Familial history of preeclampsia
        8) Diabetes mellitus
        9) Rh incompatibility
        10) Molar pregnancy
        11) History of GH

8. Manifestations of Preeclampsia (vary depending upon severity)
   a. Hypertension
   b. Proteinuria: 1+ or greater on dipstick, or 300 mg in 24-hr urine specimen
   c. CNS irritability: Headaches, hyperreflexia, positive ankle clonus
   d. Visual disturbances: Scotoma, blurred or double vision
   e. Decreased liver perfusion: Elevated liver enzyme (LDH, AST, ALT), epigastric or right–upper quadrant pain
   f. Decreased renal perfusion: Proteinuria, oliguria
   g. Decreased plasma colloid osmotic pressure: Elevated Hct, tissue edema with weight gain, pulmonary edema
   h. Elevated plasma uric acid

9. Laboratory and Diagnostic Testing
   a. Blood pressure elevation
   b. Urine studies: urinalysis for proteinuria, 24-hr urine protein
   c. Liver enzymes, serum creatinine, BUN, uric acid

10. Collaborative Care
   a. **Nursing Interventions**
      1) Monitor blood pressure.
      2) Administer medications.
      3) Discuss nutrition (balanced diet; 60 to 70 g protein, 1,200 mg calcium, 600 mcg folic acid; limit salty foods; eat foods with roughage; avoid alcohol and tobacco; limit caffeine intake).
      4) Monitor maternal daily weight, I&O, reflexes, and CNS.
      5) Obtain fetal data: Serial ultrasound, Doppler blood flow analysis, NST, CST, BPP, fetal kick count.
      6) Encourage bed rest on left side.
      7) Initiate seizure precautions (preeclampsia, eclampsia).
      8) Provide quiet environment: Private room not next to nurses' station. Dim lights.
      9) Monitor for HELLP and DIC (severe preeclampsia, eclampsia).

NOTE: Immediately after a seizure, the client can be confused and combative. Restraints can be temporarily needed. Do not leave the client alone.

   b. Medications
      1) Antihypertensive medications to keep blood pressure less than 160/110 mm Hg
      2) Magnesium sulfate: Anticonvulsant
         a) Administer IV magnesium sulfate, which is the medication of choice for prophylaxis or treatment; reduces seizure threshold (depression of the CNS). Secondary side effect is decreased blood pressure as it relaxes smooth muscles.
         b) **Nursing Interventions**
            (1) Use an infusion control device to maintain a regular flow rate.
            (2) The client might initially feel flushed, hot, and sedated with the magnesium sulfate bolus. Nausea/vomiting can occur.
            (3) Monitor vital signs (blood pressure, pulse, respirations), CNS, level of consciousness, headache or visual disturbances, reflexes, renal perfusion, output of indwelling urinary catheter, epigastric pain, and FHR.
            (4) Place the client on fluid restriction of 100 to 125 mL/hr, and maintain a urinary output of 30 mL/hr or greater.
            (5) Monitor for signs of magnesium sulfate toxicity.
               (a) Absence of patellar deep tendon reflexes
               (b) Urine output less than 30 mL/hr
               (c) Respirations less than 12/min
               (d) Decreased level of consciousness
               (e) Cardiac dysrhythmias

NOTE: If magnesium toxicity is suspected, discontinue magnesium infusion immediately. Administer calcium gluconate and notify the provider. Take actions to prevent respiratory or cardiac arrest.

C. **Diabetes Mellitus**
   1. Types
      a. Pregestational diabetes mellitus: Client had diabetes prior to pregnancy.
      b. Gestational diabetes mellitus: An impaired tolerance to glucose with the first onset or recognition during pregnancy. The ideal blood glucose level during pregnancy is 70 to 110 mg/dL. Client develops diabetes mellitus during pregnancy, usually in the second or third trimester.
   2. Contributing Factors
      a. Obesity
      b. Maternal age older than 25 years
      c. Family history of diabetes mellitus
      d. Previous delivery of an infant who was large or stillborn
   3. Manifestations
      a. Hypoglycemia (nervousness, headache, weakness, irritability, hunger, blurred vision, tingling of mouth or extremities)
      b. Hyperglycemia (thirst, nausea, abdominal pain, frequent urination, flushed dry skin, fruity breath)

4. Laboratory Testing and Diagnostic Procedures
   a. Routine urinalysis with glycosuria
   b. Glucose tolerance test (50 g oral glucose load, followed by plasma glucose analysis 1 hr later performed at 24 to 28 weeks of gestation—fasting not necessary; a positive blood glucose screening is 140 mg/dL or greater; additional testing with a 3-hr glucose tolerance test is indicated)
      1) 3-hr glucose tolerance test (following overnight fasting, avoidance of caffeine, and abstinence from smoking for 12 hr prior to testing; fasting glucose is obtained; 100 g glucose load is given; serum glucose levels are determined at 1, 2, and 3 hr following glucose ingestion)
   c. Monitor HbA1c.
   d. Monitor for ketones.
   e. BPP to ascertain fetal well-being
   f. Amniocentesis with alpha-fetoprotein
   g. NST to determine fetal well-being
5. Collaborative Care
   a. Risks to newborn increase with poor glucose control.
      1) Congenital anomalies
      2) Spontaneous abortions
      3) Macrosomia: Birth trauma and dystocia
      4) Death
      5) Hypoglycemia after birth
   b. **Nursing Interventions**
      1) Diet
      2) Exercise
      3) Blood glucose monitoring
      4) Insulin if medication required
   c. Medications
      1) Oral hypoglycemic, such as glyburide, is occasionally used for gestational diabetes.
         a) Can require insulin.
         b) Insulin needs decrease during the first trimester.
         c) Insulin needs increase during the second and third trimester due to an increase in hormones.
D. **Hyperemesis Gravidarum:** Excessive pregnancy-related nausea and/or vomiting. Hospitalization can be necessary due to dehydration and weight loss.
   1. Begins first or second month of pregnancy
   2. Contributing Factors
      a. High levels of human chorionic gonadotropin (hCG) and estrogen
   3. Decreased gastric motility and gastroesophageal reflux
   4. Manifestations
      a. Loss of 5% or more of prepregnancy body weight
      b. Dehydration, causing ketosis and constipation
      c. Nutritional deficiencies
      d. Metabolic imbalances

5. Collaborative Care
   a. **Nursing Interventions**
      1) Monitor psyche; refer as needed.
      2) Monitor weight.
      3) Monitor for dehydration, electrolyte imbalance, and metabolic alkalosis.
      4) Monitor I&O.
      5) Administer IV fluids.
      6) Small meals per client preference.
   b. Medications
      1) Antiemetics such as ondansetron
      2) Vitamin B$_6$, no more than 100 mg daily used solo or in combination with doxylamine
   c. Therapeutic Measures
      1) Acupressure; relaxation techniques
   d. Client Education
      1) Nausea and vomiting usually peak between 2 and 12 weeks of pregnancy and go away by the second half of pregnancy.
      2) **Eat small, frequent meals**; eating dry foods such as crackers can help relieve uncomplicated nausea.
      3) Increase fluid intake to prevent dehydration. Increase fluids during the times of the day when the client feels the least nauseated. Seltzer, ginger ale, or other sparkling waters can be helpful.

II Placental and Cervical Problems

A. **Abruptio Placentae**
   1. Contributing Factors
      a. Trauma
      b. Preeclampsia
      c. Multiparity
      d. Cocaine use
B. **Placenta Previa**
   1. Contributing Factors
      a. Placenta implants completely or partially over cervical os.

PLACENTA PREVIA AND ABRUPTIO PLACENTAE

	PLACENTA PREVIA	ABRUPTIO PLACENTAE
Vaginal bleeding	Usually bright red in color. Can range from minimal to severe and life-threatening	Usually dark red Can range from absent to moderate dependent on the grade of abruption
Pain	Often none	Abdomen "boardlike" and very tender
Maternal effect	Hemorrhage, shock, death	
Fetal effect	Anoxia, CNS trauma, death	
Treatment	Partial previa might be treated with bed rest. Complete previa will be treated as with abruptio placentae.	Emotional support Immediate cesarean birth Blood transfusions Monitor for DIC.

NOTE: Vaginal exams are contraindicated with vaginal bleeding.

C. **Hydatidiform Mole/Molar Pregnancy:** Benign abnormal growth of chorionic villi. Appears as avascular transparent grapelike clusters. Can develop choriocarcinoma (rare).

1. Contributing Factors

   a. Previous use of ovulation-stimulating drugs

   b. Age extremes: Early teens or over 40

   c. History of spontaneous abortion

   d. Poor nutrition

   e. Often unknown

2. Manifestations

   a. Vaginal bleeding; brown, grapelike clusters; anemia

   b. Rapid uterine growth (increase in fundal height); cramping

   c. Extreme nausea

   d. Hyperthyroidism

   e. Preeclampsia prior to 24 weeks

3. Diagnostic Testing

   a. Ultrasound

   b. Persistent high hCG levels

4. Collaborative Care

   a. Monitor psyche.

   b. Spontaneous expulsion

   c. Elective expulsion

      1) Curettage

      2) Induction not recommended

      3) Rho(D) immune globulin postexpulsion if Rh-negative

      4) Postexpulsion

         a) Follow postpartum protocol.

         b) Continue to monitor hCG levels.

         c) Follow up to rule out choriocarcinoma.

         d) Discuss contraception. Clients should avoid pregnancy for 1 year or until hCG levels return to normal.

D. **Abortion:** Expulsion of the fetus prior to viability

1. Types

   a. Spontaneous

   b. Therapeutic

   c. Elective

2. Collaborative Care

   a. Provide psychological support.

   b. Assist with ultrasound.

   c. Save all passed tissue for examination.

   d. Monitor for signs of hemorrhage. (Perform pad count. Monitor Hgb and Hct.)

   e. Monitor for signs of shock.

   f. Prepare for D&C.

   g. Administer Rho(D) immune globulin to clients who are Rh-negative.

3. Discharge Teaching

   a. Notify provider if signs of infection occur, bleeding increases, or signs of depression develop.

   b. Discuss future pregnancy plans and birth control.

   c. Provide follow-up exam.

E. **Cervical Insufficiency (Incompetent Cervix):** Premature dilation of the cervix, usually in second trimester

1. Contributing Factors

   a. Congenital

   b. Acquired

      1) History of cervical trauma

      2) Previous spontaneous delivery in second trimester

2. Manifestations

   a. Increase in pelvic pressure

   b. Pink-stained vaginal discharge or bleeding

   c. Uterine contractions

3. Diagnostic and therapeutic procedures

   a. Ultrasound showing short cervix (less than 25 mm long)

   b. Prophylactic cervical cerclage; removed at 36 to 37 weeks

4. Collaborative Care

   a. Emotional support

   b. If able to maintain pregnancy

      1) Bed rest

      2) Monitoring of client and fetus

      3) Tocolytics

      4) Hydration

      5) Cerclage (purse string suture)

F. **Ectopic Pregnancy:** Fertilized ovum implants outside of uterus (pelvis, abdomen, often fallopian tubes)

1. Contributing Factors

   a. Narrowing or scarring of fallopian tube: previous STI or PID; IUD; endometriosis; tubal surgery

2. Manifestations

   a. Delayed or missed irregular menses

   b. Unilateral stabbing pain and tenderness in lower abdomen

   c. Bleeding

   d. Shock (symptoms: hypotension, tachycardia, pallor).

3. Collaborative Care

   a. Provide psychological support.

   b. Replace fluids.

   c. Administer methotrexate (MTX).

   d. Prepare for surgery and postoperative care.

Labor and Delivery

Labor and Delivery

Labor and delivery include the period during which the neonate and placenta are delivered and up to 1 to 2 hr after delivery.

A. **Labor and Delivery Processes**—Six major factors (P's)

1. **Psyche**—The mother's psychological response to labor

2. **Powers**—Uterine contractions

   a. Uterine contractions: Act to dilate and efface the cervix

      1) Frequency—from the beginning of one contraction to the beginning of the next contraction. Contraction frequency less than 2 min is hyperstimulation.

      2) Duration—from the beginning to end of the same contraction. Contraction duration greater than 90 seconds is hyperstimulation.

      3) Intensity—strength of the uterine contraction. Can only be accurately measured with an internal uterine pressure catheter (IUPC).

   b. Effacement—shortening and thinning of the cervix. The goal is 100% effacement.

   c. Dilation—opening of the cervix. The diameter of the cervix ranges from 0 cm (closed) to 10 cm (fully dilated).

3. **Passenger**—the fetus and placenta

4. **Presentation**—the part of the fetus that enters the pelvic inlet first

   a. The three primary presentations are cephalic, breech, and shoulder. Breech and shoulder presentations are indications for cesarean birth.

   b. Station—the relationship of the presenting part to the maternal ischial spines that measures the degree of descent of the fetus

      1) Negative stations are above ischial spines (−1, −2).

      2) Zero station is at the ischial spines, or engaged (0).

      3) Positive stations are below the ischial spines (+1, +2, +3). Delivery is typically sooner.

5. **Position**—relationship of presenting part (occiput, mentum, sacrum) to the maternal pelvic inlet. Clients with fetus in persistent occiput posterior position (POP) have increase back (labor) pain and longer labors.

6. **Passageway**—birth canal, pelvis, cervix, pelvic floor and vagina

   a. Cephalopelvic disproportion—When the fetus has a head size, shape, or position that does not allow for passage through the pelvis. This can also occur secondary to maternal pelvic structure or associated problems.

B. **Manifestations of False vs. True Labor**

FALSE VS. TRUE LABOR

FALSE LABOR	TRUE LABOR
Uterine contractions	
Braxton Hicks: Irregular, do not increase in frequency or intensity	Can begin irregularly but become regular in frequency, become stronger and last longer.
Usually felt in the lower back or the abdomen above the umbilicus	Walking can increase contraction intensity.
Decrease with walking or position changes	Contractions continue despite comfort measures.
Often cease with sleep, comfort measures, oral hydration, and emptying of bladder	Usually felt in the lower back radiating to the abdomen.
Cervical dilation and effacement	
No significant change in dilation or effacement.	Cervical dilation and effacement steadily progress.
Cervix often stays in posterior position.	
Bloody show	
Usually not present	Present as cervix dilates
Fetus	
Presenting part not engaged in pelvis	Presenting part engages in pelvis

C. **Nursing Care During Labor and Delivery**

1. Admission data collection includes prenatal and medical and surgical history.

2. Obtain informed consent.

3. Review birth plan.

4. Active labor is considered an emergency medical condition by the Emergency Medical Treatment and Active Labor Act (EMTALA).

5. Monitor maternal and fetal status.

   a. Vital signs and physical data collection

   b. FHR

      1) Normal rate is 110 to 160/min; varies with fetal age

      2) Variability best indicator of fetal well-being. Moderate = 6 to 25/min

      3) External: Auscultation, ultrasound transducer

      4) Internal: Spiral electrode

         a) Requires ruptured membranes

NOTE: Any internal monitoring increases the risk of infection.

   c. Uterine contractions

      1) External: Manual or tocotransducer

      2) Internal: IUPC

   d. Vaginal discharge

   e. Cervix

      1) Cervical exams are done with sterile gloves.

      2) Limit exams, especially if a vaginal infection is suspected or if ROM has occurred.

NOTE: Try to limit the frequency of vaginal exams secondary to the risk of infection.

NURSING CARE: STAGES OF LABOR

First Stage

Cervix dilates from 0 to 10 cm.

Three phases

> Latent Phase: 0 to 3 cm
  » Contractions:
    > Irregular, mild to moderate
    > Frequency 5 to 30 min
    > Duration 30 to 45 seconds
  » Client talkative and excited
> Active Phase: 4 to 7 cm
  » Contractions
    > Regular, moderate to strong
    > Frequency 3 to 5 min
    > Duration 40 to 70 seconds
  » Client anxious and in pain
> Transitional phase: 8 to 10 cm
  » Contractions
    > Regular, very strong
    > Frequency 2 to 3 min
    > Duration 45 to 90 seconds
  » Client can have nausea/vomiting and can become irritable.

NURSING INTERVENTIONS

Admission data collection. Review birth plan; determine pain goals. In all stages, include maternal/fetal data collection, fluid intake, frequent urination.

Monitor amniotic fluid status. Nitrazine is paper used for suspected ROM. It will turn blue in the presence of alkaline amniotic fluid (pH 6.5 to 7.5).

Continue monitoring maternal and fetal status. Assist with nonpharmacological pain management. Provide analgesia if requested.

Second Stage

Pushing stage. From complete dilation through delivery of baby.

NURSING INTERVENTIONS

Monitor FHR at least every 15 min.

Assist with pushing, breathing (prevent hyperventilation), and comfort.

Record delivery time, medications, and episiotomy/laceration.

Third Stage

After delivery of baby until delivery of placenta. Contractions are usually mild. Client is usually focused on the baby.

NURSING INTERVENTIONS

Monitor vital signs, bleeding, and fundus.

Provide immediate care of newborn: ABC, Apgar score, warm environment, safety measures, infection control.

Fourth Stage

1 to 2 hr after delivery of the placenta.

NURSING INTERVENTIONS

Encourage breastfeeding and promote bonding.

Monitor vital signs, fundus, and lochia every 15 min x 4; every 30 min x 2; and in 60 min.

Hemorrhage is priority concern.

D. **Fetal Data Collection During Labor**

1. Indications for monitoring of FHR
   a. On admission and regular intervals as indicated by hospital protocol
   b. Before and after any procedure (medication, anesthesia, ROM, vaginal exam, ambulation)
   c. Throughout labor (in cases of high-risk pregnancy, use of oxytocic agents, fetal distress)
2. Interpretation of Findings
   a. FHR Classification System
      1) Category I tracings are normal (reassuring).
      2) Category III tracings are abnormal and associated with fetal hypoxemia.

THREE-TIER FHR CLASSIFICATION SYSTEM

Category I (normal)

Baseline FHR of 110 to 160/min

Baseline FHR variability: moderate heart rate fluctuations (6 to 25/min)

Accelerations: Present or absent

Early decelerations: Present or absent

Variable or late decelerations: Absent

Category II

All FHR tracings not categorized as Category I or III

Category III (abnormal)

Sinusoidal pattern

Absent baseline FHR variability and any of the following
> Recurrent variable decelerations
> Recurrent late decelerations
> Bradycardia

   b. Periodic FHR changes
      1) Accelerations (reassuring) 15/min change lasting 15 seconds (term fetus)
      2) Decelerations: Early, late, variable

PERIODIC FHR CHANGES

Name: VEAL	Cause: CHOP	Management: MINE
Variable	Cord compression	Move client
Early	Head compression	Identify labor progress
Acceleration	Other (okay)	No action needed
Late	Placental insufficiency	Execute actions immediately

EARLY DECELERATION

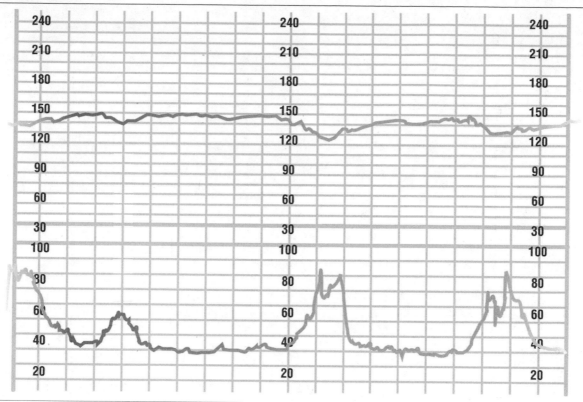

VARIABLE DECELERATION

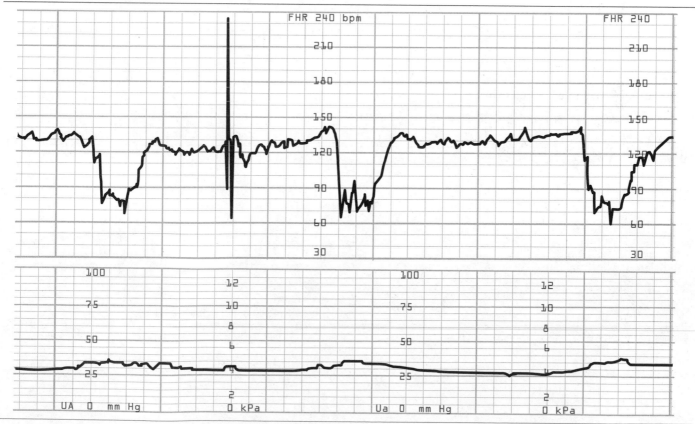

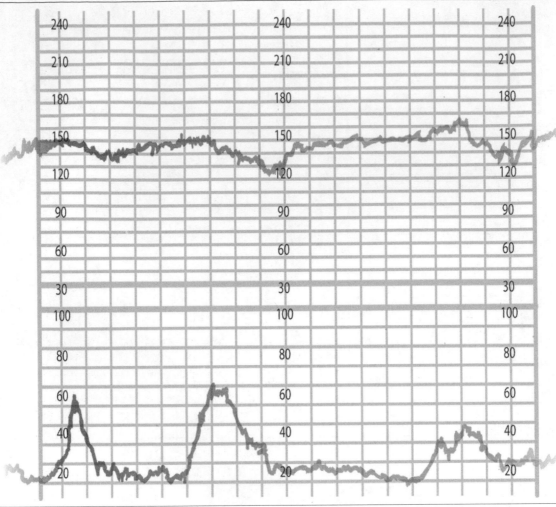

E. **Medications used in labor and delivery**

MEDICATIONS USED IN LABOR AND DELIVERY

MEDICATION	USE	NURSING INTERVENTIONS
Oxytocin	Stimulate uterine contractions May be used in all stages of labor	Monitor contractions and FHR. Monitor vital signs. Administer by IV infusion pump through secondary line. Stop immediately for late decelerations or tachysystole (hyperstimulation). Have tocolytic (such as terbutaline) immediately available for tachysystole.
Methylergonovine maleate	Stimulate uterine contractions after delivery Treat postpartum hemorrhage	Monitor bleeding and uterine tone. Obtain baseline blood pressure. Massage fundus. Administer 0.2 mg IM or PO as prescribed.
Calcium gluconate	Antidote for magnesium sulfate toxicity	Administer calcium gluconate 1 g (10 mL 10% solution) IV for signs of toxicity. Dilute with equal amounts of NS and administer 0.5 to 1 mL/min.

MEDICATION	USE	NURSING INTERVENTIONS
Terbutaline, ritodrine HCl	Tocolytic used for preterm labor	Monitor contractions and FHR. Monitor vital signs. Administer terbutaline subcutaneous 0.25 mg every 20 min as needed. Monitor for adverse effects: Tremors, dizziness, headache, tachycardia, hypotension, anxiety. Do not administer if client reports chest pain. Notify provider for blood pressure less than 90/60 mm Hg, pulse rate greater than 130/min, signs of pulmonary edema, or FHR greater than 180/min. Administer beta blocking agent as antidote.
Indomethacin	May be used as tocolytic for preterm labor	Monitor contractions and FHR. Monitor vital signs (can mask maternal fever). Administer with food to decrease side effect of GI distress. Only administer if gestational age is less than 32 weeks.
Magnesium sulfate	Tocolytic used for preterm labor CNS depressant to prevent seizure in preeclampsia	Preterm Labor > Monitor contractions and FHR. > Monitor fetal movement and FHR variability. > Monitor vital signs and urine output. Preeclampsia > Monitor vital signs, urine output, DTRs, and LOC. > Monitor magnesium levels (therapeutic range 4 to 8 mg/dL). > Administer via infusion pump in diluted form. > Use indwelling catheter to monitor urinary elimination. > Stop immediately for respirations less than 12/min, altered LOC, magnesium levels greater than 10 mEq/L or 9 mg/dL. > Administer calcium gluconate 1 g (10 mL of 10% solution) for signs of toxicity. > Observe neonate for signs of respiratory depression, hypotonia, lethargy, and hypocalcemia. > Contraindicated for clients who have myasthenia gravis.
Naloxone HCl	Antidote for opioid induced respiratory depression Reverse pruritus from epidural opioid	Monitor respiratory effort. Do not administer if mother has opioid dependency. Newborn: Administer 0.1 mg/kg IV, IM, SQ, or ET tube. Adult: Administer 0.4 to 2 mg IV. Can repeat IV at 2 to 3 min intervals up to 10 mg. Can also administer IM or SQ.
Betamethasone	Preterm labor (24 to 32 weeks) > Prevent or reduce neonatal respiratory distress syndrome in preterm infants > Stimulate production or release of lung surfactant in preterm fetus	Monitor for signs of preterm labor. Administer 12 mg deep IM for two doses 24 hr apart. Monitor blood glucose levels and lung sounds.
Misoprostol, dinoprostone	Preinduction cervical ripening (Bishop score 4 or less)	Obtain informed consent. Monitor contractions and FHR. Monitor vital signs. Evaluate Bishop score. Use cautiously in clients who have a history of asthma; glaucoma; or renal, hepatic, or cardiovascular disorders. Contraindicated in presence of fetal distress or vaginal bleeding.

LABOR AND DELIVERY MEDICATIONS WORKSHEET

Match the medication in the first column with the related information in second column.

____ 1. oxytocin
____ 2. misoprostol
____ 3. penicillin G
____ 4. methylergonovine
____ 5. terbutaline sulfate
____ 6. betamethasone
____ 7. methotrexate
____ 8. indomethacin

A. Contracts the uterus after delivery. Used to treat postpartum hemorrhage. Need baseline blood pressure before administering.
B. Induces labor or contracts the uterus after delivery. Stop immediately in the presence of late decelerations.
C. Stimulates fetal lung maturation between 24 to 32 weeks gestation.
D. Softens and thins the cervix.
E. Prostaglandin synthetase inhibitor. Can be used as tocolytic in preterm labor.
F. Used during labor when client is positive for group B Strep.
G. May be used with ectopic pregnancy to stop the growth of the embryo to save the tube.
H. Beta adrenergic agonist. Last resort for preterm labor. Call provider for heart rate greater than 130/min.

Answer key: 1. B; 2. D; 3. F; 4. A; 5. H; 6. C; 7. G; 8. E

F. **Pain Management in Labor and Delivery**

1. Nonpharmacological pain management

   a. Childbirth preparation methods (Lamaze, Bradley, Dick-Read, pattern breathing methods) are used to promote relaxation and pain relief.

   b. Sensory stimulation strategies (based on the gate-control theory) to promote relaxation and pain relief
      1) Aromatherapy
      2) Breathing relaxation techniques
      3) Visual imagery and use of focal points
      4) Music

   c. Cutaneous strategies (based on the gate-control theory) to promote relaxation and pain relief
      1) Back rubs, massage, counterpressure
      2) Effleurage: Light, gentle, circular stroking of the abdomen with fingertips
      3) Acupressure and acupuncture
      4) Water therapy

   d. Frequent maternal position changes
      1) Semi-sitting
      2) Squatting
      3) Kneeling
      4) Rocking
      5) Supine (must have wedge under one hip to tilt the uterus to avoid supine hypotension syndrome)

2. Pharmacological pain management: Analgesia and anesthesia

   a. When given early in labor, can slow or stop labor.

   b. Opioid analgesics given late in labor can cause newborn respiratory depression.

   c. Butorphanol tartrate and nalbuphine HCl should not be given to clients who have opioid dependency.

   d. Fentanyl citrate and sufentanil citrate have a short duration of action. Commonly administered with epidural and intrathecal anesthesia.

   e. Naloxone should be available as an antidote. Do not give to a client or newborn if the client is opioid-dependent.

   f. **Regional blocks** are most commonly used. They include pudendal, epidural, and intrathecal blocks.

   g. **Pudendal block** provides local anesthesia to the perineum, vulva, and rectal areas during delivery. It is administered 10 to 20 min before delivery.

   h. **Epidural block** consists of a local anesthetic along with an analgesic morphine or fentanyl injected into the epidural space at the level of the fourth or fifth lumbar vertebra. Continuous infusion or intermittent injections can be administered through an indwelling epidural catheter. Client-controlled epidural analgesia is a favored method of acute pain relief management for labor and birth. Hypotension is the most common adverse effect.

      1) **Nursing Interventions**
         a) Client should receive 1 L IV fluid bolus before epidural anesthesia.
         b) Monitor platelet count prior to initiation of epidural.
         c) Assist in sitting or side-lying position.
         d) Monitor blood pressure frequently.
         e) Monitor for bladder distention.
         f) Continue to monitor level of pain.
         g) Assist client to turn side to side every hour.
         h) Promote safety.
         i) Keep catheter insertion site clean and dry.
         j) Monitor return of sensation in legs.
         k) Assist with standing and walking first time after sensation returns.

      2) Contraindications to subarachnoid and epidural blocks.
         a) Maternal hypotension
         b) Coagulopathy (receiving anticoagulant therapy; history of bleeding disorder)
         c) Infection at injection site
         d) Increased intracranial pressure
         e) Maternal inability to cooperate

G. **Therapeutic Procedures to Assist with Labor and Delivery**

1. **Amniotomy:** The artificial rupture of the amniotic membranes (AROM) to initiate or improve contractions. Labor typically begins within 12 hr after the membranes rupture. The client is at an increased risk for cord prolapse or infection.

   a. **Nursing Interventions**

      1) Record baseline FHR prior to, continuously during, and after the procedure.

      2) Observe for changes in FHR: Bradycardia, variable decelerations, or late decelerations (cord compression or prolapse).

      3) Monitor the amount, color, consistency, and odor of amniotic fluid.

      4) Implement comfort measures (perineal care, clean pads).

      5) Monitor temperature every 2 hr.

2. **Amnioinfusion:** Intrauterine infusion of an isotonic solution (0.9% sodium chloride or lactated Ringer's) to reduce severity of variable decelerations caused by cord compression.

   a. **Nursing Interventions**

      1) Explain the procedure to the client.

      2) Assist with the amniotomy and insertion of IUPC if not already present.

      3) Warm fluid using a blood warmer prior to infusion.

      4) Maintain comfort and dryness of the client.

         a) Monitor the client continuously to prevent uterine overdistention and increased uterine tone.

         b) Continually monitor intensity and frequency of uterine contractions.

         c) Continually monitor FHR.

3. **Induction/Augmentation of Labor:** The process of chemically or mechanically initiating or strengthening uterine contractions

   a. Indications

      1) Maternal issues: History of rapid labors, preeclampsia, diabetes mellitus, severe Rh isoimmunization, chronic kidney disease, pulmonary disease

      2) Fetal/placental issues: IUGR, PROM, chorioamnionitis, postdates, fetal demise

      3) Inadequate uterine contractions (oxytocin used to augment labor)

   b. Contraindications for induction of labor

      1) Cephalopelvic disproportion (CPD)

      2) Nonreassuring FHR

      3) Placenta previa or vasa previa

      4) Prior classical uterine incision or uterine surgery

      5) Active genital herpes

      6) HIV

      7) Cervical cancer

   c. Medications

      1) Chemical methods used to soften cervix

         a) Prostaglandin E2 (placed transvaginally near cervix). Client must remain supine with wedge or in side-lying position for 30 min after insertion of gel. Delay pitocin use for 6 to 12 hr after last gel insertion.

         b) Prostaglandin E1 administered intravaginally or PO tabs.

      2) Medication used to initiate induction

         a) IV oxytocin

      3) **Nursing Interventions**

         a) Obtain informed consent. Monitor FHR and uterine activity every 15 min and with every change in dose.

         b) Observe for and report uterine tachysystole (more than 5 contractions in 10 min) or fetal distress.

         c) Obtain vital signs every 30 min and with every oxytocin change in dose.

         d) Administer pain management.

         e) Prior to administration of oxytocin vaginal exam performed for effacement, dilation, and station. (Fetus must be engaged at 0 station.)

         f) Oxytocin should be connected piggyback to the main IV line at closest infusion port to the client.

         g) Discontinue oxytocin with signs of fetal distress or uterine tachysystole (hyperstimulation).

            (1) Contraction frequency more often than one every 2 min or 5 in 10 minutes

            (2) Contraction duration longer than 90 seconds

            (3) Contraction intensity greater than 90 mm Hg with IUPC

            (4) No relaxation of uterus between contractions

            (5) Prepare to administer terbutaline 0.25 mg subcutaneously, to decrease uterine activity.

4. **Vacuum Assisted Delivery:** Attachment of a vacuum cup to the fetal head to assist in birth of the head

   a. Indications

      1) Maternal exhaustion and ineffective pushing

      2) Fetal distress during second stage of labor

   b. **Nursing Interventions**

      1) Place in lithotomy position and support with pushing.

      2) Monitor and record FHR before and during vacuum application.

      3) Check for bladder distention before application.

      4) Document number of pulls, pressure, and pop offs.

      5) Observe neonate for bruising and caput succedaneum.

      6) Inform parents caput can resolve within 24 hr or could last up to 5 days.

5. **Forceps**: Obstetric instrument used to aid in delivery of the fetal head
   a. Indications
      1) Poor progress during second stage
      2) Fetal distress
      3) Persistent occiput posterior position
      4) Abnormal presentation
   b. **Nursing Interventions**
      1) Monitor the neonate for intracranial hemorrhage, facial bruising, and facial palsy.
      2) Check FHR before traction is applied.
   c. Complications
      1) Lacerations to cervix or vagina
      2) Bladder or urethral injury
      3) Urine retention resulting from bladder or urethral injuries
      4) Hematoma formation in the pelvic soft tissues

6. **Episiotomy:** An incision that is made into the perineum to enlarge the vaginal outlet during delivery
   a. **Nursing Interventions**
      1) Monitor for pain, healing, infection, laceration of the anal sphincter (fourth-degree tear), and hemorrhage.
      2) Encourage Kegel exercises to improve and restore perineal muscle tone.
      3) Apply ice packs.
      4) Reinforce education on perineal care and to use sitz baths.

7. **Cesarean Birth:** Birth of fetus through a transabdominal incision of the uterus
   a. Types
      1) Low transverse: decrease chance of uterine rupture with future pregnancies; less bleeding after delivery
      2) Classic: rarely used
   b. Indications
      1) Previous cesarean birth
      2) Failure to progress in labor
      3) Fetal factors: Malpresentation, fetal distress, cephalopelvic disproportion, multiple fetuses, macrosomia, prolapsed cord
      4) Maternal factors: Positive HIV, active genital herpes, complete placenta previa or abruption
   c. **Nursing Interventions**
      1) Obtain informed consent.
      2) Perform preoperative data collection and surgical checklist.
      3) Administer preoperative medications.
      4) Insert IV and Foley catheter.
      5) Perform postoperative and postpartum data collection.
      6) Monitor for bleeding at site and lochia.
      7) Obtain routine postoperative vital signs.
      8) Monitor effects of anesthesia.
      9) Monitor need for pain management.
      10) Monitor for thrombophlebitis.

NCLEX ALERT: LABOR AND DELIVERY

1. It is never good to be late. (Late decelerations are bad.)
2. Absent variability (a straight line) for FHR is critical.
3. Never place a laboring client flat on her back (supine hypotension/vena cava syndrome).
4. Unexplained pain in a labor and delivery client is not good (preterm labor, abruptio placentae, amniotic fluid embolism, uterine rupture).
5. Never provide fundal pressure with shoulder dystocia (suprapubic pressure okay, also assist with McRoberts maneuver).
6. OB client with tachycardia: Think hemorrhage first.
7. Medications for postpartum hemorrhage include oxytocin, methylergonovine, and carboprost tromethamine.
8. Quick onset of epigastric pain is often the aura to seizure activity (implement safety precautions).
9. Oxygen administration should be at 8 to 10 L/min via nonrebreather face mask.
10. Nonpharmacological measures should be used in combination with pharmacological interventions.

SECTION 5

Complications During Labor and Delivery

A. **Preterm Labor:** Uterine contractions with cervical changes that occur between 20 and 37 weeks of gestation
   1. Contributing Factors
      a. Demographic factors
         1) Age younger than 15 and older than 35
         2) Low socioeconomic status
      b. Biophysical factors
         1) Previous preterm labor or birth
         2) Multifetal pregnancy
         3) Second trimester bleeding
         4) Infection
      c. Behavioral factors
         1) Lack of prenatal care
         2) Poor nutrition
         3) Substance use disorder
   2. **Nursing Interventions**
      a. Obtain vaginal swab for fetal fibronectin testing.
      b. Assist with collection of cervical cultures.
      c. Activity restriction (bed rest with bathroom privileges, left lateral position).
      d. Ensure hydration.
      e. Monitor for signs of infection: UTI, vaginal drainage including odor.
      f. Monitor maternal vital signs including temperature.
      g. Monitor FHR and contraction pattern.
      h. Administer tocolytic medications and betamethasone.

B. **Fetal Distress**

1. FHR baseline less than 110/min or greater than 160/min
2. Absent FHR variability
3. Category III FHR pattern (See the table on the FHR Classification System in this unit.)
4. Fetal blood pH less than 7.2
5. Contributing Factors
   a. Uteroplacental insufficiency
      1) Acute uteroplacental insufficiency
         a) Excessive uterine activity associated with use of oxytocin
         b) Maternal hypotension: Epidural, vena caval compression, supine position, hemorrhage
         c) Placental separation: Abruptio, placentae previa
      2) Chronic uteroplacental insufficiency
         a) Gestational hypertension
         b) Chronic hypertension
         c) Tobacco or illicit drug use
         d) Diabetes mellitus
         e) Postmaturity
6. **Nursing Interventions**
   a. Stop oxytocin.
   b. Administer oxygen at 8 to 10 L/min by nonrebreather face mask.
   c. Reposition the client.
   d. Increase IV fluids.
   e. Notify the provider.
   f. Perform fetal scalp stimulation or vibroacoustic stimulation per protocol.

C. **Umbilical Cord Problems**

1. Contributing Factors
   a. Cord compression: Pressure on the umbilical cord during pregnancy, labor, or delivery that reduces blood flow from the placenta to the fetus
      1) Causes: Abnormal presentation, inadequate pelvis, presenting part at high station, multiple gestations, prematurity, premature rupture of membranes, polyhydramnios
      2) Complications: Fetal asphyxia
   b. Nuchal cord (cord around neck)
   c. Prolapsed cord
2. **Nursing Interventions**
   a. Prolapsed cord
      1) Call for assistance immediately.
      2) Notify the provider.
      3) Using a sterile-gloved hand, insert two fingers into the vagina, and apply finger pressure on either side of the cord to the fetal presenting part to elevate it off of the cord.
      4) Reposition the client in a knee-chest or Trendelenburg position.
      5) Administer oxygen at 8 to 10 L/min by nonrebreather face mask.

      6) If the cord is protruding from the vagina, wrap it loosely in a sterile saline-soaked towel.
      7) Closely monitor FHR for variable decelerations and bradycardia.
      8) Prepare for immediate birth: Vaginal or cesarean.
   b. Cord compression
      1) Position change is priority.
      2) Administer oxygen at 8 to 10 L/min by nonrebreather face mask.
      3) Prepare to assist with amnioinfusion.

D. **Emergency Childbirth**

1. Contributing Factors
   a. Precipitous delivery
2. **Nursing Interventions**
   a. Encourage the mother to pant, unless the fetus is in breech presentation.
   b. Support the perineum.
   c. Rupture the membranes if they have not yet ruptured.
   d. Feel for the cord around the neonate's neck, and gently slip it over his head.
   e. Keep the neonate dry and warm.
   f. Do not cut the cord.
   g. Deliver the placenta. Expect a gush of blood and a lengthening of the cord.
   h. Save the placenta.
   i. Massage the fundus. Encourage breastfeeding to contract the uterus.

E. **Amniotic Fluid Emboli** (Anaphylactoid Syndrome of Pregnancy)

1. Rupture in the amniotic sac or maternal uterine veins accompanied by a high intrauterine pressure
2. Amniotic fluid enters maternal circulation and travels to and obstructs pulmonary vessels, which causes respiratory distress and circulatory collapse.
3. Manifestations
   a. Respiratory distress (restlessness, cyanosis, dyspnea, pulmonary edema, respiratory arrest)
   b. Circulatory collapse (tachycardia, hypotension, shock, cardiac arrest)
   c. Hemorrhage (bleeding from incisions and venipuncture sites, petechiae, ecchymosis, uterine atony)
   d. Seizure activity
4. **Nursing Interventions**
   a. Administer 10 L oxygen via face mask.
   b. Prepare client for intubation.
   c. Initiate or assist with CPR.
   d. Administer IV fluids.
   e. Administer blood or blood products.
   f. Prepare for an emergency birth.
   g. Prepare for an emergency cesarean birth if fetus is not yet delivered.

F. **Dystocia: Dysfunctional, Abnormal labor**
1. Contributing Factors
   a. Dysfunction of uterine contractions
   b. Abnormal position
   c. Fetopelvic disproportion
   d. Maternal exhaustion
   e. Macrosomia
2. **Nursing Interventions**
   a. Monitor fetus and status of labor.
   b. Encourage the client to void and ambulate regularly.
   c. Assist in positioning and coaching during contractions.
   d. Prepare for a possible forceps, vacuum-assisted, or cesarean birth.
   e. Shoulder dystocia: McRoberts maneuver and suprapubic pressure (not fundal pressure).

NCLEX ALERT: STANDARDS OF CARE FOR THE OBSTETRIC CLIENT

1. Never perform a vaginal exam in the presence of unexplained vaginal bleeding.
2. Establish IV access if client has excessive bleeding.
3. Rho(D) immune globulin is given to Rh-negative clients after a miscarriage, at 28 weeks gestation, and within 72 hr after delivery if newborn is Rh positive and rho(D) immune globulin is indicated.
4. Clients who are unstable should be assigned rooms close to the nurses' station.

SECTION 6

Postpartum

I **Postpartum/Puerperium**
A. **Approximate duration:** 6 weeks
B. **Main goal:** Prevent postpartum hemorrhage
C. **Greatest risks:** Hemorrhage, shock, and infection
D. **Includes physiological and psychological adjustments**
E. **Changes after delivery of the placenta:** Hormones (estrogen, progesterone, and placental enzyme insulinase [HCS]) decrease causing decreased blood glucose (HCS), diaphoresis and diuresis (estrogen). Oxytocin increases (contractions, breast milk, involution).
F. **Physical Data Collection**
1. Vital signs, Hgb, Hct, CBC, estimated blood loss in delivery
2. Pain
   a. Monitor location and intensity of pain.
   b. Examine location of pain.
   c. Implement nonpharmaceutical measures.
   d. Implement pharmaceutical measures.
      1) Consider safety of medications related to breastfeeding.
         a) Hydrocodone/acetaminophen
         b) Ibuprofen
         c) PCA (morphine sulfate, fentanyl)

3. Breasts
   a. Colostrum
      1) Transitions to milk 48 to 96 hr
      2) High nutrition
   b. Milk production occurs about day 2 or 3
      1) Sucking stimulates uterine contractions, promotes uterine involution, and increases milk production.
      2) Supplementing with formula can decrease production.
      3) Breast milk actively supports the immune system. It protects against many bacterial, viral, and protozoal infections. IgA is major immunoglobulin in human milk that provides passive immunity.
   c. Engorgement
      1) About 48 hr postpartum
      2) Can cause slight rise in temperature
      3) Client is not breastfeeding
         a) Avoid nipple stimulation.
         b) Cold compress
         c) Pain medication
         d) Supportive bra
      4) Client is breastfeeding
         a) Manually express some milk to facilitate latch.
         b) Frequent feeding or pumping
         c) Warm shower
         d) Breast massage
         e) Supportive bra
         f) Administer maternal medications immediately after breastfeeding to minimize crossover to breast milk.

NOTE: For engorgement, breastfeed every 2 to 3 hr. Encourage a warm shower immediately prior to breastfeeding. Immediately after and between feedings, apply cold compresses or ice-cold green cabbage leaves to breasts.

NOTE: Know the differences between mastitis and engorgement.

4. Uterus
   a. Involution
      1) Firm
      2) Fundus near umbilicus after delivery
      3) Descends approximately 1 cm/day
      4) Breastfeeding enhances
      5) Full bladder impedes involution
   b. Subinvolution
      1) Massage
      2) Frequent voiding
      3) Oxytocin

c. Lochia: Note color, amount (scant to moderate), presence of clots, and odor (fleshy).

   1) Color

      a) Rubra—bright red, can contain small clots. Transient flow increases during breastfeeding and upon rising. Lasts 1 to 3 days.

      b) Serosa—brownish red or pink. Lasts from day 4 to day 10.

      c) Alba—yellowish-white creamy color. Lasts from day 11 up to and beyond 6 weeks postpartum.

d. Reinforce teaching about return of menses.

   1) Ovulation can occur prior to first menses.

   2) Nonlactating client: 6 to 8 weeks

   3) Breastfeeding exclusively: can be up to 6 months

   4) Need for birth control

5. Perineum

   a. Monitor perineum using REEDA.

      1) **R**—Redness

      2) **E**—Edema

      3) **E**—Ecchymosis

      4) **D**—Drainage

      5) **A**—Approximation

   b. Comfort and healing

      1) Cold compress first 24 hr

      2) Sitz bath

      3) Positioning

      4) Perineal hygiene

      5) Kegel exercises

      6) Medication

NOTE: Saturation of one perineal pad in 15 min or less, numerous large clots, and pooling of blood under the buttocks are indicators of excessive blood loss.

6. Bladder

   a. Potential problem due to effects of anesthesia and hormones

      1) Distended bladder increases potential for uterine atony and bleeding. Fundus will deviate to the side and above the umbilicus.

      2) Assist with frequent urination.

      3) Provide noninvasive measures to promote urination.

      4) Perform bladder scan.

      5) Catheterize if retention persists.

7. Bowel

   a. Bowel movement in 1 to 2 days.

   b. Monitor for hemorrhoids.

      1) Promote fiber, activity, and fluids.

      2) Administer stool softener.

      3) Provide sitz bath.

      4) Apply topical anesthetic.

8. Edema and DTRs

   a. Monitor for pitting edema.

   b. Excessive use of oxytocin increases risk for edema.

   c. 2+ DTRs is normal.

9. Deep-vein thrombosis

   a. Prevention is key. Encourage early ambulation.

   b. Monitor for pain, redness, or swelling of lower extremities.

10. Infection

   a. Temperature is normally elevated to 38° C (100.4° F) first 24 hr after delivery.

   b. WBCs can be elevated to 20,000 to 25,000/mm³ the first 10 to 14 days.

   c. Do not assume "normal."

   d. Monitor possible sources of infection.

G. **Psychological Adaptations**

   1. Support systems

   2. Self-concept

   3. Bonding

      a. Initial contact within 60 min after birth

      b. Client exploration of infant

         1) Fingertips, then palms

         2) Extremities, then trunk

         3) En face position

      c. Collaborative Care

         1) Minimize pain, fatigue, and hunger to enhance bonding.

         2) Describe newborn behaviors.

   4. Maternal Role Adaptation

PHASES OF MATERNAL ADJUSTMENT

	CHARACTERISTICS	COLLABORATIVE CARE
Taking in	24 to 48 hr after birth: dependent, passive, focuses on own needs, excited, talkative	Assist with care. Provide comfort, nutrition, and hygiene. Listen. Review labor and delivery.
Taking hold	Second to tenth day postpartum, or up to several weeks: focuses on maternal role and care of newborn; eager to learn; can develop postpartum blues	Reinforce teaching. Provide written material, follow-up appointments, and community resources. Monitor emotional status. Discuss postpartum blues.
Letting go	Focuses on family and individual roles	Monitor progress. Discuss community resources.

5. Postpartum blues and depression

POSTPARTUM BLUES AND DEPRESSION

	Postpartum Blues	Postpartum Depression
CONTRIBUTING FACTORS	Fatigue, hormonal changes, role change, family tension, finances	History of depression*; low socioeconomic status; unwanted pregnancy; lack support systems; newborn health problems
OCCURRENCE	50% to 60% of postpartum clients	10% to 15% of postpartum clients
ONSET	1 to 10 days postpartum	1 year or more after delivery
SIGNS/ SYMPTOMS	Emotionally labile	Persistent depression; feeling overwhelmed, anxious, hopeless; inability to care for self and/or infant; thoughts of suicide
COLLABORATIVE CARE	Reinforce teaching. > Need for sleep, exercise, adequate nutrition > Seek support and assistance with newborn care > Community resources.	Use depression screening tools. Reinforce teaching. > Recognize manifestations. > Seek assistance. > Needs rapid intervention

*Note: Medications used to treat depression, such as SSRIs, are frequently Category C or D drugs and might be discontinued during pregnancy. A nurse ensures that the medications are resumed as needed after delivery.

H. **Provide focused data collection:** BUBBLE HERV

1. **B**—Breasts
2. **U**—Uterus (fundal height, uterine placement, and consistency)
3. **B**—Bowel and GI function
4. **B**—Bladder function
5. **L**—Lochia (color, odor, consistency, and amount [COCA])
6. **E**—Episiotomy (redness, edema, ecchymosis, drainage, approximation [REEDA])
7. **H**—Hemorrhoids
8. **E**—Emotions
9. **R**—Rubella (prevent pregnancy at least 1 month after receiving), rho(D) immune globulin
10. **V**—Vaccines (influenza, pneumonia, Tdap [needed only once as adult to prevent pertussis; not given if received tetanus–diphtheria vaccine within 2 years])

NOTE: Clients who receive rubella immunization should prevent pregnancy for 1 month. Clients who receive both Rho(D) immune globulin and rubella vaccine should have a titer drawn at 3 months to verify immunity.

Complications During Postpartum

A. **Hemorrhage:** Blood loss greater than 500 mL with vaginal delivery or greater than 1,000 mL with cesarean birth
   1. Contributing Factors
      a. Uterine atony
      b. Lacerations and hematomas
      c. Complications during pregnancy (placenta previa, abruptio placentae)
      d. Complications during labor (prolonged labor, rapid labor, administration of magnesium sulfate, use of forceps, retained placenta)
      e. Overdistended uterus (macrosomia, multiple fetuses)
      f. Coagulopathies (DIC)
   2. Manifestations
      a. Saturation of one or more pads in 15 min
      b. Large clots (uterine atony) or spurting of bright red blood (cervical or vaginal laceration)
      c. Formation of hematomas
      d. Boggy uterus (uterine atony)
      e. Persistent lochia rubra beyond day 3 (retained placental fragments)
      f. Change in level of consciousness
      g. Manifestations of shock
   3. **Nursing Interventions**
      a. Identify source of bleeding.
         1) Fundus: Massage if boggy.
         2) Perineum: Notify provider for laceration, episiotomy site, or hematomas.
      b. Monitor vital signs and oxygen saturation.
      c. Monitor bladder.
      d. Maintain isotonic IV fluids.
      e. Administer oxytocin.
      f. Administer other medications as needed (methylergonovine, misoprostol, carboprost tromethamine).

B. **Rh Incompatibility**

RHO(D) IMMUNE GLOBULIN

MOTHER	NEONATE	MATERNAL COOMBS'	GIVEN?
Rh⁺	Rh⁺	Not checked	No
Rh⁺	Rh⁻	Not checked	No
Rh⁻	Rh⁺	Negative	Yes
Rh⁻	Rh⁺	Positive	No
Rh⁻	Rh⁻	Not checked	No

   1. **Nursing Interventions**
      a. Observe newborn for hyperbilirubinemia.
      b. Reinforce teaching about Rh, Rho(D) immune globulin.
         1) Prevents (does not reverse) formation of antibodies
         2) Given prenatally with any invasive procedure at 28 weeks and after delivery
      c. Administer Rho(D) immune globulin.
         1) IM
         2) Given within 72 hr after delivery

C. **Thromboembolic Disorder**

1. Contributing Factors
   a. Venous stasis and hypercoagulation
   b. Immobility
   c. Pelvic pressure during labor/delivery
   d. History of thrombosis, varicosities, heart disease
2. Manifestations
   a. Pain, heat, redness, swelling in lower leg or extremity
3. **Nursing Interventions**
   a. Monitor extremities (peripheral pulses; measuring and comparing circumferences of both legs).
   b. Homan's sign is not recommended.
   c. Venous Doppler to rule out DVTs. If DVT is suspected:
      1) Bed rest and analgesia
      2) Elevation of affected extremity
      3) Antithrombotic stockings
      4) Anticoagulant therapy
D. **Puerperal Infections** (endometritis, mastitis, wound infections)
   1. Elevated temperature of at least 38° C (100.4° F) for 2 or more consecutive days, excluding the first 24 hr.
   2. Endometritis usually begins on the second to 5th day postpartum.
      a. More common after cesarean birth.
      b. Pelvic pain, uterine tenderness, foul smelling or profuse lochia; plus fever, tachycardia, and elevated WBC and RBC sedimentation rate.
   3. Mastitis is usually unilateral, occurring 2 to 4 weeks after delivery.
      a. Symptoms include chills, fever, malaise, and local breast tenderness and erythema.

SECTION 8

Newborn

I **Neonatal Period: From Birth Through 28 Days**

A. **Initial Care:** Immediately after birth
   1. Airway, Breathing, Circulation (ABCs)
   2. Thermoregulation
   3. Umbilical cord
      a. Inspect for two arteries and one vein. Observe for any bleeding from the cord, and ensure that the cord is clamped securely to prevent hemorrhage.

4. Apgar
   a. Collect data at 1 and 5 min.

APGAR: FIVE CATEGORIES

	0	1	2
Heart rate	Absent	Less than 100/min	Greater than 100/min
Respiratory effort	Absent	Slow, weak cry	Good cry
Muscle tone	Flaccid	Some flexion of extremities	Well-flexed extremities
Reflex irritability	No response	Grimace	Cry
Color	Blue, pale	Centrally pink with blue extremities	Completely pink

   b. Ratings
      1) 7 to 10 is within normal limits
      2) 4 to 6 is moderately distressed
      3) 0 to 3 is severely distressed
   5. Vital signs

VITAL SIGN DATA COLLECTION

Heart Rate

NORMAL FINDINGS	100 to 160/min
NORMAL VARIATIONS	100/min when sleeping 180/min when crying
DEVIATIONS FROM NORMAL	Persistent tachycardia 160/min or greater Persistent bradycardia 100/min or less
NURSING INTERVENTIONS	Monitor all pulses bilaterally. They should be equal and strong. Monitor apical pulse for 1 min. Monitor for murmurs.

Respirations

NORMAL FINDINGS	40 to 60/min
DEVIATIONS FROM NORMAL	Bradypnea: less than 25/min Tachypnea: greater than 60/min
NURSING INTERVENTIONS	Monitor rate, rhythm, and adventitious breath sounds. Respirations will often be shallow and irregular in the newborn. Note any signs of distress (nasal flaring, grunting, intercostal retractions, see-saw breathing).

Temperature

NORMAL FINDINGS	Axillary 37° C (98.6° F)
NORMAL VARIATIONS	36.5 to 37.2° C (97.7 to 98.9° F) axillary
DEVIATIONS FROM NORMAL	Temperature not stabilized after 10 hr
NURSING INTERVENTIONS	Prevent heat loss. (Dry infant thoroughly. Cover head. Place in warm, dry environment. Encourage skin to skin contact with mother.)

VITAL SIGN DATA COLLECTION (CONTINUED)

Blood Pressure

NORMAL FINDINGS	60 to 80 systolic; 40 to 50 diastolic
NORMAL VARIATIONS	Variations occur with crying or sleeping.
DEVIATIONS FROM NORMAL	**Hypotension** = potential sepsis or hypovolemic **Hypertension** in upper extremities = potential coarctation of aorta
🩺 NURSING INTERVENTIONS	Monitor in all four extremities on admission to nursery if problem suspected. Check arm and leg for significant differences between the lower and upper extremities (can be an indication of coarctation of the aorta).

NOTE: Rectal temperatures are contraindicated.

6. Safety
   a. Footprints and identification bands are applied in the presence of the parents and before the infant leaves delivery room. Security system is explained and initiated.
B. **Ongoing Newborn Care:** Admission to Discharge
   1. Physical Data Collection

PHYSICAL DATA COLLECTION

	FINDINGS
Posture	General flexion Spontaneous movement
Head	Circumference 2 to 3 cm greater than chest circumference Fontanels Posterior: Triangle shape, closes at 8 to 12 weeks Anterior: Diamond shape, closes at 18 months, pulse visible Observe for bulge or depression Shape Molding Caput succedaneum Cephalohematoma
Eyes	Vision best within 12 inches Strabismus; pseudostrabismus Subconjunctival hemorrhage Congenital cataracts
Ears	Responds to voice and other sounds Check for low-set ears.
Nose	Patent nares Preferential nose breather

PHYSICAL DATA COLLECTION (CONTINUED)

	FINDINGS
Skin	Pink Acrocyanosis Erythema Jaundice Hyperpigmentation Milia Café au lait spots (giraffe spots) Nevus flammeus (port-wine stains) Telangiectatic nevi (stork bites) Vernix Lanugo
Mouth	Symmetry of lip movement Soft/hard palate intact Epstein pearls
Chest	Symmetrical chest movement Nipples prominent, well formed Nipple buds are sign of maturity
Abdomen	Umbilical cord Liver might be palpable
Musculoskeletal	Evaluate joints for full range of motion Note presence of asymmetrical gluteal folds Spine straight and easily flexed Clavicles intact
Genitalia	Female: prominent labia, pseudomenstruation Male: scrotum large, palpable testes on each side, meatus at tip of penis, foreskin
GI/GU	Voiding within 24 hr Void 6 to 10 times a day after 4 days of life Meconium passed 24 to 48 hr after birth Breastfed babies have more frequent stools that appear yellow and seedy.

REFLEXES

	EXPECTED FINDING	EXPECTED AGE
Sucking and rooting	Elicited by stroking the newborn's cheek or edge of their mouth. Normal response: Newborn turns head toward the side that is touched and starts to suck.	Birth to 4 months
Palmar grasp	Elicited by placing an object in the newborn's palm. Normal response: Newborn grasps the object.	Present at birth and until 3 to 6 months
Plantar grasp	Elicited by touching the sole of the newborn's foot. Normal response: Newborn curls toes downward.	Birth to 8 months
Moro reflex (startle)	Elicited by striking a flat surface that the newborn is lying on, or allowing the head and trunk of the newborn in a semisitting position to fall backward to an angle of at least 30°. Normal response: Newborn's arms and legs extend and abduct symmetrically; fingers form a "C."	Birth to 4 months

	EXPECTED FINDING	EXPECTED AGE	
Tonic neck reflex (fencer position)	The newborn extends the arm and leg on the side when the head is turned to that side with flexion of the arm and leg of the opposite side.	Birth to 3 to 4 months	
Babinski	Elicited by stroking outer edge of sole of foot toward toes. Normal response: Toes fan upward and out.	Birth to 1 year	

2. Reactivity
   a. Observe for periods of reactivity in the newborn.
      1) **First period of reactivity:** The newborn is alert and exhibits exploring activity, makes sucking sounds, and has a rapid heartbeat and respiratory rate. Lasts 15 to 30 min after birth.
      2) **Period of relative inactivity:** Sleep. Heart rate and respirations decrease. Lasts from 30 min to 2 hr after birth.
      3) **Second period of reactivity:** Reawakens. Often gags and chokes on mucus that has accumulated in their mouth. This period usually occurs 2 to 8 hr after birth but can last 10 min to several hours.

C. **Gestational Age Data Collection:** New Ballard Score
   1. Provides maturity rating. Performed within 48 hr after birth.
   2. Components of Gestational Age Data Collection
      a. Physical Components
         1) Skin
         2) Lanugo
         3) Plantar surfaces
         4) Breasts
         5) Eyes/ears
         6) Genitals
      b. Neuromuscular
         1) Posture
         2) Square window
         3) Arm recoil
         4) Popliteal angle
         5) Scarf sign
         6) Heel to ear
   3. Medications
      a. Eye prophylaxis
         1) Erythromycin or tetracycline administered within 1 hr after birth.
      b. Vitamin K IM administered within 1 hr of birth.
      c. Hepatitis vaccine administered within 12 hr of birth
   4. Diagnostic and Therapeutic Procedures
      a. Cord blood: ABO blood type and Rh-status if the mother's blood type is O or she is Rh-negative.
      b. CBC (anemia, polycythemia, infection, clotting problems)
      c. Glucose level
      d. Serum bilirubin
      e. Newborn metabolic screen
      f. PKU
      g. Newborn hearing screen
      h. Pulse oximetry

5. Collaborative Care
   a. **Nursing Interventions**
      1) Monitor for signs and symptoms of respiratory distress.
      2) Promote patent airway.
         a) Perform oral and nasal suction only if needed.

NOTE: When using bulb syringe, remember M before N.

NOTE: Newborns delivered by cesarean birth are more susceptible to fluid remaining in the lungs than newborns who were delivered vaginally.

      3) Promote thermoregulation.
         a) Maintain body temperature of 36.5°C (97.7°F) axillary.
         b) Prevent heat loss.
      4) Monitor glucose levels.

NOTE: Identify potential risks and prevent heat loss by evaporation, conduction, convection, or radiation.

   b. Monitor nutrition.
      1) Initiate feedings immediately after birth (breast milk or formula).
         a) Maintain a fluid intake of 100 to 140 mL/kg/24 hr.
         b) Monitor for normal weight gain. (Both breast milk and formula provide 20 kcal/oz.)
   c. **Nursing Interventions** to promote successful breastfeeding
      1) Explain breastfeeding techniques to the mother. Have the mother wash her hands, get comfortable, and have fluids to drink during breastfeeding.
      2) Offer the newborn the breast immediately after birth and feed every 2 to 3 hr.
      3) Explain the let-down reflex (stimulation of maternal nipple releases oxytocin that causes the letdown of milk).
      4) Reassure the mother that uterine cramps are normal during breastfeeding, resulting from oxytocin.
      5) Express a few drops of colostrum or milk and spread it over the nipple to lubricate the nipple and entice the newborn.
      6) Show the mother the proper latch-on position.
   d. Formula-feeding
      1) Feed every 3 to 4 hr.
      2) **Nursing Interventions** to promote successful formula feeding
         a) Always hold the bottle. Never prop it.
         b) Avoid supine position during feeding (danger of aspiration).
         c) Hold newborn close and at 45° angle during feeding.
         d) Reinforce teaching with parents about how to prepare formula, bottles, and nipples.

e) Check the flow of formula from the bottle to ensure it is not coming out too slowly or quickly.

f) Place the nipple on top of the newborn's tongue.

g) Keep the nipple filled with formula to prevent the newborn from swallowing air.

h) Burp the newborn several times during a feeding, usually after each ½ to 1 oz of formula.

i) Discard unused formula when the newborn is finished feeding and after open for 1 hr due to an increased possibility of bacterial contamination.

e. Monitor elimination.

1) Document number of voidings and stools.

2) Keep the perineal area clean and dry. Should have first void and stool within 24 hr.

f. Provide skin care.

1) Cord care: Cleanse with neutral-pH cleanser and sterile water. The cord should be kept clean and dry to prevent infection.

NOTE: The Association of Women's Health, Obstetric and Neonatal Nurses (2013) recommendations for cord care include cleaning the cord with water (using cleanser sparingly if needed to remove debris) during the initial bath of the newborn.

2) First bath after temperature stabilizes

NOTE: When handling the newborn, providers should wear gloves until after the first bath.

g. Promote bonding.

1) Encourage mothers and family members to hold the newborn.

h. Promote safety and security for the newborn and family.

1) Verify that identification bands are correctly placed according to facility protocol.

2) Follow identity verification protocol each time the newborn is taken to a parent.

3) All facility staff who assist in caring for the newborn are required to wear identification badges.

i. Provide circumcision care.

1) Before the procedure, identify any family history of bleeding tendencies; hypospadias; epispadias; ambiguous genitalia; illness; or infection.

2) Obtain informed consent.

3) Monitor for complications: bleeding or swelling with urine retention.

4) Reinforce teaching with parents to change diapers at least every 4 hr. Clean the penis with warm water. With clamp procedures, apply petroleum jelly with each diaper change for at least 24 hr. Expect a yellowish mucus over the glans by day 2; do not wash it off. Avoid premoistened towelettes (which contain alcohol) to clean the penis, which heals within 2 weeks.

6. Client Education

a. Safety

1) Position on back to sleep

2) Thermoregulation

3) Nutrition and weight gain (healthy newborn needs 100 to 140 mL/kg/24 hr; no water supplement; loss of 5% to 10% immediately after birth is normal, to be regained in 10 to 14 days)

4) Elimination (voiding 6 to 8 diapers a day)

5) Avoid submerging in water until cord falls off (around 10 to 14 days after birth)

6) CPR

7) Newborn behaviors

8) Car seat regulations

9) Oral and nasal suctioning

10) Sudden infant death syndrome (no exposure to secondhand smoke)

11) Signs of illness to report

12) Newborn follow-up care and immunization schedule

13) Crib safety: Space between mattress and sides of crib should be less than 2 fingerbreadths; slats on crib should be no more than 2.5 inches apart.

Q&A

1. What would be included in discharge teaching about bathing a newborn?

2. Identify priority nursing interventions following circumcision.

Answer Key: 1. Should be performed before feeding. Use mild soap without hexachlorophene; no lotions, oils, or powders. No tub bath until cord falls off and is healed. 2. Observe the newborn for bleeding. Check site every 15 min for 1 hr and then every hour for at least 12 hr. Also check for voiding and swelling.

SECTION 9

Complications of the Newborn

It is essential for a nurse to immediately identify complications and implement appropriate interventions.

A. **Maternal Substance Use**

1. General Information

a. Intrauterine alcohol and drug exposure can cause anomalies, neurobehavioral changes, and signs of withdrawal in the neonate.

b. Response is dependent on specific drug, dose, metabolism and excretion by the mother and fetus, timing of exposure, and length of exposure.

2. Fetal alcohol syndrome (FAS)

a. Contributing Factors

1) Amount and duration of consumption (chronic or periodic intake)

2) Daily intake increases the risk of FAS

b. Manifestations (will have signs in three categories)

1) Growth restriction

2) CNS alterations (intelligence deficit, attention deficit disorder, diminished fine motor skills, poor speech)

3) Craniofacial features (microcephaly, small eyes or short palpebral fissures, thin upper lip, flat midface)

4) Other signs

a) Feeding problems

b) Increased wakefulness

c) Hearing loss

3. Tobacco use during pregnancy

a. Manifestations

1) Prematurity, low birth weight

2) Increased risk for sudden infant death syndrome

3) Increased risk for asthma, pneumonia

4) Developmental delays

4. Drug and alcohol withdrawal syndrome in the newborn

a. Objective data: Use a neonatal abstinence scoring system.

1) CNS

a) Increased wakefulness

b) High-pitched, shrill cry; incessant crying

c) Irritability, tremors

d) Hyperactive with an increased Moro reflex. Heroin withdrawal causes decreased Moro reflexes and hypothermia or hyperthermia.

e) Increased deep-tendon reflexes, increased muscle tone

f) Seizures

2) Skin

a) Abrasions and/or excoriations on the face and knees

3) Metabolic, vasomotor, and respiratory findings

a) Nasal congestion with flaring

b) Frequent yawning, skin mottling

c) Tachypnea greater than 60/min

d) Sweating and a temperature greater than 37.2°C (99°F)

4) Gastrointestinal

a) Poor feeding, regurgitation (projectile vomiting)

b) Diarrhea

c) Excessive, uncoordinated, constant sucking

5) Vital organ anomalies

a) Heart defects (atrial and ventricular septal defects, tetralogy of Fallot, patent ductus arteriosus)

b. Medications

1) Phenobarbital: anticonvulsant

a) It is prescribed to decrease CNS irritability and control seizures for neonates who have alcohol or opioid use disorder.

c. Diagnostic Procedures

1) Laboratory tests: Blood tests should be done to differentiate between neonatal drug withdrawal and central nervous system irritability.

a) CBC

b) Blood glucose

c) Calcium and magnesium

d) TSH, T_4, T_3

e) Drug screen of urine or meconium to reveal the agent used

f) Hair analysis

2) Diagnostic Procedures

a) Chest x-ray to rule out congenital heart defects

d. Collaborative Care

1) **Nursing Interventions** include normal newborn care plus the following.

a) Perform a neonatal abstinence scoring system assessment.

b) Monitor newborn reflexes.

c) Monitor ability to feed and digest intake.

d) Monitor fluid and electrolytes, skin turgor, fontanels, and I&O.

e) Observe behavior (crying, sleep patterns, tremors).

f) Maintain IV.

g) Reduce external stimuli (swaddle; do not place next to nurses' desk).

h) Small, frequent feedings with high-calorie formula (can need gavage feedings).

i) If sucking is a problem, use preterm nipples and nipples with larger holes.

j) Have suction immediately available (risk for aspiration).

k) For newborns who are addicted to cocaine, avoid eye contact and use vertical rocking and a pacifier.

l) Initiate a consult with Child Protective Services.

m) Consult lactation services to evaluate if breastfeeding is desired and not contraindicated.

B. **Hypoglycemia:** A serum glucose level of less than 40 mg/dL

1. Contributing Factors

a. Maternal diabetes mellitus

b. Preterm infant

c. LGA or SGA

d. Stress at birth (cold stress, asphyxia)

2. Manifestations

a. Objective data: physical findings

1) Poor feeding

2) Jitteriness/tremors

3) Hypothermia

4) Diaphoresis

5) Weak cry

6) Lethargy

7) Flaccid muscle tone

8) Seizures/coma

3. Diagnostic Laboratory Tests and Procedures

   a. Two consecutive plasma glucose levels less than 40 mg/dL in a newborn who is term; less than 25 mg/dL in a newborn who is preterm

4. Collaborative Care

   a. **Nursing Interventions**

     1) Perform heel stick for blood glucose within 2 hr of birth.

     2) Provide frequent oral or gavage feedings.

     3) Monitor the neonate's blood glucose level closely per facility protocol.

     4) Monitor IV if the neonate is unable to orally feed.

C. **Respiratory Distress Syndrome (RDS)**

1. RDS occurs as a result of surfactant deficiency in the lungs and is characterized by poor gas exchange and ventilatory failure.

2. Surfactant is a phospholipid that assists in alveoli expansion.

3. Surfactant keeps alveoli from collapsing and allows gas exchange to occur.

4. Contributing Factors

   a. Preterm gestation

   b. Perinatal asphyxia (meconium staining, cord prolapse, nuchal cord)

   c. Stress/asphyxia during labor (maternal hypotension, UPI)

5. Manifestations: Physical Data Collection

   a. Objective data

     1) Tachypnea (respiratory rate greater than 60/min)

     2) Nasal flaring

     3) Expiratory grunting

     4) Intercostal and substernal retractions

     5) Labored breathing

     6) Fine rales on auscultation

     7) Cyanosis

     8) Unresponsiveness, flaccidity, and apnea with decreased breath sounds (manifestations of worsened RDS)

6. Diagnostic Procedures and Laboratory Tests

   a. Culture and sensitivity of the blood, urine, and cerebrospinal fluid (rule out sepsis)

   b. Blood glucose and serum calcium

   c. ABGs reveal hypercapnia (excess of carbon dioxide in the blood) and respiratory or mixed acidosis.

   d. Chest x-ray

7. **Nursing Interventions**

   a. Administer lung surfactant (beractant for preterm infant).

   b. Avoid suctioning ET tube for 1 hr after administration of medication.

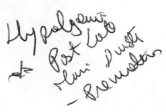

D. **Preterm Newborn:** Birth occurs after 20 weeks and before 38 weeks gestation.

1. Contributing Factors

   a. Maternal gestational hypertension

   b. Multiple pregnancies

   c. Adolescent pregnancy

   d. Lack of prenatal care

   e. Substance use disorder

   f. Smoking

   g. Previous history of preterm delivery

   h. Abnormalities of the uterus or cervix

   i. Premature rupture of the membranes

2. Manifestations: Physical Data Collection

   a. Objective data

     1) New Ballard assessment shows a physical and neurological assessment totaling less than 37 weeks of gestation.

     2) Episodes of apnea.

     3) Signs of increased respiratory effort or respiratory distress.

     4) Physical characteristics: Typically has low birth weight; minimal subcutaneous fat; head large in comparison to body; wrinkled features; weak grasp reflex; before 34 weeks has inability to coordinate suck and swallow; and weak or absent gag, suck, and cough reflex.

3. **Nursing Interventions**

   a. Perform rapid initial assessment.

   b. Transfer to high-risk nursery.

   c. Maintain thermoregulation.

   d. Administer respiratory support.

   e. Administer parenteral or enteral nutrition and fluids (less than 34 weeks).

   f. Provide nonnutritive sucking.

   g. Minimize stimulation (cluster care, smooth and light touch, dim lighting, noise reduction).

E. **Postterm Infant**

1. Contributing Factors

   a. Gestational age more than 42 weeks

2. Manifestations: Physical Data Collection

   a. Dry, parchment-like skin

   b. Longer, harder nails

   c. Profuse scalp hair

   d. Absent vernix

   e. Hypoglycemia

3. Complications

   a. Progressive aging of placenta

   b. Difficult delivery

   c. High perinatal mortality

   d. Jaundice (hyperbilirubinemia)

4. **Nursing Interventions**

   a. Early and frequent heel sticks (glucose testing)

   b. Initiate early feeding

   c. Observe for birth injuries (from shoulder dystocia—fractured clavicle, brachial plexus injury, facial paralysis)

F. **Hyperbilirubinemia**

1. Physiologic Jaundice (benign)

   a. Caused by breakdown of fetal RBCs, excessive bruising, and liver immaturity.

   b. Jaundice appears after 24 hr of age.

2. Pathologic Jaundice (underlying disease; increased RBC production or breakdown)

   a. Appears before 24 hr of age or is persistent after day 7.

   b. Usually caused by blood group incompatibility (Rh- or ABO incompatibility) or an infection.

   c. Kernicterus (bilirubin encephalopathy): Bilirubin levels at or higher than 25 mg/dL. Can lead to anemia and brain damage.

3. Manifestations

   a. Yellowish tint to skin, sclera, and mucous membranes.

   b. Jaundice is identified best by blanching skin on the cheek or sternum.

   c. Note time of onset to distinguish between physiologic and pathologic jaundice.

   d. Identify the underlying cause by reviewing the maternal prenatal, family, and newborn history.

4. Diagnostic and Laboratory Procedures

   a. Monitor the infant's bilirubin levels every 4 hr until the level returns to normal.

   b. Identify maternal and newborn blood type to determine if there is a presence of ABO-incapability. This occurs if the newborn has blood type A, B, or AB, and the mother is type O.

   c. Review Hgb and Hct.

   d. A direct Coombs' test reveals the presence of antibody-coated (sensitized) Rh-positive RBCs in the newborn.

   e. Monitor electrolyte levels for indications of dehydration during phototherapy.

   f. Transcutaneous level is a noninvasive method to measure an infant's bilirubin.

5. **Nursing Interventions**

   a. Phototherapy, sunlight, or exchange transfusion is administered to the newborn.

   b. Monitor vital signs.

   c. Maintain an eye mask over the newborn's eyes for protection of corneas and retinas.

   d. Keep newborn undressed. Cover male genitalia to prevent testicular damage from heat and light waves.

   e. Avoid applying lotions or ointments to the infant because they absorb heat and can cause burns.

   f. Remove the newborn from phototherapy every 4 hr and unmask the newborn's eyes, checking for signs of inflammation or injury.

   g. Reposition the newborn every 2 hr to expose all of the body surfaces to the phototherapy lights and prevent pressure sores. Check the lamp energy with a photometer per unit protocol.

   h. Turn off the phototherapy lights before drawing blood for testing.

   i. Observe the newborn for side effects of phototherapy.

      1) Bronze discoloration: not a serious complication

      2) Maculopapular skin rash: not a serious complication

      3) Development of pressure areas

      4) Dehydration (symptoms: poor skin turgor, dry mucous membranes, decreased urinary output)

      5) Elevated temperature

   j. Monitor elimination and daily weights, watching for signs of dehydration.

   k. Monitor the newborn's axillary temperature every 4 hr during phototherapy because temperature can become elevated.

   l. Feed the newborn early and frequently—every 3 to 4 hr to promote bilirubin excretion in the stools.

   m. Continue to breastfeed the newborn. Supplementing with formula can be prescribed.

   n. Maintain adequate fluid intake to prevent dehydration.

   o. Reassure parents that most newborns experience some degree of jaundice.

   p. Explain hyperbilirubinemia, its causes, diagnostic tests, and treatment to parents.

   q. Explain that the newborn's stool contains some bile that will be loose and green.

   r. Administer an exchange transfusion for infants who are at risk for kernicterus.

SECTION 10

Women's Health

A. **Contraception:** Methods of contraception include natural family planning, barrier, hormonal, and intrauterine methods, as well as surgical procedures.

1. Monitor the client's need/desire for contraception.

2. Thoroughly discuss benefits, risks, and alternatives of each method.

3. Support clients in making the decision that is best for their individualized situations.

4. Refer to contraception methods table in Unit Four: Pharmacology in Nursing.

B. **Infertility:** Inability to conceive despite engaging in unprotected sexual intercourse for at least 12 months

1. Contributing Factors

   a. Structural or hormonal disorders (tubal occlusion, endometriosis, obesity)

   b. Decreased or abnormal sperm

   c. STIs (See the table on sexually transmitted infections in this unit.)

   d. Exposure to radiation or toxic substances

2. Diagnostic Procedures
   a. Infertility procedures
      1) Semen collection
      2) Pelvic examination
      3) Ultrasonography
      4) Hysterosalpingography
      5) Hysteroscopy
      6) Laparoscopy
3. Collaborative Care
   a. Perform infertility data collection.
   b. **Nursing Interventions**
      1) Encourage couples to express and discuss their feelings.
      2) Monitor for adverse effects associated with medications to treat female and male infertility.
      3) Advise that the use of medications to treat female infertility can increase the risk of multiple births by more than 25%.
      4) Provide information regarding assisted reproductive therapies.
   c. Referrals to support groups
      1) Genetic counseling

C. **Vaginal Infections**
1. Normal vaginal secretions are clear to cloudy, nonirritating, and nonoffensive in odor, with pH of 4 to 5.
2. Most common vaginal infections: Bacterial vaginosis (BV), candidiasis, trichomoniasis
3. Most common causes: Irritations (bath salts or bubble bath), tight-fitting clothing (especially jeans), or anything that disrupts the normal vaginal flora (douching, sexual activity, contamination by feces)
4. Reinforce preventive measures. (Perform genital hygiene. Avoid douching. Use condoms. Void before and after intercourse. Decrease dietary sugar. Drink yeast-active milk. Eat yogurt with lactobacilli.)
   a. If at risk for STIs, clients should not use an IUD or diaphragm for contraception.
5. Bacterial vaginosis: Etiology unknown. Associated with preterm labor and birth.
   a. Manifestations
      1) Increased thin vaginal discharge and fishy odor.
   b. **Collaborative Care and Nursing Interventions**
      1) Administer metronidazole.
      2) Treatment of partner is not routinely recommended.
6. *Vulvovaginal candidiasis* (yeast infection): Most common organism is *Candida albicans*
   a. Contributing Factors
      1) Use of oral contraceptives, frequent use of antibiotics, frequent douching, diabetes mellitus, immunosuppression
      2) Ensure that both partners are treated.
   b. Manifestations
      1) Yellow or gray discharge
      2) Discomfort with urination and intercourse
      3) Irritation and itching
7. Sexually transmitted infections (See the table on sexually transmitted infections in this unit.)

D. **Cancer**
1. **Cervical Cancer:** Forms in the tissue of the cervix
   a. Contributing Factors
      1) Human papillomavirus is responsible for most cervical cancer
      2) Multiple partners with initial sex before age 18
      3) History of STIs
      4) Immunosuppression
      5) Cigarette smoking
   b. Manifestations
      1) Abnormal bleeding
      2) Pelvic pain or pain during intercourse
   c. Diagnostic Screening
      1) Pap test
      2) HPV, DNA test
   d. Collaborative Care/Treatment
      1) Conization, laser surgery, loop electrocautery excision procedure, cryosurgery, hysterectomy, radiation, and/or chemotherapy
      2) Prevention
         a) Delay initial intercourse.
         b) Avoid smoking.
         c) Practice safe sex.
         d) The human papillomavirus quadrivalent vaccine is given as three injections over 6 months. Initiate as early as age 11 or up to 26 years.
2. Endometrial Cancer: Often detected at an early stage, as it produces early vaginal bleeding between menstrual cycles or after menopause
   a. Contributing Factors
      1) Obesity
      2) Nulliparity
      3) Late menopause
   b. Manifestations
      1) Postmenopausal bleeding
      2) Abnormal bleeding
   c. Diagnostic Screening
      1) There is no specific screening. Endometrial biopsy is performed for diagnosis.
      2) At the time of menopause, all clients should be informed about the risks and symptoms of endometrial cancer.
   d. Collaborative Care
      1) Radium
      2) X-ray therapy
      3) Hysterectomy
   e. **Nursing Interventions**
      1) Monitor for grieving.
      2) Reinforce preoperative teaching.
      3) Provide postoperative care.
      4) Explore psychosexual needs.

3. Ovarian Cancer: Cancerous growth originating from different parts of the ovary
   a. Contributing Factors
      1) Age older than 40 years
      2) Nulliparity
      3) Family history of ovarian, breast, or colon cancer
      4) History of dysmenorrhea or heavy bleeding
      5) Hormone replacement therapy
      6) Use of infertility medications
   b. Manifestations
      1) Early symptoms are not obvious.
      2) Later symptoms can include the following.
         a) Pressure or pain in the abdomen, pelvis, back, or legs
         b) Swollen or bloated abdomen, nausea, indigestion, constipation, diarrhea, fatigue, shortness of breath, frequent urination, vaginal bleeding
   c. Diagnostic Screening
      1) CA 125 blood test: more than 35 u/mL is abnormal.
      2) Intravaginal ultrasound
      3) Pelvic exam
   d. Collaborative Treatment
      1) Chemotherapy
      2) Radiation
      3) Surgery

4. **Breast Cancer:** Abnormal growth of breast tissue
   a. Contributing Factors
      1) Family history (first-degree relative)
      2) Early menarche (younger than 12 years) and late menopause (older than 51 years)
      3) Nulligravida
      4) Early or prolonged use of oral contraceptives
      5) Long-term use of HRT
      6) Overweight
      7) Lifestyle: sedentary, excessive alcohol intake
   b. Manifestations
      1) Lump in breast or axilla region
      2) Thickening, dimpling, redness, pain, or asymmetry in breasts
      3) Pulling, discharge, or pain in nipple area
   c. Diagnostic Screening
      1) Mammogram: Women 40 and older should get a mammogram every 1 to 2 years.
      2) Clinical breast exam: Women should receive this exam annually.
      3) Breast self-exam: Women should perform this monthly, 1 week after menses.
      4) BRCA1 and BRCA2 gene test: Cannot be done within 3 months of a blood transfusion.
   d. Treatment
      1) Surgery (mastectomy) postoperative care
         a) Head of the bed elevated 30° when awake and arm supported on pillow.
         b) Position on unaffected side.
         c) Sling on affected side while ambulating.
         d) No injections, blood pressures, or blood draws from affected side. Place sign above bed with these precautions.
         e) Monitor incision and drainage tubes. (Drains are usually left in for 1 to 3 weeks.)
      2) Chemotherapy (combination therapy): cyclophosphamide, doxorubicin, fluorouracil
      3) Radiation
      4) Hormone therapy
         a) Gonadotropin-releasing hormone (GnRH)-leuprolide
         b) Selective estrogen receptor modulators (SERMs): tamoxifen and raloxifene. SERMs are used in women who are at high risk for breast cancer or who have advanced breast cancer. Tamoxifen increases risk of endometrial cancer, deep vein thrombosis, and pulmonary embolism. Raloxifene does not have these side effects.
   e. Preventive Teaching
      1) Encourage screenings.
      2) Diet should include five servings of fruits and vegetables daily.
      3) Maintain healthy weight, and exercise regularly.
      4) Limit alcohol intake, and avoid or cease smoking.

E. **Uterine Disorders**
   1. **Myomas (uterine fibroids):** Benign fibroid tumors of the uterine muscle
      a. Contributing Factors
         1) African Americans older than age 30 who have never been pregnant
      b. Manifestations
         1) Pelvic pain or pressure
         2) Hypermenorrhea
      c. Collaborative Treatment
         1) Medication
         2) Surgery
   2. **Endometriosis:** Endometrial tissue located outside of the uterus
      a. Contributing Factors
         1) Can involve retrograde menstruation
         2) Hereditary factors
         3) Impaired immune function
      b. Manifestations
         1) Severe dysmenorrhea
         2) Lower abdominal pain; pain during intercourse; back and rectal pain
         3) Abnormal bleeding
      c. Collaborative Treatment
         1) Oral contraceptives (hormone therapy), surgery, or pregnancy

F. **Menopause:** Complete cessation of menstruation for 1 year

1. Manifestations

   a. Vasomotor symptoms: hot flashes

   b. Genitourinary: atrophic vaginitis, vaginal dryness, incontinence

   c. Psychological: mood swings, changes in sleep patterns, decreased REM sleep

   d. Skeletal: decreased bone density

   e. Cardiovascular: decreased HDL, increased LDL

   f. Dermatologic: decreased skin elasticity, loss of hair on head and in the pubic area

   g. Reproductive: breast tissue changes, irregular menses

2. Collaborative Care and **Nursing Interventions**

   a. Monitor the client's psychosocial response.

      1) Discuss menopausal hormone therapy (HT)

      2) Reinforce teaching about self-administration of HT.

      3) Advise clients to immediately quit smoking if applicable.

      4) Reinforce teaching about how to prevent and monitor for development of venous thrombosis.

   b. Reinforce teaching about alternate hormone therapies (dong quai, black cohosh, vitamin E). These decrease hot flashes in some women.

   c. Older adult clients can decrease risk of osteoporosis by performing regular weight-bearing exercises; increasing intake of high-protein and high-calcium foods; avoiding alcohol, caffeine, and tobacco; and taking calcium with vitamin D supplements.

   d. Reinforce teaching about health promotion.

      1) Schedule annual exams (physical, pelvic, mammogram).

      2) Schedule bone density test.

      3) Reinforce teaching about atypical manifestations of MI.

      4) Discuss diet, exercise, and alternative therapies.

PRENATAL AND LABOR & DELIVERY COMPLICATIONS WORKSHEET

This worksheet reviews basic knowledge of prenatal and labor and delivery complications. (Answers can be used only once. Some answers will not be used.)

____ 1. amniotic fluid emboli	A. Benign abnormal growth of chorionic villi. Persistent, high, hCG levels. Birth control x 1 year after D&C.
____ 2. abruptio placentae	B. Low implantation of the placenta. Completely or partially covers cervical os. Usually painless. Bright red bleeding.
____ 3. cardiac disease	C. Hemolytic disease of the newborn: Rh-incompatibility. Occurs when a mother who is Rh-negative has a newborn who is Rh-positive. Direct Coombs' test has antibody coated Rh-positive RBCs in the newborn.
____ 4. eclampsia	
____ 5. ectopic pregnancy	
____ 6. erythroblastosis fetalis	
____ 7. gestational trophoblastic disease (hydatidiform mole)	D. Very tender, boardlike abdomen. Can have absent to moderate dark red bleeding.
	E. Excessive pregnancy-related nausea and/or vomiting. Believed to be caused by high levels of hCG.
____ 8. HELLP syndrome	F. Expanding maternal plasma volume and increased cardiac output in the presence of preexisting heart condition can cause this problem.
____ 9. hyperemesis gravidarum	G. Hematologic condition that coexists with severe preeclampsia involving hepatic dysfunction.
____ 10. placenta previa	H. Most important action with this disorder is to perform a sterile vaginal exam to support the presenting part to increase blood flow to the fetus.
____ 11. prolapsed cord	
____ 12. preterm labor	I. Life-threatening event in which amniotic fluid, fetal cells, hair, or other debris enters the maternal circulation, resulting in respiratory distress, circulatory collapse, hemorrhage, and possible seizure activity.
	J. Fertilized egg implants outside of the uterus. Cardinal sign includes sharp unilateral abdominal pain.
	K. Severe preeclampsia symptoms with the onset of seizure activity.
	L. Contractions with cervical change between 20 and 37 weeks gestation. Use tocolytics to stop contractions and betamethasone to promote fetal lung maturity.

Answer Key: 1. I; 2. D; 3. F; 4. K; 5. J; 6. C; 7. A; 8. G; 9. E; 10. B; 11. H; 12. L

SEXUALLY TRANSMITTED INFECTIONS

SYMPTOMS IN WOMEN	SYMPTOMS IN MEN	COMPLICATIONS	TREATMENTS

Chlamydia
If symptoms appear, usually not until several weeks after infected.

SYMPTOMS IN WOMEN	SYMPTOMS IN MEN	COMPLICATIONS	TREATMENTS
Vaginal discharge Vaginal bleeding Painful/frequent urination Abdominal pain Fever/nausea Usually asymptomatic	Small amounts of clear or cloudy penile discharge Painful/frequent urination Swollen/tender testicles	Can pass to sexual partners and to neonate during childbirth (conjunctivitis, pneumonia) PID Can lead to infertility in women and sterility in men	Oral antibiotics, usually azithromycin or doxycycline. Preventive treatment in newborn: erythromycin ointment in eyes within 1 hr of birth.

Genital herpes
Transmission most commonly occurs from infected partner who has no visible lesion.

SYMPTOMS IN WOMEN	SYMPTOMS IN MEN	COMPLICATIONS	TREATMENTS
Most are asymptomatic. Initial outbreak: painful blisters and possible systemic symptoms (fever, body aches, enlarged lymph nodes). Recurrences: mild tingling or shooting pains hours to days before herpetic eruption. Blisters last 7 to 21 days.	Some have no symptoms. Blisters on mouth or genital region. Blisters can reoccur.	No cure. Symptoms are treated. Can pass to sexual partners and to neonate during childbirth.	Caused by a virus. Antiviral medications (acyclovir, famciclovir, valacyclovir) can shorten and prevent outbreaks. Cesarean birth indicated if active lesions present during the last 2 weeks before delivery. Antiviral medication (acyclovir) started at 36 weeks gestation to prevent outbreak before delivery.

Gonorrhea (GC)
Symptoms can appear 2 to 21 days after infection.

SYMPTOMS IN WOMEN	SYMPTOMS IN MEN	COMPLICATIONS	TREATMENTS
Yellow/gray vaginal discharge Vaginal bleeding between periods Symptoms mild and nonspecific Pelvic or lower abdominal pain	Yellow/green penile discharge Painful urination/bowel movement Frequent urination Swollen/tender testicles (epididymitis)	Transmitted to sexual partner and to the neonate in uterus/during childbirth (ophthalmia neonatorum) Can lead to infertility in women and sterility in men Untreated GC can cause urogenital, anorectal, conjunctival, and pharyngeal infections. Can also spread to the blood and cause disseminated gonococcal infection (DGI). DGI is usually characterized by arthritis, tenosynovitis, and/or dermatitis.	First-line treatment is single intramuscular injection of ceftriaxone 250 mg. Ceftriaxone is routinely accompanied by azithromycin or doxycycline to address the likelihood of coinfection with chlamydia Because of high reinfection rates, patients should be retested in 3 to 6 months. Preventive treatment of newborn: erythromycin ointment in eyes.

HIV
Symptoms can appear months to several years after infection.

Acute retroviral syndrome is characterized by nonspecific symptoms (fever, malaise, lymphadenopathy, skin rash). Frequently occurs in the first few weeks after HIV infection, before antibody test results become positive.

SYMPTOMS IN WOMEN	SYMPTOMS IN MEN	COMPLICATIONS	TREATMENTS
Can be infected for several years without symptoms Weight loss/fatigue Recurring vaginal yeast infections Diarrhea/flu-like symptoms Oral thrush	Can be infected for several years without symptoms Weight loss/fatigue Diarrhea/flu-like symptoms Oral thrush	There is no cure for HIV, but treatment is available. Can be passed by sexual contact, contaminated needles, during childbirth, or during breastfeeding	HIV is a virus that progressively depletes CD4 lymphocytes. Prevention counseling is key. Screening with early detection is critical. Medication includes antiretroviral therapy (HAART) Management for obstetrical clients includes antiretroviral regimens and obstetrical interventions (zidovudine, nevirapine) and elective Cesarean birth at 38 weeks of pregnancy, and education to avoid breastfeeding.

SEXUALLY TRANSMITTED INFECTIONS (CONTINUED)

SYMPTOMS IN WOMEN	SYMPTOMS IN MEN	COMPLICATIONS	TREATMENTS

Human papillomavirus (HPV)
There are multiple strains. Some can cause genital warts and others have been linked to cervical cancer. Symptom appearance time varies.

SYMPTOMS IN WOMEN	SYMPTOMS IN MEN	COMPLICATIONS	TREATMENTS
Genital warts, also referred to as condylomas Appear as small, flesh-colored or gray swelling in the genital area Can clump together and form a cauliflower shape Itching/burning around the genitalia Abnormal pap test	Genital warts that can recur Itching/burning around the genitalia	Can pass to sexual partners and neonate during childbirth. Warts can spread. Some strains can lead to cancer. A rare complication is recurrent respiratory papillomatosis (RRP).	HPV vaccines recommended for 11- or 12-year-old boys and girls. May be given to girls beginning at age 9. Medications to treat genital warts include imiquimod and podophyllin.

Pelvic inflammatory disease (PID)
Several different bacteria can cause PID. Many cases have been related to chlamydia and gonorrhea.

SYMPTOMS IN WOMEN	SYMPTOMS IN MEN	COMPLICATIONS	TREATMENTS
Lower abdominal pain Can have unpleasant odor Painful intercourse/urination Abnormal vaginal discharge (yellow or green) with unpleasant odor Fever, chills, nausea, and vomiting	PID does not occur in males.	Can cause ectopic pregnancy Can lead to infertility Can cause chronic pain in abdominal area	Depending on the severity of PID, the following can be used for treatment. > Antibiotics > Hospitalization/bed rest > Outpatient intensive treatment

Syphilis
There are three stages of syphilis. Stage 1 symptoms can appear 1 week to 3 months after infection.

SYMPTOMS IN WOMEN	SYMPTOMS IN MEN	COMPLICATIONS	TREATMENTS
Stage 1: Primary > Sore(s) on genitalia or mouth > Sore(s) can last 2 to 6 weeks Stage 2: Secondary > Rash on body > Flu-like symptoms Stage 3: Tertiary (last) Stage > Neurological/cardiovascular complications	Stage 1: Primary > Sore(s) on genitalia or mouth > Sore(s) can last 2 to 6 weeks Stage 2: Secondary > Rash on body > Flu-like symptoms Stage 3: Tertiary (last) Stage > Neurological/cardiovascular complications	Can pass to sexual partners and to the neonate during pregnancy Can cause miscarriage Can cause heart disease, blindness, or brain damage Can lead to death	Caused by bacteria. Penicillin G is the medication of choice.

Trichomoniasis (Trich)
Symptoms can appear 3 days to 2 weeks after infection.

SYMPTOMS IN WOMEN	SYMPTOMS IN MEN	COMPLICATIONS	TREATMENTS
Can be asymptomatic Common symptom: yellowish to greenish, frothy, mucopurulent, copious, malodorous discharge Dysuria and dyspareunia Vaginal irritation and pruritus	Often no symptoms White, watery penile discharge Painful/frequent urination	Can pass to sexual partners Can lead to prostate infection	Recommended treatment is metronidazole or tinidazole unless the client is in the first trimester of pregnancy. Partners should also be treated.

Nursing Care of Children

Foundations of Nursing Care of Children

Family

A. Identify the legal guardian.

B. Build a relationship with the family and child.

C. Monitor family dynamics.

D. Collaborative Care

1. **Nursing Interventions**

   a. Respect family diversity.

   b. Monitor parent-child interactions.

   c. Assist families to understand growth and development needs.

   d. Assist families to adapt to the needs of a child who has a health problem.

   e. Assist families to participate in care as appropriate.

   f. Use community resources for family adaptation.

Growth and Development

Expected Growth and Development of the Infant (1st Year of Life)

A. **Physical Development**

1. Fontanels

   a. Posterior closes by 6 to 8 weeks of age

   b. Anterior closes by 12 to 18 months of age

2. Dentition

   a. First tooth appears between ages 6 and 10 months.

   b. Six to eight teeth appear by the end of first year.

   c. For children younger than 2 years: Age of the child in months – 6 = Number of teeth

   d. Pain relief for teething

      1) Cold

         a) Refrigerated pacifier

         b) Cold teething ring

         c) Acetaminophen; ibuprofen if older than 6 months (do not use more than 3 days)

         d) Over-the-counter teething gels

   e. Tooth care

      1) Clean teeth with cool, wet cloth.

   f. Do not give bottles to infants when they are falling asleep.

3. Vision

   a. Infant vision is undeveloped, improves gradually.

   b. At birth, can focus on objects 8 to 10 inches away.

   c. Best able to discern shapes with contrast such as black/white and bright colors.

   d. Red reflex should be present.

4. Measurements of growth

   a. Height, weight, and head circumference plotted on graph

      1) Measure recumbent length. (Do not use tape measure.)

      2) Measure weight to the nearest 10 g (0.35 oz). Infants should be nude. Document devices, such as arm boards.

      3) Measure head circumference at the widest point.

   b. Identify issues

      1) Measurements below 5th percentile or above 95th percentile

   c. Rules of thumb

      1) Newborns can lose up to 10% of birth weight by 3 to 4 days of age.

      2) Birth weight is reattained by 2 weeks of age.

      3) Birth weight doubles by 5 months of age.

      4) Birth weight triples by 12 months of age.

      5) Birth length increases approximately 2.5 cm (1 in) per month for the first 6 months.

      6) Birth length increases 50% by 12 months of age.

MOTOR SKILL DEVELOPMENT OF THE INFANT

AGE	GROSS MOTOR SKILLS	FINE MOTOR SKILLS
1 month	Demonstrates head lag	Strong grasp reflex
2 months	Lifts head off mattress when prone	Holds hands in an open position, grasp reflex disappearing
3 months	When in prone position, will raise head and shoulders Has slight head lag Bears weight on forearms	No longer has grasp reflex Actively holds rattle Keeps hands loosely open
4 months	Rolls from back to side	Holds object with both hands
5 months	Rolls from front to back	Able to grasp objects voluntarily Takes objects directly to mouth
6 months	Rolls from back to front	Holds bottle Picks up object if dropped
7 months	Bears full weight on feet Sits, leaning forward on both hands	Moves objects from hand to hand
8 months	Sits unsupported	Uses thumb and index finger in crude pincer grasp

MOTOR SKILL DEVELOPMENT OF THE INFANT (CONTINUED)

AGE	GROSS MOTOR SKILLS	FINE MOTOR SKILLS
9 months	Creeps on hands and knees instead of crawling Pulls to a standing position	Pincer grasp is more precise
10 months	Changes from a prone to sitting position	Grasps rattle by its handle
11 months	Walks while holding onto something	Neat pincer grasp Deliberately drops objects for them to be picked up Places objects into a container
12 months	Sits down from a standing position without assistance Walks with one hand held	Tries to build a two-block tower without success Can turn pages in a book (many at a time)

INFANT DEVELOPMENT MILESTONES

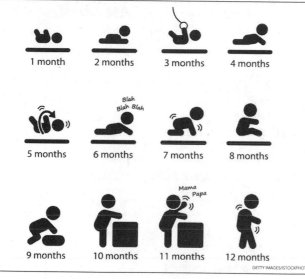

GETTY IMAGES/ISTOCKPHOTO

B. **Cognitive Development**

1. Piaget: Sensorimotor phase (birth to 24 months)

   a. Separation: Learns to separate from other objects in the environment

   b. Object permanence: Learns that objects exist when hidden out of view

      1) Occurs at approximately 9 to 10 months of age

   c. Mental representation: Recognizes and uses symbols

2. Language

   a. Crying is the first form of verbal communication

   b. Coos and babbles; turns head to the sound of a rattle by 3 months

   c. Laughs aloud by 4 months

   d. Comprehends "no" by the age of 9 months

   e. Three to five words other than "dada" or "mama" by 12 months of age

C. **Psychosocial Development**

1. Erikson: Trust vs. Mistrust

   a. Trust develops as needs are met.

   b. Mistrust develops when needs are inadequately or inconsistently met, or if needs are met before vocalized by the infant.

2. Social Development

   a. Bonding

   b. Separation anxiety (4 to 8 months)

   c. Fear of strangers (6 to 8 months)

3. Body-Image Changes

   a. Discovers mouth produces pleasure.

   b. Discovers smiling causes others to react.

   c. Hands and feet are objects of play.

D. **Age-Appropriate Activities**

1. Solitary play

2. Shaking rattles

3. Looking in mirrors

4. Chewing on teething toys

5. Playing pat-a-cake

6. Playing with blocks

7. Listening to someone read

E. **Health Promotion for Infants**

1. Newborn infants require a medical visit with a provider within 72 hr of discharge.

   a. Immunizations

      1) CDC recommendations for healthy infants (younger than 12 months of age)

         a) Birth: hepatitis B (Hep B)

         b) 2 months: diphtheria and tetanus toxoids and pertussis (DTaP), rotavirus vaccine (RV), inactivated poliovirus (IPV), *Haemophilus influenzae* type B (Hib), pneumococcal vaccine (PCV), and Hep B

         c) 4 months: DTaP, RV, IPV, Hib, PCV

         d) 6 months: DTaP, IPV (6 to 18 months), PCV, and Hep B (6 to 18 months); RV; Hib

         e) 6 to 12 months: seasonal influenza vaccination yearly (The trivalent inactivated influenza vaccine is available as an intramuscular injection.)

NOTE: Always refer to the CDC website (www.cdc.gov) for the latest immunization requirements and schedules.

2. Nutrition

   a. Breastfeeding provides a complete diet for the first 6 months of life.

      1) Iron-fortified formula is an acceptable alternative to breast milk. No other forms of milk or milk products (cow, goat, almond, evaporated) should be used during the first 12 months.

      2) Vitamin D supplements within first few days of life.

      3) Iron supplements after 4 months of age for infants who are exclusively breastfed.

      4) Juice and water are not needed during the first 4 months.

      5) Fruit juice should not be provided to children younger than 1 year of age.

b. Solid foods are introduced around 4 to 6 months of age.
  1) Introduce new foods one at a time and evaluate tolerance.
  2) Introduce iron-fortified cereal first.
  3) Introduce fruits and vegetables at 6 to 8 months.
  4) Nutritious finger foods such as cheese and raw fruit (no grapes) may be introduced at 8 to 9 months of age.
  5) Chopped, cooked, and unseasoned table foods are appropriate by 12 months of age.
  6) No citrus fruits, eggs, or meat until after 6 months; no honey until after 12 months.
c. Weaning
  1) Begin when infant shows signs of readiness and can drink from a cup. Usually occurs after 6 months.
  2) Stop bedtime feeding last.

3. Sleep Patterns
  a. Nocturnal sleep pattern is established by 3 to 4 months of age.
  b. Sleeps through the night and takes one to two naps during the day by age 12 months.

II Safety for Infants

A. **Aspiration**
  1. Provide age-appropriate toys.
  2. Avoid small objects (grapes, coins, candy).
  3. Check clothing and household objects for safety hazards (loose buttons, draw strings).

B. **Suffocation**
  1. Keep plastic bags and balloons out of reach.
  2. Remove pillows from crib.
  3. Remove mobiles from crib by 4 to 5 months of age.
  4. Use firm crib mattresses with a snug fit.
  5. Crib slats no farther apart than 6 cm (2 3/8 in).

C. **Bodily Harm**
  1. Keep sharp objects out of reach.
  2. Anchor furniture and heavy objects.
  3. Do not leave infants unattended with animals.
  4. Monitor infants for shaken baby syndrome.

D. **Burns**
  1. Check temperature of bath water.
  2. Set hot water thermostats at or less than 49° C (120° F).
  3. Keep working smoke detectors in the home.
  4. Turn handles of pots and pans to the back of stoves.
  5. Use physical coverings and apply sunscreen if infants will be exposed to the sun.
  6. Cover electrical outlets.
  7. Do not heat breast milk or formula in the microwave.

E. **Drowning**
  1. Do not leave infants unattended around water sources (tubs, toilets, cleaning buckets)
  2. Secure fencing around swimming pools.
  3. Close bathroom doors.

F. **Falls**
  1. Keep infant seats on the ground or floor if used outside the car.
  2. Place safety gates at top and bottom of stairs.
  3. Position crib mattresses in the lowest position with rails all the way up.

G. **Poisoning**
  1. Keep the poison control number readily available.
  2. Avoid exposure to lead paint.
  3. Keep toxins and plants out of reach. Use safety locks on cabinets.
  4. Store medications in childproof containers out of reach.
  5. Maintain working carbon monoxide detectors at home.

H. **Motor Vehicle Injuries**
  1. Newborns should be placed in a federally approved car seat at a 45 degree angle; secure with safety belt.
  2. Rear-facing in back seat.
  3. Place shoulder harnesses in slots at or below level of infant's shoulders.
  4. Place retainer clip at axillary level of infant.
  5. Rear-facing until 2 years of age or the height recommended by the manufacturer.
  6. If air bags are near the infant (such as in a vehicle without a rear seat), the passenger seat air bag should be inactivated.

I. **Sudden Infant Death Syndrome (SIDS)**
  1. Contributing Factors
    a. Male sex
    b. Age younger than 1 year (peak: 2 to 3 months)
    c. Prematurity
    d. Low birth weight
    e. Low Apgar scores
    f. Low socioeconomic status
    g. Family history of SIDS
    h. Maternal smoking or secondhand smoke
    i. Twin or multiple birth
    j. Co-sleeping
  2. Prevention
    a. Place infants on their backs for sleep.
    b. Encourage breastfeeding.
    c. Offer a pacifier when sleeping.
    d. Prevent overheating.
    e. Do not place pillows and blankets in the crib. Keep the infant's head uncovered during sleep.
    f. Maintain up-to-date immunizations.

III Expected Growth and Development of the Toddler (Ages 1 to 3 Years)

A. **Physical Development**

1. Anterior fontanel closes by 18 months of age.
2. Weight: Four times birth weight at 30 months of age.
3. Height: Toddlers grow about 7.5 cm (3 in) per year.
4. Head circumference: Equal to chest circumference by 1 to 2 years of age.

MOTOR SKILL DEVELOPMENT OF THE TODDLER

AGE	GROSS MOTOR SKILLS	FINE MOTOR SKILLS
15 months	Walks without help Creeps up stairs	Uses a cup well Builds a tower of two blocks
18 months	Runs clumsily; falls often Throws ball overhand Jumps in place with both feet Pulls and pushes toys	Manages a spoon without rotation Turns pages in a book, two or three at a time Builds tower of three or four blocks
2 years	Walks up and down stairs by placing both feet on each step Runs with wide stance Kicks ball forward without falling	Builds a tower of six or seven blocks Turns pages in a book, one at a time
2.5 years	Jumps across the floor, or off a chair or step using both feet Takes a few steps on tiptoe Stands on one foot momentarily	Draws circles and crosses Has good hand-finger coordination

TODDLER DEVELOPMENT MILESTONES

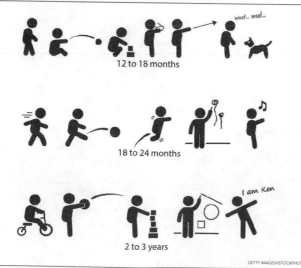

12 to 18 months

18 to 24 months

2 to 3 years

GETTY IMAGES/ISTOCKPHOTO

B. **Cognitive Development**

1. Piaget: The sensorimotor phase transitions to the preoperational phase around 19 to 24 months of age.
   a. Object permanence is developed.
   b. Memory develops.
   c. Preoperational thought allows the toddler to use symbols to represent objects.
2. Language
   a. 1 year: one-word sentences
   b. 2 years: two- to three-word sentences
   c. 3 years: simple sentences
3. Psychosocial Development
   a. Erikson: Autonomy vs. Shame and Doubt
   b. Independence
   c. Negativism
   d. Temper tantrums
   e. Ritualism
   f. Separation anxiety peaks.
4. Moral Development
   a. Egocentric
   b. Sense that good behavior is rewarded and bad behavior is punished
5. Self-Concept Development
   a. See themselves as separate from parents
6. Body Image Changes
   a. Appreciates the usefulness of various body parts
   b. Develops gender identity by 3 years of age

C. **Age-Appropriate Activities**

1. Solitary play evolves to parallel play.
   a. Filling and empty containers
   b. Playing with blocks
   c. Looking at books
   d. Push-pull toys
   e. Scribbling with crayons
2. Toilet training
   a. Begins when the toddler is able to recognize the urge to urinate or defecate.
   b. Nighttime continence usually develops last.
3. Discipline
   a. Consistent with well-defined boundaries

D. **Health Promotion for Toddlers**

1. Immunizations
   a. CDC recommendation for toddlers (1 to 3 years of age)
      1) 12 to 15 months: inactivated poliovirus (third dose between 6 to 18 months); *Haemophilus influenzae* type B; pneumococcal conjugate vaccine; measles, mumps, and rubella; and varicella
      2) 12 to 23 months: hepatitis A (Hep A), given in two doses at least 6 months apart
      3) 15 to 18 months: diphtheria, tetanus, and acellular pertussis
      4) 12 to 36 months: yearly seasonal trivalent inactivated influenza vaccine (TIV); live, attenuated influenza vaccine (LAIV) by nasal spray (must be 2 years or older)

2. Nutrition
   a. Avoid snacks high in fat, sugar, and sodium.
   b. Serving size is about 1 tbsp per year of age.
   c. Should consume 24 to 28 oz milk per day. Change from whole milk to low-fat milk after 2 years of age.
   d. Limit juice to 4 to 6 oz per day.
   e. Include 1 cup of fruit daily.
   f. Do not eat or drink during play or when lying down.
   g. Prefer finger foods.
   h. Picky eaters. Physiologic anorexia occurs.
3. Sleep and Rest
   a. Average 11 to 12 hr of sleep per day and one nap
   b. Resists going to bed
4. Dental Care
   a. Establish a dental provider by 1 year of age.
   b. An adult caregiver should brush and floss the toddler's teeth after meals and at bedtime.

IV Safety for Toddler

A. **Aspiration**
   1. Avoid small objects (coins, candy) and toys with small parts.
   2. Avoid common causes of choking: hot dogs, nuts, grapes, peanut butter, raw carrots, tough meat, popcorn.
   3. Keep away from balloons.
   4. Check clothing for drawstrings and loose buttons.
   5. Reinforce teaching with parents about emergency procedures for choking.

B. **Bodily Harm**
   1. Keep sharp objects out of reach.
   2. Store firearms in locked boxes or cabinets.
   3. Do not leave toddlers unattended with animals.
   4. Reinforce teaching about stranger safety.

C. **Burns**
   1. Check temperature of bath water.
   2. Set hot water thermostats at or less than 49° C (120° F).
   3. Keep working smoke detectors in the home.
   4. Turn handles of pots and pans to the back of stoves.
   5. Cover electrical outlets.
   6. Apply sunscreen when exposed to the sun.

D. **Drowning**
   1. Do not leave unattended in bathtubs.
   2. Keep toilet lids closed.
   3. Supervise closely when near pools or water.
   4. Teach toddlers how to swim.

E. **Falls**
   1. Keep doors and windows locked.
   2. Position crib mattresses in the lowest position with rails all the way up.
   3. Place safety gates at top and bottom of stairs.

F. **Motor Vehicle Injuries**
   1. Remain in rear-facing car seat until the age of 2 years or the height recommended by manufacturer.
   2. Forward-facing car seat for toddlers older than 2 years, or who exceed the height recommendation.
   3. The back seat is the safest area.
   4. If the vehicle does not have a rear seat, the passenger seat air bag should be inactivated.

G. **Poisoning**
   1. Keep poison control number readily available.
   2. Avoid exposure to lead paint.
   3. Place safety locks on cabinets that contain cleaners and other chemicals.
   4. Store medications in childproof containers out of reach.
   5. Maintain working carbon monoxide detectors at home.

H. **Suffocation**
   1. Keep plastic bags out of reach.
   2. Do not place pillows in the crib.
   3. Crib mattresses should fit tightly.
   4. Crib slats no farther apart than 6 cm (2 3/8 in).
   5. Remove doors from unused appliances (such as refrigerators).

V Expected Growth and Development of the Preschooler (Ages 3 to 6 Years)

A. **Physical Development**
   1. Weight: Gains 2 to 3 kg (4.4 to 6.6 lb) per year.
   2. Height: Grows 6.5 to 9 cm (2.5 to 3.5 in) per year.
   3. Fine and gross motor skills improve.

MOTOR SKILLS OF THE PRESCHOOLER

AGE	GROSS MOTOR SKILLS	FINE MOTOR SKILLS
3 years	Alternates feet when going up and down stairs	Builds a tower of nine to 10 cubes
	Rides a tricycle	Imitates cross when drawing
	Jumps off bottom step	Cannot draw a stick figure; might draw a circle with facial features
	Stands on one foot for a few seconds	
4 years	Skips and hops on one foot	Uses scissors
	Throws a ball overhead	Laces shoes
	Catches ball reliably	Copies square, traces cross and diamond
5 years	Jumps rope	Ties shoelaces
	Walks backward with heel to toe	Use pencil well
	Moves up and down stairs easily	Prints some letters
	Throws and catches ball with ease	Draws most of a stick figure

B. **Cognitive and Language Development**

1. Piaget
   a. Preoperational phase transitions to intuitive thought.
   b. Makes judgments based on visual appearances.
2. Variations in thinking
   a. Magical thinking: Thoughts can cause events to happen.
   b. Animism: Inanimate objects are alive.
   c. Centration: Focuses on one aspect instead of the whole.
   d. Time: Understands sequence of daily events.
3. Language Development
   a. Enjoys talking.
   b. Speaks in three- to five-word sentences.

C. **Psychosocial Development**

1. Erikson—Initiative vs. Guilt
   a. Energetic learners but lack physical abilities to be successful at everything.
   b. Guilt can occur if they misbehave or are unable to accomplish a task.
2. Self-Concept Development
   a. Feels good about mastering skills which promote independence (such as dressing self).
   b. Can regress (bedwetting, sucking thumb) during times of stress, insecurity, or illness.
3. Body-Image Change
   a. Recognizes differences in appearances.
   b. Begin to compare themselves with others.
   c. Intrusive experiences (injections, cuts) are traumatic due to poor understanding of anatomy.
4. Moral Development
   a. Early preschoolers take actions based on the result of reward or punishment.
5. Social Development
   a. Older preschoolers take actions to satisfy personal needs.
   b. Begins to understand fairness.
   c. Prolonged separation (such as hospitalization) can cause anxiety.
   d. Favorite toys and appropriate play should be used.
   e. Does not exhibit stranger anxiety.
   f. Pretend play; can develop imaginary friends.

D. **Age-Appropriate Activities**

1. Associative play with some cooperation
2. Common activities
   a. Playing ball
   b. Puzzles
   c. Riding tricycles
   d. Pretend play and dress-up
   e. Painting
   f. Reading books
   g. Electronic games and TV—limit screen time to 2 hr

E. **Health Promotion for Preschoolers**

1. Immunizations
   a. CDC recommendations for preschoolers (3 to 6 years old)
      1) 4 to 6 years: DTaP; measles, mumps, and rubella (MMR); varicella; and IPV
      2) 3 to 6 years: Yearly seasonal influenza vaccine; TIV; or LAIV by nasal spray
2. Nutrition
   a. Consume half the amount of adults (1,800 kcal).
   b. Can continue to be picky eaters, but more willing to try different foods at 5 years of age.
   c. Provide a diet with adequate protein, calcium, iron, folate, vitamins A & C.
   d. Consume five servings of fruits and vegetables per day.
   e. Do not consume sweetened beverages.
3. Dental Health
   a. Eruption of primary teeth is finalized.
   b. Parents should assist and supervise brushing and flossing.
   c. Dental trauma is common and should be immediately assessed by dentist.
4. Sleep and Rest
   a. Require about 12 hr of sleep per day.
   b. Can require daytime nap.
   c. Sleep disturbances are common.

VI. Safety for Preschoolers

A. **Bodily Harm**

1. Place all firearms and ammunition in locked cabinets or containers.
2. Reinforce teaching about stranger safety.
3. Wear protective equipment (such as a helmet) on bicycles, skateboards, and scooters.

B. **Burns**

1. Set hot water thermostats at or less than 49° C (120° F).
2. Keep working smoke detectors in the home.
3. Apply sunscreen when outside.

C. **Drowning**

1. Do not leave unattended in bathtubs.
2. Supervise closely when near pools or any body of water.
3. Teach water safety and how to swim.

D. **Motor Vehicle Injuries**

1. Use a federally approved car restraint according to manufacturer recommendations.
2. Transition to a booster seat when forward-facing car seat is outgrown.
3. An approved car restraint system is recommended until a height of 145 cm (4 feet, 9 in) is achieved or 8 to 12 years of age.
4. Safest area for children is back seat.
5. If vehicle does not have a rear seat, passenger seat air bag should be inactivated.

E. **Poisoning**

1. Keep poison control number readily available.
2. While this age group is more aware of dangers, poisoning is still a concern. Continue to implement precautions.

VII Expected Growth and Development of the School-Age Child (Age 6 to 12 Years)

A. **Physical Development**

1. Weight: Gains 2 to 3 kg (4.4 to 6.6 lb) per year.

2. Height: Grows 5 cm (2 in) per year.

3. Prepubescence

   a. Physiological changes in females around the age of 9 years.

   b. Visible sexual maturation in males is minimal.

4. Permanent teeth erupt.

5. Bones continue to ossify.

B. **Cognitive and Language Development**

1. Piaget: Concrete Operations

   a. Learns to tell time.

   b. Masters concept of conservation; mass is understood first.

   c. Sees the perspective of others.

   d. Solves problems.

2. Language

   a. Defines many words and understands rules of grammar.

   b. Understands that a word can have multiple meanings.

C. **Psychosocial Development**

1. Erikson—Industry vs. Inferiority

   a. A sense of industry is achieved through development of personal and interpersonal skills, which allows the child to contribute to society.

   b. A sense of inferiority can occur if previous stages have not been mastered or if the child is unable or not ready to assume responsibilities.

2. Moral development

   a. Early school-age years

      1) Does not understand reasoning behind rules and expectations

      2) Believe they are wrong and others are right

      3) Judgment guided by rewards and punishment

      4) Can interpret accidents as punishment

   b. Later school-age years

      1) Can judge the intentions of an act rather than the consequences

      2) Understands different points of view

      3) Conceptualizes treating others as they like to be treated

3. Self-concept development

   a. Develops an awareness of themselves in relation to others

   b. Understands personal values, abilities, and physical characteristics

   c. Gains confidence by establishing a positive self-concept

   d. Influenced by parents; by middle-childhood, peers and teachers are more valuable

4. Body image changes

   a. Curiosity about sexuality should be addressed with education.

   b. Knowledgeable about the body.

   c. Compares body to peers.

   d. Aware of physical disabilities in others.

   e. Might be excluded if different.

   f. More modest than preschoolers and place more emphasis on privacy issues.

5. Social development

   a. Peers are important. Peer pressure begins.

   b. Clubs and best friends are popular.

   c. School-age children prefer the company of same-gender companions, but can begin developing an interest in other genders toward the end of the school-age years.

   d. Most relationships come from school associations.

   e. Bullying can occur in an attempt to cause harm or to control.

   f. Conformity becomes evident.

D. **Age-Appropriate Activities**

1. Play is competitive and cooperative.

2. Common activities

   a. Board games

   b. Jump rope

   c. Collecting

   d. Bicycles

   e. Organized sports

   f. Crafts

E. **Health Promotion for School-Age Children**

1. Immunizations

   a. CDC recommendations for school-age children (6 to 12 years of age)

      1) If not given between 4 and 5 years of age, children should receive the following vaccines by 6 years of age: DTaP; inactivated poliovirus; MMR; and varicella.

      2) Yearly seasonal influenza vaccine: TIV or LAIV by nasal spray.

      3) 11 to 12 years: tetanus and diphtheria toxoids and pertussis vaccine (Tdap); human papillomavirus vaccine–HPV2 or HPV4 in three doses for females, HPV4 for males; and meningococcal (MCV4).

2. Nutrition

   a. Eat adult portions by the end of school-age years.

   b. Obesity is a concern. Parents should avoid using food as a reward and emphasize physical activity.

   c. Do not skip meals.

3. Sleep and Rest

   a. Variable; depends on age, level of activity, and health status.

   b. Approximately 9 hr of sleep at age 11 years.

4. Health screenings

   a. Scoliosis

   b. Dental health

      1) Obtain regular checkups; fluoride treatments if necessary.

      2) Brush after meals and snacks, and at bedtime.

VIII Safety for School-Age Children

A. **Bodily Harm**
   1. Keep firearms locked in cabinets or boxes.
   2. Identify safe play areas.
   3. Teach stranger safety.
   4. Teach to wear protective equipment (helmets, pads).

B. **Burns**
   1. Teach fire safety and burn hazards.
   2. Teach safety precautions for cooking.
   3. Keep working smoke detectors in the home.
   4. Use sunscreen when outside.

C. **Drowning**
   1. Supervise when swimming or when near a body of water.
   2. Teach water safety and how to swim.
   3. Check depth of water prior to diving.

D. **Motor Vehicle Injuries**
   1. Use an approved car restraint system until a height of 145 cm (4 feet, 9 inches) is achieved or 8 to 12 years of age.
   2. Teach to use a seat belt when a car restraint system or booster seat is no longer required.
   3. Lap belts should lay across upper thighs (not the stomach).
   4. Shoulder belts should lay across chest (not the neck).
   5. Do not ride in the bed of a pickup truck.
   6. Teach pedestrian safety.

E. **Poisoning/Substance Use**
   1. Keep cleaners and chemicals locked and placed out of reach.
   2. Teach to say "no" to drugs and alcohol.

IX Expected Growth and Development of the Adolescent (12 to 20 Years)

A. **Physical Development**
   1. Females
      a. Height: grow 5 to 20 cm (2 to 8 in)
      b. Weight: gain 7 to 25 kg (15.5 to 55 lb)
      c. Growth stops about 2 years after menarche.
   2. Males
      a. Height: grow 10 to 30 cm (4 to 12 in)
      b. Weight: gain 7 to 30 kg (15.5 to 66 lb)
      c. Growth stops around 18 to 20 years of age.
   3. Sexual maturation occurs.

B. **Cognitive and Language Development**
   1. Piaget—Formal Operations
      a. Able to think of more than two categories of variables at the same time
      b. Can evaluate own thinking
      c. Imaginative and idealistic
      d. More capable of using formal logic to make decisions
      e. Understands how actions can influence others

C. **Psychosocial Development**
   1. Erikson—Identity vs. Role Confusion
      a. Develops personal identity; views themselves as unique
      b. Peer groups greatly influence behavior
      c. Sees themselves as invincible
   2. Sexual identity
      a. Intimate relationships can develop
      b. Masturbation
   3. Moral development
      a. Uses internalized moral principles to solve dilemmas
      b. Questions existing moral values to society and individuals
   4. Self-concept development
      a. Progresses from viewing themselves in relation to similarities with peers to recognizing unique individual characteristics
   5. Body image changes
      a. Normality is based on comparison with peers.
      b. Image established during adolescence is retained throughout life.
   6. Social development
      a. Peers are a support system.
      b. Friendships with best friends are stronger and last longer.
      c. Parent-child relationships change to allow independence.

D. **Age-Appropriate Activities**
   1. Nonviolent video games
   2. Nonviolent music
   3. Sports
   4. Caring for a pet
   5. Career training programs
   6. Reading
   7. Social events (going to movies, school dances)

E. **Health Promotion for Adolescents**
   1. Immunizations
      a. CDC recommendations for clients 13 to 18 years old
         1) Include catch-up doses of any recommended immunizations not received at 11 to 12 years old.
         2) Yearly seasonal influenza vaccine: TIV or LAIV by nasal spray.
         3) 16 to 18 years: MCV4 booster is recommended if first dose was received between ages 13 and 15 years. A booster dose is not needed if the first dose is received at age 16 or older.
   2. Screenings
      a. Scoliosis
      b. Growth and development (physical health, self-image, physical activity)
      c. Social and academic (relationships, grades)
      d. Emotional well-being (mental health, sexuality)
      e. Risk reduction (tobacco, alcohol, other drugs)
      f. Violence and injury prevention

3. Nutrition
   a. Need additional calcium, iron, protein, and zinc.
   b. Intake of folic acid, vitamin B_6, vitamin A, iron, calcium, and zinc can be inadequate.
   c. Yearly assessments of height, weight, and BMI to identify issues.
      1) Overeating—avoid using food as a reward.
      2) Undereating
4. Sleep and Rest
   a. Sleep habits change due to increased metabolism and rapid growth.
   b. Need for sleep increases.
   c. Can stay up late and sleep later in the morning than previously.
5. Dental health
   a. Corrective appliances are common.
   b. Brush after meals, snacks, and at bedtime.
   c. Floss daily.
   d. Regular checkups.
   e. Regular fluoride treatments if necessary.
6. Sexuality
   a. Provide accurate information.
   b. Emphasize abstinence.
   c. Education: Prevent sexually transmitted infections and pregnancy.

x Safety for Adolescents

A. **Bodily Harm**
1. Keep firearms unloaded and locked in a cabinet or box.
2. Teach proper use of sporting equipment.
3. Insist on using protective equipment (helmets, pads) during activities like riding a bicycle or skiing.
4. Be aware of changes in mood. Monitor for the following.
   a. Poor school performance
   b. Lack of interest
   c. Social isolation
   d. Disturbances in appetite or sleep
   e. Expression of thoughts of suicide

B. **Burns**
1. Teach fire safety.
2. Apply sunscreen when outside.
3. Avoid tanning beds.

C. **Motor-vehicle injuries**
1. Encourage drivers' education courses.
2. Emphasize use of seat belts.
3. Discourage use of cell phones and driving.
4. Teach dangers of drinking and driving.
5. Role model desired behavior.

D. **Substance use**
1. Monitor for signs of substance use.
2. Teach to say "no" to harmful substances and alcohol.

xi Child Maltreatment: Neglect and Abuse

A. Occurs across all economic and educational backgrounds and racial/ethnic/religious groups
B. **Types**
1. Physical: Causing pain or harm (shaken baby syndrome, fractures)
2. Sexual: Occurs when sexual contact takes place without consent, regardless of the victim being able to give consent. Includes any sexual behavior toward a minor and dating violence.
3. Emotional: Humiliating, threatening, or intimidating behavior
4. Neglect: Failure to provide physical (food, clothes) or emotional (affection, nurturing) needs

C. **Contributing Factors**
1. Parental
   a. Poor self-esteem
   b. Victim of abuse
   c. Lack of knowledge: parenting skills
   d. Young or single parent
   e. Social isolation
   f. Substance use disorder
2. Child
   a. 1 year old or younger
   b. Unwanted
   c. Premature
   d. Hyperactive
   e. Physical or mental disability
3. Environment
   a. Chronic stress
   b. Socioeconomic factors (unemployment, divorce)

D. **Manifestations of Abuse and Neglect**
1. Expected Findings
   a. Inconsistencies between the parent's and child's report
   b. Inconsistency between nature of injury and developmental level of child
   c. Repeated injuries requiring emergency treatment
   d. Inappropriate responses from the parents or child
2. Physical and emotional neglect
   a. Failure to thrive; lack of social smile in infant
   b. Lack of hygiene
   c. Frequent injuries; delay in seeking health care
   d. Dull affect; withdrawn
   e. School absences
   f. Enuresis
   g. Suicide attempt
   h. Self-stimulating behaviors
3. Physical abuse
   a. Bruises in various stages of healing
   b. Burns, fractures, lacerations
   c. Fear of parents
   d. Lack of emotion; withdrawal
   e. Aggression

4. Shaken baby syndrome
   a. Poor feeding; vomiting
   b. Bulging fontanels; retinal hemorrhages
   c. Seizures; posturing
   d. Respiratory distress
5. Sexual abuse
   a. Bruising, lacerations, or bleeding of the genitals, anus, or mouth
   b. STI; frequent UTI
   c. Sudden change in behavior or personality; regressive behavior
6. Collaborative Care
   a. **Nursing Interventions**
      1) Identify abuse as soon as possible. Mandatory reporting is required of suspected or actual cases of child abuse.
      2) Do not leave child unattended. Use language the child understands.
      3) Monitor for unusual bruising on abdomen, back, or buttocks.
      4) Document findings objectively. Include diagrams and pictures.
      5) Interview the child and parents separately.
   b. Diagnostic Procedures
      1) Imaging: X-ray, computerized tomography (CT), magnetic resonance imaging (MRI)
      2) Laboratory: CBC, urinalysis, test for sexually transmitted infection

SECTION 3

Adapting Nursing Care for the Child

EXPECTED VITAL SIGNS

Expected reference ranges vary by age and—in some instances—by sex.

Changes in vital signs occur with activity, medication, and illness.

At birth, heart rate and respirations are higher than adults. Blood pressure is lower than adults.

As the child ages, heart rate and respirations decrease and the blood pressure increases.

The data below provides general ranges. The nurse must consider all factors when analyzing findings.

AGE	BLOOD PRESSURE	HEART RATE	RESPIRATORY RATE
0 to 30 days	65 to 75/ 40 to 50 mm Hg	110 to 160/min	30 to 60/min
1 month to 1 year	75 to 100/ 40 to 55 mm Hg	100 to 150/min	30 to 50/min
1 to 2 years	85 to 105/ 40 to 60 mm Hg	90 to 130/min	24 to 40/min
3 to 5 years	90 to 110/ 45 to 70 mm Hg	80 to 110/min	20 to 30/min
6 to 12 years	100 to 120/ 60 to 80 mm Hg	70 to 100/min	18 to 25/min
13 to 18 years	110 to 130/ 60 to 80 mm Hg	55 to 90/min	12 to 20/min

Stress of Hospitalization

A. Families and children can experience major stress. The child's cognitive ability and stage of development influence their response.
B. **Stages of Separation anxiety**
   1. Protest (screaming, physical aggression)
   2. Despair (withdrawal, developmental regression)
   3. Detachment (interacts with strangers, appears happy)
C. **Family Responses**
   1. Fear and guilt
   2. Frustration
   3. Alteration in family roles
   4. Worry (finances, missed work, other children)
D. **Nursing Interventions**
   1. Recognize stress, and intervene as soon as possible.
   2. Consider families of children who are ill as clients.
   3. Reinforce teaching with the child and family about what to expect.
   4. Maintain a routine as much as possible.
   5. Encourage parents or family members to stay with child.
   6. Encourage independence and provide choices.
   7. Explain treatments and procedures.
   8. Provide developmentally appropriate activities.

AGE-RELATED NURSING INTERVENTIONS

AGE	INTERVENTIONS
Infant	Place infants whose parents are not in attendance close to nursing stations so that their needs can be met quickly.
	Provide consistency in assigning caregivers.
Toddler	Provide consistency in assigning caregivers.
	Encourage parents to provide routine care (changing diapers, feeding).
	Encourage the child's autonomy by giving appropriate choices.
Preschooler	Explain all procedures using simple, clear language. Avoid terms that can be misinterpreted by the child.
	Promote independence by encouraging the child to provide self-care.
	Encourage the child to express feelings.
	Validate fears and concerns.
	Provide toys that allow for emotional expression, such as a pounding board to release feelings of protest.
	Give choices when possible, such as "Do you want to take the pink or purple medicine first?"
	Allow younger children to handle equipment if it is safe.
School-age	Provide factual information.
	Encourage the child to express feelings.
	Maintain a normal routine for long hospitalizations, including time for school work.
	Encourage contact with peer group.
Adolescent	Provide factual information.
	Include in the planning of care to relieve feelings of powerlessness and lack of control.
	Encourage contact with peer group.

II Therapeutic Play

A. Purpose

1. Encourages acting out of various feelings
2. Allows the ability to learn coping strategies
3. Assists in gaining cooperation for medical treatment

B. Data Collection

1. Developmental level
2. Motor skills
3. Level of activity tolerance
4. Preferences

C. Nursing Interventions

1. Select safe toys. Encourage parents to bring toys from home. (Consider isolation precautions.)
2. Select activities to enhance development.
3. Observe for clues to fears or anxieties.
4. Use dolls or stuffed animals to demonstrate procedures before they are performed.
5. Allow the child to go to playroom if able.
6. Involve a child life specialist in planning activities.

EFFECT OF HOSPITALIZATION ON CHILDREN

Infant

LEVEL OF UNDERSTANDING	Unable to describe illness and follow directions
	Lacks understanding of the need for therapeutic procedures
EFFECT OF HOSPITALIZATION	Displays physical behaviors as expressions of discomfort due to inability to verbalize
	Exaggerated stranger anxiety (6 to 18 months)
	Can experience sleep deprivation due to strange noises, monitoring devices, and procedures

Toddler

LEVEL OF UNDERSTANDING	Limited ability to describe illness
	Poorly developed sense of body image and boundaries
	Limited understanding of the need for therapeutic procedures
	Limited ability to follow directions
EFFECT OF HOSPITALIZATION	Experiences separation anxiety
	Can have regression of behavior
	Can exhibit an intense reaction to any type of procedure due to the intrusion of boundaries

Preschooler

LEVEL OF UNDERSTANDING	Limited understanding of the cause of illness, but knows what illness feels like
	Limited ability to describe symptoms
	Fears related to magical thinking
EFFECT OF HOSPITALIZATION	Can experience separation anxiety
	Can harbor fears of bodily harm
	Might believe illness and hospitalization are a punishment

EFFECT OF HOSPITALIZATION ON CHILDREN (CONTINUED)

School-age child

LEVEL OF UNDERSTANDING	Beginning awareness of body functioning
	Ability to describe pain
	Increasing ability to understand cause and effect
EFFECT OF HOSPITALIZATION	Fears loss of control
	Seeks information as a way to maintain a sense of control
	Might sense when not being told the truth
	Can experience stress related to separation from peers and regular routine

Adolescent

LEVEL OF UNDERSTANDING	Increasing ability to understand cause and effect
	Perceptions of illness severity are based on the degree of body image changes
EFFECT OF HOSPITALIZATION	Develops body image disturbance
	Attempts to maintain composure, but is embarrassed about losing control
	Experiences feelings of isolation from peers
	Worries about outcome and effect on school/ activities
	Might not adhere to treatments/medication regimen due to peer influence

III Pain Management

A. Assessment of pain depends on cognitive, emotional, and physical development. Children younger than 4 years of age are unable to report pain accurately.

TOOLS USED IN PAIN ASSESSMENT

Faces, Legs, Activity, Cry, and Consolability (FLACC) Pain Tool *2 months to 7 years*	Pain rated on a scale of 0 to 10 Assess behaviors of child. > F: Face > L: Legs > A: Activity > C: Cry > C: Consolability
FACES Pain Rating Scale *3 years and older*	Rating scale uses drawings of happy and sad faces to depict levels of pain. Numeric Scale: 5 years and older Child rates pain on scale of 0 to 5. Can substitute numbers and convert to 0 to 10 scale. Child reports a number or points to level of pain on a visual scale.

TOOLS USED IN PAIN ASSESSMENT (CONTINUED)

Oucher *3 to 13 years old*	Pain rated on a scale of 0 to 5 using six photographs Can substitute numbers and convert to a 0 to 10 scale Child organizes photographs in order of no pain to worst pain and chooses picture that best describes their feeling
Noncommunicating children's pain checklist *3 years and older*	Observe behaviors for 10 min. Score each category using 0 to 3 scale. > Vocal > Social > Facial > Activity > Body and limbs > Physiological

B. **Collaborative Care**

1. **Nursing Interventions**

   a. Use an appropriate pain tool to assess pain. Reassess frequently.

   b. Include parents/provider in the assessment of pain.

   c. Administer medications in a timely manner and evaluate effectiveness.

   d. Include nonpharmacological measures.

      1) Distraction: Play therapy, tell a story

      2) Relaxation: Hold, rock, swaddle, reposition

      3) Imagery: Guide child to use imagination

      4) Behavioral: Stickers, contracts

      5) Sensory: Massage, skin to skin, pacifier

   e. Use treatment room for painful procedures. Allow parents to remain with child.

   f. Use appropriate terminology for developmental level.

   g. Provide choices.

2. Pharmacological Measures

   a. Two-step approach is recommended.

      1) First step: Non-opioid for mild pain in children 3 months of age or older

         a) Nonsteroidal anti-inflammatory drugs are frequently used.

      2) Second step: Strong opioid for moderate or severe pain.

         a) Morphine is the medication of choice.

ANALGESIA FOR CHILDREN

ROUTE	NURSING IMPLICATIONS
Oral	Preferred route Takes 1 to 2 hr to reach peak analgesic effects Not recommended for rapid pain relief or fluctuating pain
Topical/ transdermal	Eutectic mixture of local anesthetics (EMLA) contains equal quantities of lidocaine and prilocaine in the form of a cream or disk. > Use for any procedure in which the skin will be punctured (IV insertion, biopsy) 60 min prior to a superficial puncture and 2½ hr prior to a deep puncture. > Place an occlusive dressing over the cream after application. > Remove the dressing and clean the skin prior to procedure. Reddened or blanched skin indicates an adequate response. > Tap skin to demonstrate to child that skin is not sensitive. > Tell parents to apply at home prior to coming to a health care facility for a procedure. Fentanyl > For children older than 12 years of age > Provides continuous pain control > Onset of 12 to 24 hr and a duration of 72 hr > Can use immediate-release opioid for breakthrough pain > Treat respiratory depression with naloxone
Continuous Intravenous	Provide steady blood levels
Bolus	Rapid pain control in approximately 5 min
Patient-controlled analgesia (PCA)	Self-administration of medication Lockouts prevent overdosing
Family-controlled analgesia	Same concept as PCA Parent or caregiver manages child's pain

IV Safe Medication Administration

A. Growth and organ system maturity affect metabolism and excretion of medications in infants and children. Dosage is based on age, body weight, and body surface area (BSA).

B. **Collaborative Care**

1. **Nursing Interventions**

   a. Calculate the safe dosage. Notify the provider if medication is outside the safe dose range.

   b. Ask a second nurse to verify dosing for high-risk and facility-regulated medications

   c. Follow Rights of Medication Administration.

      1) Use two client identifiers prior to administration: client name and date of birth.

      2) Use parent(s) for verification of infants or nonverbal children.

NOTE: Two identifiers from the ID band must be confirmed (client name, date of birth, hospital identification number).

3) Determine parents' level of involvement with administration.

4) Provide choices (e.g., left vs. right arm).

5) Prepare child according to developmental stage and age.

d. Routes of Medication Administration

1) Aerosol Medications

a) Use a mask for younger children.

2) Oral Medications

a) Place or hold the child in an upright position.

b) Use the smallest measuring device for liquid medication (dropper, dosing syringe, medication cup).

c) Do not use a teaspoon or tablespoon for measuring.

d) Allow the infant to suck medication through a nipple, syringe, or dropper. (Do not mix in a bottle of formula or juice.)

e) Determine ability to swallow pills.

f) Ask the child to hold nose before, during, and after administration.

g) Mix medication in small amount of sweet fluid or food (such as applesauce) or add flavoring.

3) Optic Medications

a) Position the child supine or sitting.

b) Extend the child's head and ask the child to look up.

c) Pull the lower eye lid down and apply medication in the pocket.

d) Administer ointments before nap or bedtime.

e) Apply light pressure to the lacrimal punctum for 1 min (prevents unpleasant taste)

f) Apply medication in the nasal corner if eyes shut tight.

4) Otic Medications (should be at room temperature)

a) Place the child in prone or supine position the with affected ear up.

b) Younger than 3 years of age: Pull pinna down and back.

c) Older than 3 years of age: Pull pinna up and back.

5) Nasal Medications

a) Position the child with head extended. Hold an infant in the football position.

b) Insert tip vertically, then angle prior to administration.

6) Rectal Medications

a) Insert quickly (beyond rectal sphincters).

b) Hold buttocks together for 5 to 10 min.

7) Injections

a) Factors influencing injection sites

(1) Amount and viscosity

(2) Type of medication

(3) Muscle mass (amount, condition)

(4) Frequency and number of medications

(5) Access for contamination risk

8) Intradermal

a) Administer on inside surface of the forearm.

b) Use TB syringe with 26- to 30-gauge needle with intradermal bevel.

c) Insert at 15° angle.

d) Do not aspirate.

9) Subcutaneous (SQ)

a) Common sites: lateral aspect of upper arm, abdomen, anterior thigh

b) Inject volumes less than 0.5 mL.

c) Use 1 mL syringe with 26- to 30-gauge needle.

d) Insert at 90° angle; 45° angle for children who are thin.

10) Intramuscular (IM)

a) Common site: vastus lateralis (infants/small children).

b) Apply EMLA to the site for 60 min prior to injection.

c) Use 22- to 25-gauge, ½- to 1-inch needle (smallest possible).

d) Volume to be injected: 0.5 mL or less for infants; up to 2 mL for children.

e) Identify the need for assistance, and secure the child firmly prior to procedure.

11) Intravenous (IV)

a) Apply EMLA to the site 60 min prior to the procedure.

b) Use 20- to 24-gauge catheter (smallest possible).

c) Use transilluminator.

d) Attach extension tubing.

e) Keep equipment out of sight until ready to use.

f) Avoid using the child's dominant hand, or hand used for sucking.

V Nursing Care of Children: Death and Dying

A. Incorporate physical, psychological, spiritual, and emotional needs.

B. **Palliative care:** Focus is on dying instead of prolonging life when a cure is not available.

1. Nursing: Manage symptoms and provide supportive care.

C. **Hospice care:** Specialized in care of a client who is dying.

1. Nursing: Focus on pain control and comfort. Allow client to die with dignity.

2. Provide support to family who is grieving.

3. Provide honest information regarding prognosis, disease progression, treatment options, and effects of treatments.

4. All health care personnel must be aware of child's and family's decisions.

5. Nurses can experience personal grief during this time.

D. **Types of Grief**

1. Anticipatory: Death is expected or a possible outcome.
2. Complicated: Extends for more than 1 year following the loss.
   a. Intense thoughts
   b. Feelings of loneliness
   c. Distressing yearning, emotions, and feelings
   d. Disturbances in personal activities
   e. Counseling can be required
3. Parental: Intense, long-lasting, and complex
   a. Secondary losses related to absence of hopes and dreams
   b. Differences in maternal and paternal grief

E. **Factors Influencing Grief, Loss, and Coping**

1. Interpersonal relationships and social support
2. Type and significance of loss
3. Culture and ethnicity
4. Spiritual and religious beliefs
5. Prior experience with loss
6. Socioeconomic status

F. **Collaborative Care**

1. **Nursing Interventions**: Children Who Have Terminal Illnesses
   a. Allow an opportunity for anticipatory grieving.
   b. Provide consistency among nursing personnel.
   c. Encourage parents to stay with the client.
   d. Attempt to maintain a normal environment.
   e. Communicate honestly.
   f. Encourage independence.
   g. Stay with the client as much as possible.
   h. Administer analgesics to control pain.
   i. Assist with arranging religious or cultural rituals as requested.
   j. Allow for visitation of family and friends as desired.
   k. Provide opportunities for the client and family to ask questions.
   l. Remain neutral and accepting.
   m. Recognize and support differences in grieving.
   n. Give families privacy.
   o. Encourage discussion of special memories.
2. After death
   a. Allow family to stay with the body as long as they desire.
   b. Allow family to rock or hold the client if desired.
   c. Offer family the option to assist with preparation of the body.
   d. Assist with preparations involving the death ritual.
   e. Encourage parents to prepare the client's siblings for the funeral.
   f. Remain with the family and provide support.
   g. Allow family to share stories about the client's life.
   h. Refer to the client by name.
   i. Allow all family members to communicate feelings.

CHILDREN'S RESPONSE TO DEATH/DYING

AGE	RELEVANT FACTORS
Infants/toddlers (birth to 3 years)	Little to no concept of death
	Egocentric thinking prevents toddlers from understanding death
	Mirror parental emotions (sadness, anger, depression, anxiety)
	Respond according to changes due to hospitalization (change in routine, painful procedures, immobilization, separation)
	Can regress to an earlier stage of behavior
Preschool children (3 to 6 years)	Egocentric thinking
	Magical thinking allows preschoolers to believe thoughts can cause an event such as death; can feel guilt or shame
	Interpret separation from parents as punishment for bad behavior
	View death as temporary
	Lack concept of time (gone to sleep)
School-age children (6 to 12 years)	Start to respond to logical or factual explanations
	Begin to have an adult concept of death (inevitable, irreversible, universal). This generally applies to older school-age children (9 to 12 years).
	Experience fear of the disease process, death process, unknown, and loss of control
	Fear is often displayed through uncooperative behavior.
	Can be curious about funeral services and what happens to the body after death
Adolescents (12 to 20 years)	Adult-like concept of death
	Can have difficulty accepting death because they are discovering who they are, establishing an identity, and dealing with issues of puberty
	Rely more on their peers rather than the influence of their parents, which can cause the reality of a serious illness to make adolescents feel isolated
	Might be unable to relate to peers and communicate with their parents
	Can become more stressed by changes in physical appearance from the medications or illness than the prospect of death
	Can experience guilt and shame

SECTION 4

Nursing Care of the Child Who Has a Congenital Anomaly

A. **Congenital Heart Disease**

1. Contributing Factors
   a. Maternal factors
      1) Infection in early pregnancy
      2) Alcohol or substance use during pregnancy
      3) Diabetes mellitus
   b. Genetic factors
      1) Family history of congenital heart disease
      2) Presence of other congenital anomalies or syndromes

CONGENITAL HEART ANOMALIES

ANOMALY	HEMODYNAMICS	MANIFESTATIONS	TREATMENT
Defects with Increased Pulmonary Blood Flow			
Patent ductus arteriosus Failure of the fetal ductus arteriosus to close within minutes or a few days after birth Defect can vary in size	Blood shunts from aorta to pulmonary artery (left-to-right shunt) Oxygenated blood (aorta) mixes with deoxygenated blood (pulmonary artery)	Respiratory distress Murmur (machine hum) Bounding pulses Widened pulse pressure Poor feeding Asymptomatic or signs of heart failure	Administration of indomethacin Administration of ibuprofen (can be used for premature infants) Insertion of coils to occlude PDA during cardiac catheterization Surgical procedure: Thoracoscopic repair
Ventricular septal defect An abnormal opening in the septum between the left and right ventricle Defect can vary in size	Blood shunts from left to right ventricle and back into pulmonary artery (left-to-right shunt) Oxygenated blood (left ventricle) mixes with deoxygenated blood (right ventricle) and is pumped back into the lungs instead of the body Increased pulmonary vascular resistance Right ventricular hypertrophy Potential enlargement of right atrium	Loud, harsh murmur auscultated at left sternal border Mild cyanosis that increases with crying Heart failure	Closure during cardiac catheterization Surgical procedure > Pulmonary artery banding > Complete repair with patch
Atrial septal defect An abnormal opening in the septum between the left and right atria Defect can vary in size	Blood shunts from left to right atria and flows back to the right side of the heart (left-to-right shunt) Oxygenated blood (left atria) mixes with deoxygenated blood (right atria) and increases total amount of blood that flows toward the lungs Blood is pumped back into the lungs instead of flowing to the left ventricle and to the rest of the body	Can be asymptomatic Can go undiagnosed until school age or adulthood Murmur Shortness of breath with activity Frequent respiratory infections Dysrhythmias Heart palpitations or skipped beats	Closure during cardiac catheterization Surgical procedure: Patch closure
Defects with Decreased Pulmonary Blood Flow			
Tetralogy of Fallot Includes four defects > Pulmonary stenosis > Ventricular septal defect (VSD) > Overriding aorta > Hypertrophy of right ventricle	Left and right ventricle pressures can be equal (because the VSD is usually large) Blood can shunt from left to right or from right to left High pulmonary vascular resistance (right-to-left shunt) High systemic vascular resistance (left-to-right shunt) Decreased blood flow to lungs and the amount of oxygenated blood returning to the left side of the heart (pulmonic stenosis) Each ventricle can distribute blood to the systemic system (depends on the position of the aorta)	Cyanosis and hypoxia (tet spell) Heart sounds vary depending on defect Cardiomegaly Heart failure Systolic murmur	Palliative shunt in infant who cannot undergo primary repair Complete repair within first year
Defects with Mixed Blood Flow			
Transposition of great vessels (TGV) The two main arteries are reversed Aorta exits the right ventricle instead of the left Pulmonary artery originates from the left ventricle instead of the right	No exchange between systemic and pulmonary circulations Aorta exits from right ventricle and carries deoxygenated blood back to the body Pulmonary artery originates from the left ventricle and carries oxygenated blood from the lungs back to the lungs Results in inadequate oxygenated blood in the body A PDA or septal defect must be present for blood to enter the systemic or pulmonary circulation	Cyanosis Heart sounds vary depending on defect Cardiomegaly Heart failure	Intravenous prostaglandin E to keep ductus arteriosus open Balloon atrial septostomy Surgical arterial switch (within first weeks of life) Other surgical procedures depending on defect present

ANOMALY	HEMODYNAMICS	MANIFESTATIONS	TREATMENT
Defects with Obstructive Blood Flow			
Coarctation of the aorta Narrowing of the lumen of the aorta, resulting in obstruction of blood flow from the ventricle	Increased pressure proximal to defect (upper extremities) Decreased pressure distal to defect (lower extremities)	Upper extremities: elevated blood pressure, bounding pulses Lower extremities: decreased blood pressure, weak/absent pulses, cool skin Dizziness Syncope Headache Epistaxis Heart failure	Infants and children: balloon angioplasty Adolescents: placement of stents Surgical procedure: Repair of defect recommended for infants younger than 6 months of age

B. **Heart failure (HF):** Impaired myocardial function

1. Data Collection

   a. Expected Findings

      1) Impaired myocardial function
      2) Sweating
      3) Tachycardia
      4) Pallor
      5) Cool extremities
      6) Weak pulses
      7) Hypotension
      8) Gallop rhythm
      9) Cardiomegaly

   b. Pulmonary congestion

      1) Tachypnea
      2) Dyspnea
      3) Retractions
      4) Nasal flaring
      5) Grunting
      6) Wheezing
      7) Cyanosis
      8) Cough
      9) Orthopnea
      10) Exercise intolerance

   c. Systemic venous congestion

      1) Hepatomegaly
      2) Peripheral edema
      3) Ascites
      4) Neck vein distention
      5) Periorbital edema
      6) Weight gain

2. Collaborative Care

   a. **Nursing Interventions**

      1) Conserve the child's energy.

         a) Frequent rest periods
         b) Cluster care
         c) Small, frequent meals
         d) Bathing PRN
         e) Keep crying to minimum in cyanotic children

      2) Monitor I&O and daily weight.
      3) Allow the child to sleep with several pillows. Maintain semi-Fowler's when awake.
      4) Allow the infant to rest during feedings, taking approximately 30 min to complete the feeding.
      5) Gavage feed the infant as needed. Use a high-calorie formula.
      6) Administer humidified oxygen.
      7) Monitor oxygen saturation every 2 to 4 hr.
      8) Suction airway as needed.
      9) Monitor family coping. Provide support.
      10) Reinforce teaching to the family to report signs of worsening of heart failure (increased sweating, decreased urinary output).

   b. Medications

      1) Digoxin: improves myocardial contractility

         a) Hold if apical pulse is less than 90/min for infants; less than 70/min for children.
         b) Observe for signs of toxicity (bradycardia, poor feeding, nausea, vomiting).
         c) If given as a PO liquid, provide oral care if teeth are present to prevent tooth decay.

      2) Captopril or enalapril
      3) Furosemide or chlorothiazide

C. **Down Syndrome**

1. Most common chromosomal abnormality of a generalized syndrome. Affects growth and development. Cognitive and sensory impairments. Associated with many anomalies.

2. Trisomy 21 seen in 97% of cases.

3. Data Collection

   a. Contributing factors

      1) Exact etiology unknown
      2) Maternal age older than 35 years
      3) Paternal age older than 55 years

   b. Expected Findings

      1) Separated sagittal suture
      2) Enlarged anterior fontanel
      3) Small head
      4) Flattened forehead
      5) Epicanthal folds
      6) Upward, outward slant to eyes

7) Small nose, depressed nasal bridge

8) Small ears

9) High-arched narrow palate

10) Protruding tongue

11) Short, broad neck

12) Shortened rib cage

13) Potential congenital heart defect

14) Protruding abdomen

15) Broad, short feet and hands with stubby toes and fingers

16) Transverse palmer crease

17) Short stature

18) Hyperflexibility, hypotonia, muscle weakness

19) Dry skin that cracks easily

c. Diagnostic Procedures

1) Prenatal: alpha-fetoprotein

2) Chromosome analysis

d. Complications

1) Cognitive impairment: Intelligence varies.

2) Social development: Can be 2 to 3 years beyond mental age. Socializing has strengths.

3) Congenital anomalies: Congenital heart disease (septal defects common), renal agenesis, Hirschsprung's disease, tracheoesophageal fistula, skeletal defects

4) Sensory: Strabismus, excessive tearing, cataracts, hearing problems

5) Other medical conditions: Upper respiratory infections, thyroid dysfunction, increased risk of leukemia

6) Growth: Reduced height and weight; prone to obesity

7) Sexual development: Delayed or incomplete

> **NOTE:** Feeding strategies for child who has Down Syndrome (to accommodate protruding tongue)
> › Use small, long, straight-handled spoon.
> › Push food toward the back and side of mouth.
> › Refeed food if thrust out.

4. Collaborative Care

a. **Nursing Interventions**

1) Support family at time of diagnosis.

2) Facilitate bonding. Assist with holding.

a) Wrap tightly in a blanket prior to picking up infant (hypotonicity).

3) Manage secretions (nasal aspiration, vaporizer, postural drainage).

4) Evaluate and monitor the following.

a) Eyesight and hearing

b) Thyroid function

c) Height and weight

d) Developmental milestones

5) Monitor for atlantoaxial instability (neck pain, weakness, torticollis).

a) Make appropriate referrals (social work, home health, school, genetic counseling, speech therapy, physical therapy, occupational therapy).

D. **Club Foot**

1. Also known as talipes equinovarus. Deformity of the ankle and foot involving bone deformity, malpositioning, and soft tissue contracture.

2. Data Collection

a. Contributing Factors

1) Positional (intrauterine crowding)

2) Presence of other disorders (cerebral palsy)

3) Heredity

4) Idiopathic

b. Expected Findings

1) Toes are turned inward, lower than the heel.

2) Portions of the foot can turn sideways or upward.

3) Limited motion and flexibility of ankle.

4) Affected foot is usually smaller and shorter.

5) If unilateral, the affected extremity is often shorter and atrophy of the calf is present.

c. Diagnostic Procedures

1) Prenatal ultrasound

2) Visible at birth if not detected prenatally

3) Hip examination (increased risk of hip dysplasia)

3. Therapeutic Procedures

a. Serial casting shortly after birth with weekly stretching of foot muscles until maximum correction is achieved

b. Placement of serial long-leg cast

c. Surgical: Percutaneous heel cord tenotomy usually performed, followed by a long-leg cast for 3 weeks

d. A Denis Browne bar and specialized shoes can be applied to maintain correction and prevent recurrence.

4. Collaborative Care

a. **Nursing Interventions**

1) Encourage parents to hold and cuddle the child.

2) Monitor and maintain the cast or corrective device.

3) Monitor neurovascular status and skin integrity.

b. Client Education

1) Reinforce teaching to the family about the importance of regular cast changes.

2) Provide information about care of the cast or corrective device.

3) Report potential complications (skin breakdown, alteration in circulation).

4) Encourage activities to promote normal growth and development.

E. **Developmental Dysplasia of the Hip (DDH)**

1. Abnormal development of hip structures: Can develop during fetal life, infancy, or childhood
2. Acetabular dysplasia: Delay in acetabular development.
3. Subluxation: Incomplete dislocation of femoral head
4. Dislocation: Femoral head loses contact with acetabulum
5. Contributing Factors
   a. Family history, sex, birth order, intrauterine position, laxity of a joint
   b. Intrauterine placement, mechanical situations (size of infant, multiple births, breech presentation), genetic factors

NOTE: Increased incidence when infants are wrapped tightly or strapped to cradle boards. Decreased incidence when mothers carry infants on their backs with legs widely abducted.

6. Expected Findings
   a. Newborn
      1) Asymmetry of gluteal and thigh folds
      2) Limited hip abduction
      3) Positive Ortolani test
      4) Positive Barlow test
   b. Child
      1) Affected leg is shorter
      2) Positive Trendelenburg sign
      3) Walks on toes on one foot
      4) Walks with a limp
7. Diagnostic Procedures
   a. Ultrasound: Should be performed at 2 weeks of age to determine the cartilaginous head of the femur
   b. X-ray: Can diagnose DDH in infants older than 4 months
8. Therapeutic Procedures
   a. Treatment varies with age and severity of findings. Initiate early for best outcomes.
9. Nonsurgical Interventions
   a. Pavlik harness
   b. Hip abduction braces
   c. Bryant traction (skin)
   d. Hip spica cast
10. Surgical Interventions
    a. Closed or closed reduction
    b. Osteotomy (pelvic, femur)
    c. Tenotomy

KEY POINT: The Barlow and Ortolani maneuvers should be performed only by an experienced clinician to prevent injury to the infant's hip.

11. Collaborative Care
    a. **Nursing Interventions**
       1) Encourage holding.
       2) Promote growth and development.
       3) Pavlik harness
          a) Maintain harness placement.
          b) Check straps every 1 to 2 weeks for adjustment.
          c) Monitor neurovascular status and skin integrity.
       4) Bryant traction (skin)
          a) Maintain alignment.
          b) Monitor neurovascular status, skin integrity, and pain.
          c) Maintain traction.
       5) Hip spica cast
          a) Change frequently to accommodate growth.
          b) Position cast on pillows. Handle with palms of hands until dry.
          c) Monitor neurovascular status, skin integrity, and pain.
          d) Turn and position. Provide range of motion of unaffected extremities.
          e) Monitor nutrition and hydration.
          f) Apply waterproof barrier around genital opening of cast to prevent soiling.
12. Client Education and Referrals
    a. Keep the Pavlik harness on continuously, except during bathing, if prescribed.
    b. Return for follow-up visits weekly at the start of therapy and then as needed.
    c. Monitor and report complications.
    d. Reinforce skin care (specific to procedure).
    e. Hold and cuddle the child.
    f. Meet the developmental needs of the child.
    g. Reinforce teaching regarding care after discharge with emphasis on using appropriate equipment (stroller, wagon, car seat) for maintaining mobility.

F. **Spina Bifida**

1. Failure of the osseous spine to close.
2. Neural tube defects (NTDs) are present at birth (might not be visible).
3. Spina bifida occulta: Protruding sac is not visible.
4. Spina bifida cystica: Protruding sac is visible.
   a. Meningocele: Sac contains spinal fluid and meninges.
   b. Myelomeningocele: Sac includes spinal fluid, meninges, and nerves.
5. Contributing Factors
   a. Maternal factors: Medications/substances taken during pregnancy, malnutrition, insufficient intake of folic acid during pregnancy, exposure to radiation or chemicals during pregnancy
   b. Genetics
   c. Presence of other syndrome or congenital anomaly

6. Expected Findings

 a. Spina bifida occulta
  1) Dimpling in lumbosacral area
  2) Port wine angioma
  3) Dark tufts of hair
  4) Subcutaneous lipoma

 b. Spina bifida cystica
  1) Protruding sac midline of the osseous spine
  2) Other findings vary widely depending on location of defect
  3) Flaccid, lower extremity paralysis
  4) Sensory deficits
  5) Urinary incontinence (dribbling)
  6) Bowel incontinence
  7) Prolapsed rectum
  8) Club foot, kyphosis, hip dislocation, or other skeletal defects

7. Diagnostic Procedures

 a. Prenatal: Ultrasound, amniocentesis
 b. Infants: MRI, ultrasound, CT scan

8. Therapeutic Procedures

 a. Surgical repair

9. Collaborative Care

 a. Interprofessional Care: Neurosurgery, neurology, urology, orthopedics, physical therapy, nutrition, occupational therapy, social services

 b. **Nursing Interventions**
  1) Initial care/Preoperative
   a) Protect the sac.
    (1) Place prone in infant warmer with hips flexed, legs abducted (without clothing).
    (2) Place sterile, moist, nonadhering dressing with 0.9% sodium chloride to sac. Change the dressing every 2 hr.
    (3) Avoid applying any pressure to the sac.
    (4) Monitor neurological status (head circumference, fontanels, cry, suck, movement, sensory).
    (5) Inspect sac for leaks, irritation, and signs of infection.
    (6) Maintain strict I&O. (Intermittent catheterization can be required.)
    (7) Obtain laboratory specimens as prescribed.
    (8) Administer IV antibiotics as prescribed.
    (9) Avoid rectal temperatures.
    (10) No diapering until defect is repaired and healed.
    (11) Monitor and promote infant–parent bonding.
    (12) Prepare infant and family for surgical procedure.

  b) Postoperative
   (1) Maintain prone position until other positions are prescribed.
   (2) Monitor neurological status (head circumference, fontanels, cry, suck, movement, sensory).
   (3) Monitor incision site and provide care (CSF leakage/infection).
   (4) Monitor I&O.
   (5) Intermittent catheterization can be required.
   (6) Resume oral feedings.
   (7) Provide range of motion to extremities.
   (8) Administer pain medication as prescribed.

  c) Complications
   (1) Skin ulceration
   (2) Latex allergy
   (3) Increased intracranial pressure
   (4) Shunt malfunction, infection, or hydrocephalus
   (5) Bladder dysfunction
   (6) Orthopedic issues

NOTE: Think BACK. Latex allergy is linked to certain foods: Bananas, Avocado, Chestnuts, Kiwi.

  c. Client Education
   1) Assist family with obtaining medical equipment/services needed at home.
   2) Provide postoperative education (incision care, signs of infection, medications, skin care, repositioning, range of motion exercises, findings to report to provider, activities to promote growth and development).
   3) Inform parents of an increased risk for latex allergy and strategies to reduce exposure.
   4) Provide list of common household items and foods that can contain latex.
   5) Reinforce teaching about signs of an allergic reaction (urticaria, wheezing, anaphylaxis).
   6) Demonstrate how to administer epinephrine and when to call 911.
   7) Demonstrate how to measure head circumference and palpate fontanel.
   8) Discuss signs of increased intracranial pressure and when to notify provider.
   9) Inform parents of an increased risk for bladder dysfunction (spasms or flaccidity); to monitor urine for foul odor, blood, or other signs of infection; and how to perform intermittent catheterization.
   10) Reinforce teaching about care of a shunt, cast, splint, or stoma (vesicostomy).

G. **Cerebral Palsy**

1. Nonprogressive, but permanent impairment of motor function affecting muscle control, coordination, and posture (spastic, dyskinetic, ataxic). Most common permanent physical disability of childhood. Can involve alterations in sensation, perception, communication, cognition, and behavior. Wide range of intelligence (50% to 60% is within normal limits).

2. Data Collection

   a. Contributing Factors
      1) Exact cause unknown.
      2) Can include prenatal, perinatal, and postnatal factors.

   b. Expected Findings
      1) Vary depending on type of CP
      2) Delayed gross motor development; failure to meet developmental milestones
      3) Abnormal motor performance
         a) Abnormal or asymmetrical crawl
         b) Stands or walks on toes; ataxia
         c) Involuntary movements (facial grimacing, writhing movements of tongue)
         d) Poor sucking and difficulty feeding
         e) Persistent tongue thrust
         f) Alterations in muscle tone
         g) Increased or decreased resistance to passive movements
         h) Poor head control
         i) Exaggerated arching of back
         j) Abnormal posture
         k) Persistence of primitive reflexes (Moro, plantar, palmar grasp, hyperreflexia, ankle clonus)

3. Diagnostic Procedures
   a. Complete neurological assessment
   b. Metabolic and genetic testing
   c. General movements assessment (children older than 2 years and younger than 5 years of age)

4. MRI

5. Collaborative Care

   a. **Nursing Interventions**
      1) Adapt interventions/communication according to child's developmental level.
      2) Communicate with the child directly. Include parents as needed.
      3) Keep head of bed elevated (especially for increased amount of oral secretions).
      4) Ensure suction is available. Suction oral secretions as needed.
      5) Identify risk for aspiration. Implement precautions.
      6) Implement safety precautions. (Pad side rails and arms of wheelchair.)
      7) Provide pulmonary hygiene.
      8) Ensure adequate nutrition. Administer gastrostomy feedings if applicable.
      9) Position correctly for feeding (head positioning/manual jaw control methods as needed).
      10) Provide high-calorie milk products for children 1 year or older.
      11) Provide diet high in fruit and fiber (prevents constipation).
      12) Monitor for pain/muscle spasms and administer medications as prescribed.
      13) Provide skin care. (Monitor skin. Turn frequently. Keep skin dry.)
      14) Monitor growth and development.
      15) Determine need for speech and hearing evaluation or other referrals.
      16) Incorporate family in plan of care.
      17) Determine family coping and support and evaluate need for respite care.

   b. Medications
      1) Baclofen: Skeletal muscle relaxant
      2) Diazepam
      3) Botulinum toxin A: Used primarily for spasticity in lower extremities
      4) Antiepileptics: Control seizure activity

   c. Therapeutic Measures
      1) Physical therapy (braces, splints, wheelchair)
      2) Occupational therapy (utensils for eating and writing)
      3) Speech-language therapy (oral-motor skills, adaptive communication techniques)
      4) Special education (early intervention programs)
      5) Behavioral therapy
      6) Can include gastrostomy, tenotomy, procedures to correct orthopedic and or dental problems.

   d. Client Education and Referrals
      1) Emphasize the need for frequent rest periods.
      2) Review feeding schedule and feeding techniques if changes were made during hospitalization.
      3) Provide information regarding expected responses, side effects, and adverse reactions to medications.
      4) Reinforce teaching about pulmonary hygiene techniques.
      5) Discuss measures to prevent skin breakdown.
      6) Encourage clients to adhere to immunization schedule.
      7) Encourage parents to provide a stimulating environment and incorporate therapeutic measures into daily activities. (Adapt environment for safety.)

   e. Complications
      1) Visual and hearing impairment
      2) Behavioral disorder
      3) Difficulty with speech and communication
      4) Cognitive impairment
      5) Orthopedic (scoliosis, hip dislocation)
      6) Nystagmus/amblyopia
      7) Otitis media
      8) Seizures

H. **Congenital Gastrointestinal Disorders**
   1. **Hypertrophic pyloric stenosis**
      a. Description and Contributing Factors
         1) Thickening of the pyloric sphincter, which causes an obstruction
         2) Most common within first 5 weeks of life
      b. Manifestations
         1) Projectile vomiting after feeding or intermittently
         2) Constant hunger
         3) Palpable olive-shaped mass in right upper abdominal quadrant
         4) No evidence of pain
         5) Possible peristaltic wave moving left to right when lying supine
         6) Signs of dehydration (sunken fontanel, no tears, decreased wet diapers, dry mouth)
         7) Failure to gain weight
      c. Diagnostic Procedures
         1) Abdominal ultrasound shows elongated mass surrounding pyloric area.
      d. **Nursing Interventions**
         1) Preoperative
            a) Monitor vital signs.
            b) Monitor for signs of dehydration.
            c) Administer IV fluids (corrects electrolyte imbalances).
            d) Insert NG tube (decompression).
            e) Maintain NPO status.
            f) Maintain strict I&O.
         2) Postoperative
            a) Monitor vital signs.
            b) Administer IV fluids.
            c) Maintain strict I&O.
            d) Monitor daily weights.
            e) Monitor for signs of infection.
            f) Clear liquid diet 4 to 6 hr after surgery. Advance to breast milk or formula as tolerated.
            g) Document tolerance to feedings (can have some vomiting during the first 24 to 48 hr after surgery).
      e. Medications
         1) Analgesics
      f. Therapeutic Measures
         1) Surgical: Laparoscopic pyloromyotomy
         2) Temporary colostomy can be required.
      g. Client Education and Referrals
         1) Report any signs of infection or intolerance of feedings.

   2. **Hirschsprung's disease (congenital aganglionic megacolon)**
      a. Description and Contributing Factors
         1) Occurs when a section of the colon is aganglionic, resulting in decreased motility and obstruction
      b. Manifestations
         1) **Newborn:** Failure to pass meconium within 24 to 48 hr, refusal to eat, episodes of vomiting bile, abdominal distention
         2) **Infant:** Failure to thrive, constipation, abdominal distention, episodes of vomiting and diarrhea
         3) **Older child:** Constipation, abdominal distention, visible peristalsis, ribbon-like stool, palpable fecal mass, malnourished appearance
      c. Diagnostic Procedures
         1) Rectal biopsy to confirm absence of ganglionic cells
      d. **Nursing Interventions**
         1) Preoperative
            a) If malnourished, provide high-protein, high-calorie, low-fiber diet. TPN can be required.
            b) Monitor for manifestations of enterocolitis or bowel perforation.
            c) Administer IV fluids.
            d) Bowel prep with saline enemas.
         2) Postoperative
            a) Monitor surgical site.
            b) Monitor bowel sounds and bowel function.
            c) Monitor for irregular passage of stool (constipation, incontinence).
      e. Medications
         1) Analgesics
         2) Antibiotics
      f. Therapeutic Measures
         1) Surgical removal of aganglionic section of bowel
         2) Temporary colostomy can be required.
      g. Client Education and Referrals
         1) Reinforce wound care and colostomy care if applicable.
         2) Monitor for signs of infection.
         3) Monitor for complications after discharge (enterocolitis, fecal incontinence, obstruction).
         4) Reinforce teaching to parents how to perform daily anal dilations (if required).
         5) Monitor for manifestations of dehydration.

   3. **Intussusception**
      a. Description and Contributing Factors
         1) The telescoping of the intestine upon itself
         2) Can progress to ischemia
         3) Common in infants and children 3 months to 6 years old

b. Manifestations

    1) Intervals of sudden abdominal pain; appears normal between episodes

    2) Empty lower right quadrant (Dance sign)

    3) Palpable, sausage-shaped mass in the right upper quadrant of the abdomen and/or a tender, distended abdomen

    4) Stools that are mixed with blood and mucus that resemble the consistency of red currant jelly

c. Diagnostic Procedures

    1) Ultrasonography

    2) Rectal examination reveals mucus and blood

d. **Nursing Interventions**

    1) Preoperative

       a) Maintain NPO status.

       b) Administer IV fluids (correct and prevent dehydration).

       c) Insert NG tube (decompression).

       d) Monitor stools.

    2) Postoperative

       a) Observe for passage of water-soluble contrast (if used).

       b) Monitor incision if surgery is required.

       c) Monitor stool patterns (intussusception can recur).

! Point to Remember

Passage of normal brown stool usually indicates intussusception has resolved itself. Report immediately; diagnostic and therapeutic procedures can be altered.

e. Medications

    1) Antibiotics as prescribed

f. Therapeutic Measures

    1) Air enema (with or without contrast) performed by radiologist

    2) Ultrasound-guided hydrostatic (saline) enema

    3) Surgery, if enema is unsuccessful

g. Client Education and Referrals

    1) Monitor stools and for manifestations of intussusception.

4. **Cleft lip (CL) and cleft palate (CP)**

a. Description and Contributing Factors

    1) Cleft lip results from incomplete fusion of the oral cavity during intrauterine life.

    2) Cleft palate results from incomplete fusion of the palatine plates during intrauterine life.

    3) Contributing factors: family history; exposure to alcohol, cigarette smoke, anticonvulsants, or steroids during pregnancy; deficiency of folate during pregnancy.

b. Manifestations

    1) Cleft lip is visible at birth.

    2) Cleft palate can be detected by visual inspection of oral cavity or by palpating the hard and soft palate with a gloved finger.

c. Diagnostic Procedures

    1) Cleft lip and cleft palate can be diagnosed prior to birth by routine ultrasound.

d. **Nursing Interventions**

    1) Preoperative

       a) Evaluate and promote bonding.

       b) Inspect lip. Palpate palate using gloved finger.

       c) Monitor ability to suck.

       d) Refer to lactation consultant/social services.

       e) Inform parents that noisy feeding is common and not a sign of choking.

       f) Tell parents to observe for facial sign that indicates feeding should be stopped briefly (raised eyebrows, wrinkled forehead, watery eyes).

       g) Cleft lip

         (1) Encourage breastfeeding.

         (2) Use wide-base nipple for bottle feeding and squeeze cheeks together to decrease width of cleft.

       h) Cleft palate or cleft lip and palate

         (1) Position the infant upright while cradling head during feeding.

         (2) Use modified bottles/feeders (one-way flow valve, squeezable bottles).

         (3) Use wide or long nipples with a cut slit.

         (4) Burp the infant after every ounce.

         (5) Transition to cup feeding prior to CP repair.

    2) Postoperative: Cleft Lip

       a) Maintain airway.

       b) Obtain vital signs.

       c) Major goal: Protect the site.

       d) Avoid prone position. Position upright in infant seat.

       e) Apply elbow restraints immediately after surgery (varies by surgeon).

       f) Monitor and supervise closely to prevent damage to sutures (fingers in mouth).

       g) Administer pain medication.

       h) Clean suture line using cotton-tip applicator. Saline, water, or diluted hydrogen peroxide can be used.

       i) Apply thin layer of antibiotic ointment to suture line.

    3) Postoperative: Cleft Palate

       a) Administer oxygen (usually by face mask).

       b) Position to prevent airway obstruction. The client can be placed on the abdomen in the immediate postoperative period.

       c) Observe closely for signs of airway obstruction, hemorrhage, and laryngeal spasm.

d) Report croup, stridor, difficulty breathing, or frequent swallowing.

e) Monitor pain. Administer medications.

f) Clear liquids for 24 hr; liquid diet for 2 weeks.

g) Use open cup for liquids.

h) Avoid placing suction catheters, pacifiers, tongue depressors, rigid spoons, straws, or hard-tipped sippy cups in the mouth.

i) Apply elbow restraints.

j) Remove restraints to allow movement. (Supervise closely.)

e. Medications

1) Analgesics

2) Antibiotics

f. Therapeutic Measures

1) Cleft lip repair typically performed between 2 and 3 months

2) Cleft palate repair typically performed between 6 and 12 months

g. Client Education and Referrals

1) Discuss proper feeding techniques.

2) Reinforce teaching with parents how to clean incision.

3) Monitor the operative site for infection, bleeding, or crusting.

4) Discuss proper positioning for sleep.

5) Discuss the proper use of restraints.

Nursing Care of the Child Who Has an Acute Condition

A. **Gastrointestinal Disorders**

1. **Acute Gastrointestinal Infections**

    a. Contributing Factors

    1) Age: The younger the child, the more susceptible and serious the condition

    2) Underlying poor health: Malnutrition, Immunocompromised

    3) Environment: Crowding, poor sanitation, lack of access to clean water

    4) Lack of knowledge: Poor food preparation and storage, inadequate hand hygiene

    5) Can be exacerbated by antibiotic and other medication therapies

    b. Expected Findings

    1) Diarrhea

    2) Vomiting

    3) Malaise

    4) Fever

    5) Poor appetite

    6) Dehydration

    7) Weight loss

    8) Stool examination; culture positive for ova, parasites, or bacteria

    9) Enzyme-linked immunosorbent assay (ELISA) positive for rotavirus or giardia

CROUP SYNDROMES

	Acute Epiglottitis	Acute Laryngotracheal Bronchitis	Acute Spasmodic Laryngitis
ETIOLOGY	Bacterial, usually *H. influenzae*	Viral (RSV, influenza A, B) *Mycoplasma pneumonia*; measles; parainfluenza types 1, 2, 3	Viral Possibly allergy-related
AGE MOST AFFECTED	2 to 5 years old	Infant, child younger than 2 years old	1 to 3 years old
ONSET	Progresses rapidly	Gradual onset of symptoms	Child goes to bed well; "midnight" or "twilight" croup awakens child
EXPECTED FINDINGS	Stridor, drooling, tripod position (chin pointing out, mouth opened, tongue protruding), high fever, dysphagia, dyspnea, muffled, frog-like voice, tachypnea, tachycardia	Inspiratory stridor, barking, brassy cough, hoarseness, restlessness, irritability, substernal retractions, low-grade fever Symptoms are usually worse at night.	Wakes suddenly with dyspnea, barking, metallic cough, stridor, hoarseness, restlessness Symptoms disappear during the day; recurrent
THERAPEUTIC PROCEDURES AND MEDICATIONS	MEDICAL EMERGENCY Possible intubation, tracheostomy, lateral neck radiograph, corticosteroids, humidified O_2, IV fluids Antibiotics (droplet precautions for first 24 hr after IV antibiotics initiated) Child is very frightened	Cool air (take outside)/cool mist for mild croup Steroids, oral/IV fluids, nebulized racemic epinephrine as prescribed Nebulized budesonide	Cool mist, steroids, racemic epinephrine, supportive care
NURSING INTERVENTIONS	Encourage position of comfort. Droplet isolation. Provide calm reassurance to child and caregiver. Monitor O_2 status. Ensure intubation equipment is at bedside. DO NOT put anything in the mouth (tongue depressor, culture swab).	Frequently monitor VS including pulse oximetry. Be alert to signs of impending respiratory obstruction (tachypnea, tachycardia, retractions, nasal flaring, restlessness). Encourage caregiver to stay with and hold child to calm. Provide reassurance.	Usually managed at home Cool mist vaporizer Encourage quiet activity

c. Laboratory Tests and Diagnostic Procedures
   1) Stool examination for blood, ova, parasites
   2) Stool culture for bacteria
   3) ELISA for rotavirus, giardia
   4) CBC
   5) Electrolytes
d. Therapeutic Procedures and Medications
   1) Antimicrobials (antibiotic, antiparasitic)
   2) Antipyretics
   3) Antiemetics if unable to tolerate anything orally

> **NOTE:** Older antiemetics (promethazine, metoclopramide) should not be routinely administered to children due to the potential for adverse effects (somnolence, nervousness, irritability, dystonic reactions).

   4) IV fluids only if unable to tolerate oral fluids
e. **Nursing Interventions**
   1) Provide oral rehydration therapy. Administer 5 to 10 mL every 1 to 5 min. Vomiting is not a contraindication unless severe.
   2) After rehydration, alternate with water, breast milk, and lactose-free formula.
   3) Reintroduce a normal diet as soon as possible (lessens severity of illness and improves weight gain).
   4) Weigh the client daily. Weight is the best indicator of fluid gains and losses.
   5) Monitor electrolytes, blood glucose, and acid-base status.
   6) Carefully monitor intake and output.
   7) Do not measure temperature rectally.
   8) If hospitalization is required, give nothing by mouth. Prepare to administer parenteral fluids.
f. Client Education
   1) Observe for signs of dehydration by counting wet diapers and voiding. Seek medical attention if dehydration is suspected (especially for infants) due to the risk for hypovolemia shock.
   2) Reinforce the importance of hand hygiene, proper food storage, and clean water.

GASTROINTESTINAL INFECTIONS OF CHILDREN

MANIFESTATIONS	TRANSMISSION
Escherichia coli (E. coli)	*bacterial*
Watery, then bloody diarrhea Abdominal cramping Can develop hemolytic uremic syndrome	Contaminated food (beef, milk, fresh produce), water Person to person
Clostridium difficile (C. diff)	*bacterial*
Mild, watery diarrhea Can develop pseudomembranous colitis	Associated with alteration in normal intestinal flora by antibiotics
Salmonella	*bacterial*
Mild to severe nausea and vomiting Abdominal cramping Bloody diarrhea	Undercooked meat, eggs, poultry Person to person

GASTROINTESTINAL INFECTIONS OF CHILDREN (CONTINUED)

MANIFESTATIONS	TRANSMISSION
Enterobius vermicularis (pinworm)	*helminthic*
Perianal itching Enuresis	Fecal-oral
Giardia lamblia	*parasitic*
Diarrhea Greasy stools Abdominal cramping Vomiting Anorexia	Contaminated food, water, animals Person to person
Rotavirus	*viral*
Most common cause of diarrhea in children younger than 5 years	
Mild-moderate fever	Often nosocomial
Vomiting followed by watery diarrhea	Fecal-oral

> **KEY POINT:** Fruit juice, carbonated drinks, gelatin, caffeine, broth, and sports drinks do not help diarrhea and vomiting. A BRAT (bananas, rice, applesauce, toast) diet is also contraindicated. All have low nutritional value and can disrupt electrolyte balance.

2. **Hyperbilirubinemia**
   a. Bilirubin is a byproduct of the breakdown of red blood cells. When the immature liver is unable to process bilirubin for excretion, excessive amounts accumulate (primarily in sclera, nails, and skin), manifesting as jaundice.
   b. Contributing Factors
      1) Prematurity
      2) Breastfeeding
      3) Liver compromise
      4) Mother who has diabetes
      5) Native American or Asian descent
      6) Birth injury that causes bruising or hematoma
      7) Decreased intake
      8) Hereditary hemolytic disease
      9) Sibling who has a history of hyperbilirubinemia
      10) Exclusive breastfeeding with excessive weight loss
      11) Rh-negative mother
   c. Expected Findings
      1) Jaundice in sclera, nails, or skin, occurring when unconjugated bilirubin levels exceed 5 mg/dL
   d. Laboratory Tests and Diagnostic Procedures
      1) Serum bilirubin
      2) Coombs (direct, indirect)
      3) Transcutaneous bilirubinometry
   e. Therapeutic Procedures and Medications
      1) Phototherapy
      2) Exchange transfusion for dangerously high bilirubin levels
      3) Immunoglobulin if caused by blood incompatibility
      4) Tin-mesoporphyrin (prevents bilirubin formation)

f. **Nursing Interventions**

1) Regularly observe for jaundice by blanching skin over bony prominences, observing sclera, mucous membranes, and nails.

2) Monitor color in natural daylight.

3) Obtain transcutaneous bilirubinometry readings (not accurate if neonate is under phototherapy).

4) Weigh the client daily.

5) Monitor voiding and stooling.

6) Monitor feeding patterns and hydration.

7) Initiate breastfeeding within 1 hr of birth.

8) Encourage rooming in.

9) For infants under phototherapy

   a) Expose as much skin as possible to light.

   b) Ensure that an opaque mask is in place over the infant's eyes. Remove the mask when the infant is taken out from under lights.

   c) Monitor for temperature instability.

g. Client Education

1) Reinforce the importance of adequate intake.

2) Leave the infant under the lights as much as possible, with mask in place.

3) Explain how to monitor for jaundice and to notify the provider if it worsens.

4) Explain the importance of monitoring urinary and stool output.

TYPES OF HYPERBILIRUBINEMIA OF THE NEWBORN

Physiologic Jaundice

CAUSE	Immature liver function Increased bilirubin load from increased number of RBCs in the newborn
ONSET	After first 24 hr
DURATION	Decreases 5th to 7th day
THERAPY	Increase feeding frequency. Monitor stool. Use phototherapy for significant increase in bilirubin.

Breastfeeding Jaundice

CAUSE	Decreased intake before mother's breast milk comes in Infrequent stooling
ONSET	3rd to 5th day
DURATION	Varies
THERAPY	Frequent breastfeeding No supplements (can decrease breast milk production) Phototherapy for significant increase in bilirubin

Hemolytic Disease

CAUSE	ABO or Rh blood incompatibility
ONSET	First 24 hr Bilirubin levels increase more than 5mg/dL/day
DURATION	Depends on severity
THERAPY	Immunoglobulin, tin-mesoporphyrin, exchange transfusion Encourage mother to pump and store breast milk for future feeding. Rh$_0$(D) immune globulin to prevent Rh incompatibility

3. **Acute Appendicitis**

a. Inflammation of the vermiform appendix caused by obstruction due to fecalith (hardened stool is most common), inflamed lymphoid tissue following a viral infection, or a parasite

b. Contributing Factors

1) Age: peak incidence is 10 years old

2) Recent viral infection

3) Intestinal helminth infection

c. Expected Findings

1) Focal abdominal tenderness in the periumbilical area, progressing to right lower quadrant

   a) McBurney's point, located two-thirds the distance between the umbilicus and anterosuperior iliac spine

   b) Rovsing's sign: tenderness in the right lower quadrant that occurs during palpation or percussion of other abdominal quadrants

2) Nausea, vomiting, anorexia, poor feeding

3) Diarrhea or constipation

4) Lethargy

5) Pain in right hip when walking

6) Low-grade fever (38° C [100.4° F])

7) Decreased or absent bowel sounds

8) Tachypnea, tachycardia

9) Rigid abdomen

10) If perforation occurs

   a) Sudden relief from pain, followed by an increase

   b) Temperature elevations of 38.9 to 39.4° C (102 to 103° F), chills

   c) Progressive abdominal distention

   d) Tachycardia, tachypnea

   e) Pallor

d. Laboratory Tests and Diagnostic Procedures

1) Complete blood count (white cell count greater than 10,000 mm^3 and elevated C-reactive protein are common, but not specific)

2) Urinalysis

3) Computerized tomography

4) Ultrasound

e. **Unruptured Appendix**

1) Therapeutic Procedures and Medications

   a) IV fluids

   b) IV antibiotics

   c) Electrolyte replacement

   d) Laparoscopic incisions to surgically remove the appendix

   e) Analgesics

2) **Nursing Interventions**

  a) Review pain assessment and continue to monitor. Tell the child to point to the area of pain. Note change in activity

  b) Prepare the child for surgery. Ensure consent forms have been signed.

  c) Monitor vital signs.

  d) Maintain NPO status.

  e) Maintain bed rest until surgery. Allow child to assume position of comfort.

  f) Avoid applying heat to the abdomen.

  g) Monitor bowel sounds. Palpation should be very gentle.

  h) After surgery, monitor oxygen status, vital signs, and level of consciousness. Administer oxygen as needed.

  i) Monitor and provide incision care as prescribed.

  j) Monitor abdomen for distention. Monitor for passage of flatus and stool.

  k) Administer analgesics as needed.

  l) Encourage early ambulation.

  m) Provide a small pillow or stuffed animal for abdominal support.

3) Client Education

  a) Reinforce teaching about incision care.

  b) Monitor for signs of infection.

f. **Ruptured Appendix**

1) Therapeutic Procedures

  a) IV fluids, antibiotics, electrolytes

  b) NG suction

  c) Surgery (wound may be left open or closed)

  d) Analgesics

2) **Nursing Interventions** are the same as for unruptured, plus the following.

  a) After surgery, provide wound care and irrigation as prescribed. Note the quantity and character of drainage.

  b) Maintain NG to low, intermittent suction.

  c) Administer analgesics on a routine schedule for the first few days after surgery.

  d) Ambulate in room. Sit in a chair at least three times per day.

  e) Due to emergent nature of surgery, encourage child and parents to express feelings and ask questions.

KEY POINT: Never administer laxatives or enemas to anyone exhibiting severe abdominal pain. These can increase risk of perforation.

4. **Necrotizing Enterocolitis**

a. Acute inflammatory disease related to ischemia of the bowel, immature GI defenses, and bacterial proliferation; causes devastating damage to the bowel wall which results in tissue death. Onset is usually 4 to 10 days after feedings are initiated.

b. Contributing Factors

  1) Prematurity

  2) Neonate who has complications (respiratory distress, birth asphyxia, shock, polycythemia, infection)

  3) Intrauterine growth restriction

  4) Neonate who has received an exchange transfusion and/or enteral feedings

c. Expected Findings

  1) Abdominal distension

  2) Lethargy

  3) High gastric residuals

  4) Apnea that worsens

  5) Hypotension

  6) Anemia

  7) Metabolic acidosis

  8) Leukopenia, leukocytosis

  9) Electrolyte imbalance

  10) Sausage-shaped dilation of the intestine

  11) Pneumatosis (bubbly appearance of thickened bowel wall)

  12) Bloody stools

  13) Bile-stained emesis

  14) Hypothermia

  15) Decreased urinary output

d. Laboratory Tests and Diagnostic Procedures

  1) Abdominal radiography

  2) CBC

  3) Arterial blood gases

  4) Blood culture

  5) Electrolyte panel

e. Therapeutic Procedures and Medications

  1) Prevent by withholding feedings for 24 to 48 hr for any neonate who has experienced complications. Minimize enteral feedings. Encourage breastfeeding.

  2) NPO

  3) NG to low, intermittent suction

  4) IV fluids and antibiotics

  5) Correction of hypovolemia, electrolyte imbalances

  6) Oxygen (intubation likely)

  7) Serial abdominal x-rays every 4 to 6 hr

  8) Surgical intervention to remove necrotized bowel; possible temporary colostomy

f. **Nursing Interventions**

1) Monitor bowel sounds, gastric residuals, and stool.

2) Monitor vital signs, including blood pressure and oxygen saturation.

3) Monitor arterial blood gases.

4) Avoid measuring temperature rectally.

5) Leave clients undiapered to prevent pressure on abdomen.

6) Position supine or on side.

7) Measure abdominal girth.

8) Institute strict handwashing. Isolate infants who have confirmed cases.

9) Maintain clients on oxygen and provide respiratory support as needed.

10) Monitor for septicemia, disseminated intravascular coagulation, and hypoglycemia.

11) If surgery is performed, provide routine postoperative care, including analgesia.

12) Perform colostomy care, if indicated.

13) Provide emotional support to parents. Encourage them to share feelings and ask questions.

g. Client Education

1) Reinforce teaching about the protective quality of breast milk (confers passive immunity, macrophages, lysozymes).

2) Prepare parents for surgical intervention as needed and for possible long-term complications (short bowel syndrome, colonic stricture, fat malabsorption, failure to thrive).

B. **Urinary Disorders**

1. **Minimal Change Nephrotic Syndrome**

a. Glomeruli become permeable to protein, primarily albumin, which reduces the serum albumin level and lowers the serum osmotic pressure. Cause is unknown.

b. Contributing Factors

1) Occurs primarily in preschool children. Peak incidence is between 2 and 3 years of age.

2) Often preceded by viral upper respiratory infection

c. Expected Findings

1) Facial puffiness, especially around the eyes, seen upon rising in the morning; dissipates through the day

2) Swelling of abdomen, genitalia, lower extremities (more prominent during the day)

3) Gradual or rapid onset of anasarca (generalized edema)

4) Ascites

5) Diarrhea, anorexia

6) Dark, frothy urine; decreased output

7) Extreme pallor

8) Fatigue, irritability

9) Muehrcke (white) lines in nails

10) Increased susceptibility to infection

11) Hypoalbuminemia

12) Hypercholesterolemia

13) Massive proteinuria, high specific gravity, hyaline casts

14) Increased platelets (500,000 to 1,000,000/mm³)

15) Hyponatremia (around 130 to 135 mEq/L)

16) Hypocalcemia

d. Laboratory Tests and Diagnostic Procedures

1) Serum protein, serum albumin

2) Electrolyte panel

3) CBC

4) Lipid panel

5) Urinalysis

6) Specific gravity

7) Renal biopsy

8) Blood urea nitrogen and creatinine

e. Therapeutic Procedures and Medications

1) Corticosteroids

2) Immunosuppressants

3) Diuretics

4) Antibiotics

5) Usual vaccines (no live vaccines) plus pneumococcal conjugate and pneumococcal polysaccharide vaccines

6) Sodium-restricted diet during periods of massive edema

f. **Nursing Interventions**

1) Engage in quiet activity.

2) Strictly monitor I&O. Monitor urine for protein.

3) Monitor edema (daily weight, daily measurement of abdominal girth).

4) Monitor skin integrity.

5) Monitor vital signs.

6) Protect clients from contact with anyone who has an infection.

7) Elevate edematous parts. Clean skin and separate with clothing, cotton, or antiseptic powder.

8) Maintain low-sodium diet. Consult with dietitian to provide palatable foods.

9) After edema subsides, allow clients to resume normal activities.

g. Client Education

1) Reinforce teaching with parents about how to check urine for protein.

2) Review requirements for a low-sodium diet.

3) Discuss medication administration and possible side effects.

4) Reassure parents that symptoms will dissipate as recovery continues.

5) Discuss ways to address social isolation and boredom.

2. **Acute Glomerulonephritis**

   a. Most commonly, a postinfectious disorder associated with pneumococcal, streptococcal, and viral infections. Thought to be a response to the deposition of immune complexes in the glomeruli.

   b. Contributing Factors

      1) Recent pneumococcal, streptococcal, or viral infection

      2) Most prevalent in summer and early fall

      3) Family history of the disease

   c. Expected Findings

      1) Edema of the face: worse in the morning; spreads to gonads, abdomen, and lower extremities throughout the day

      2) Anorexia

      3) Severely decreased urinary output

      4) Cloudy, smoky brown urine (often described as tea- or cola-colored); proteinuria, hematuria; decreased glomerular filtration rate

      5) Headache, abdominal discomfort, dysuria

      6) Lethargy, irritability, pallor

      7) Mild to moderate increase in blood pressure

      8) Azotemia

      9) Can have elevated streptococcal antibody titers

      10) Decreased glomerular filtration rate

      11) Decreased serum complement (C3) level; returns to normal 8 to 10 weeks after the disease

      12) Hyperkalemia, acidosis, hypocalcemia, hyperphosphatemia

      13) Generalized cardiac enlargement, pulmonary congestion, and pleural effusion during edematous phase

   d. Laboratory Tests Diagnostic Procedures

      1) Urinalysis

      2) Blood urea nitrogen, creatinine, glomerular filtration rate

      3) Antistreptolysin O (ASO) titer

      4) Serum complement level

      5) Electrolyte panel

      6) Chest x-ray

   e. Therapeutic Procedures and Medications

      1) Sodium and water restriction if output is significantly reduced

      2) Diuretics, unless renal failure is severe

      3) Antihypertensives

      4) Antibiotics for persistent streptococcal infection

      5) Fluid restriction if glomerular filtration rate is significantly decreased

   f. **Nursing Interventions**

      1) Encourage activity as desired.

      2) Monitor daily weight.

      3) Monitor vital signs, level of consciousness, and changes in behavior.

      4) Limit sodium in the diet. Limit potassium if oliguric. Limit protein with severe azotemia.

      5) Note volume and character of urine.

      6) Monitor intake.

      7) If fluids are restricted, evenly divide fluids while the child is awake. Serve in small cups.

      8) Monitor skin. Elevate edematous parts. Encourage frequent movement and repositioning.

      9) Refer for a dietary consult.

   g. Client Education

      1) Discuss dietary restrictions with the child and parents. Have the child identify palatable foods that are allowed.

      2) Reinforce the importance of adhering to follow-up appointments.

      3) Reinforce how to provide fluids if the child has a fluid restriction.

      4) Discuss ways to prevent infection transmission.

      5) Encourage plans for activity that allow for frequent rest.

3. **Urinary Tract Infection**

   a. An infection of the lower urinary tract (urethra, bladder), upper urinary tract (ureters, kidneys), or both. Diagnostic factors are pyuria and at least 50,000 colonies per mL of a single pathogenic organism in a clean-catch or sterile urine specimen. *Escherichia coli* is responsible for 85% of cases.

   b. Contributing Factors

      1) Female sex

      2) Caucasian

      3) Uncircumcised male

      4) Vesicoureteral reflux

      5) Sexual activity, masturbation

      6) Incomplete emptying of the bladder resulting in urinary stasis, dysfunctional voiding

      7) Inadequate fluid intake

      8) Urinary tract abnormalities

      9) Constrictive clothing or diapers, synthetic underwear, prolonged wearing of wet clothing

      10) Constipation

      11) Catheters

      12) Pinworms

      13) Bubble baths, hot tubs, whirlpool baths

      14) Beginning of toilet training

   c. Expected Findings

      1) Thick, cloudy urine with mucous strands

      2) Pyuria (at least 10 white blood cells/mL of uncentrifuged urine)

      3) Bacterial growth in urine culture

      4) Infants

         a) Irritability, lethargy

         b) Screaming with urination

         c) Poor feeding, vomiting, diarrhea

         d) Fever

         e) Newborns can exhibit fever or hypothermia, jaundice, cyanosis, tachypnea

         f) Hematuria

5) Children

   a) Abdominal, flank, back pain

   b) Dysuria, malodorous urine

   c) Hematuria

   d) Incontinence in previously toilet-trained child

   e) Enuresis

   f) Male clients can dribble urine

   g) Straining to urinate

   h) High fever, severe flank and abdominal pain, and leukocytosis are symptoms of pyelonephritis.

   i) Clients can be asymptomatic or display symptoms inconsistent with urinary tract infection (respiratory, gastrointestinal).

d. Laboratory Tests and Diagnostic Procedures

  1) Urinalysis

  2) Urine culture

  3) Ureteral catheterization

  4) Bladder washout

  5) Renography

  6) Ultrasound

  7) Voiding cystourethrogram

  8) Intravenous pyelography

  9) Dimercaptosuccinic acid scan

e. Therapeutic Procedures and Medications

  1) Antibiotics, IV for pyelonephritis

  2) Analgesics

  3) Treatment of contributing anatomic defects

f. **Nursing Interventions**

  1) Ensure that clean-catch urine specimens are collected properly.

  2) Collect first morning urine for analysis.

  3) Assist with suprapubic aspiration or collect catheterized specimen for culture.

  4) Encourage adequate fluid intake.

  5) Encourage frequent urination and complete emptying of bladder.

  6) Monitor urine output and character.

  7) Administer mild analgesia as needed.

  8) Encourage a high-fiber diet.

g. Client Education

  1) Reinforce teaching with female clients to wipe from front to back.

  2) Reinforce teaching about double voiding (urinate, stop, and attempt to urinate again) to ensure adequate emptying.

  3) Reinforce the importance of wearing cotton underwear and nonrestrictive clothing.

  4) Demonstrate how to retract and clean foreskin, if uncircumcised.

  5) Discuss the need to promptly change out of wet clothing.

  6) Avoid bubble baths, whirlpool tubs, and hot tubs.

  7) Emphasize importance of adequate fluid intake.

  8) Encourage sexually active adolescents to void immediately after intercourse.

  9) Emphasize the importance of completing antibiotic regimens.

C. **Respiratory Disorders**

1. **Tonsillitis**

  a. Tonsillitis refers to inflamed tonsils, which are usually accompanied by pharyngitis and often caused by a virus or bacterium.

  b. Contributing Factors

    1) Exposure to pathogenic organism

    2) Increased susceptibility in younger children due to immature immune systems

  c. Expected Findings

    1) Halitosis

    2) Snoring

    3) Nasal-sounding voice

    4) Difficulty swallowing, breathing

    5) Mouth-breathing

    6) Edema, inflammation, erythema

    7) Difficulty hearing due to blocked Eustachian tubes

    8) Throat pain that worsens with swallowing

    9) Fever

    10) Persistent cough

    11) Possible positive throat culture for Group A beta-hemolytic streptococcus

  d. Laboratory Tests

    1) Throat culture

    2) CBC

    3) Clotting times

  e. Therapeutic Procedures and Medications

    1) Antibiotics, if positive for Group A beta-hemolytic streptococcus

    2) Antipyretics

    3) Analgesics

    4) Topical anesthetics

    5) Antiemetics

    6) Tonsillectomy

  f. **Nursing Interventions**

    1) Tonsillitis

      a) Soft or liquid diet

      b) Cool-mist vaporizer

      c) Cool liquids

      d) Warm saline gargles

    2) Tonsillectomy

      a) Prepare the child and parents for surgery. Ensure consent forms are signed.

      b) Note bleeding tendencies. Note clotting times.

      c) Obtain baseline vital signs.

      d) Report any symptoms of an upper respiratory infection.

      e) Report loose teeth.

3) Postoperatively

    a) Discourage coughing, clearing throat, and blowing nose.

    b) Monitor for signs of hemorrhage (frequent swallowing, repeated throat clearing, hematemesis).

    c) Monitor for airway obstruction, stridor, drooling, restlessness, agitation, tachypnea, and cyanosis.

    d) Position the client to facilitate drainage. Elevate the head of the bed.

    e) Restrict food and fluid until swallowing with no signs of hemorrhage are observed.

    f) Offer ice chips, sips of water, cool liquids, and ice pops.

    g) Refrain from offering red or brown foods that can be mistaken for blood.

    h) Apply ice collar.

    i) Advance to soft foods.

    j) Administer narcotic analgesics on a regular schedule.

g. Client Education

1) Provide information about what to expect on admission and after surgery.

2) Avoid irritating or spicy foods.

3) Avoid gargles and vigorous tooth-brushing.

4) Discuss strategies for continued pain management.

5) Identify the signs of hemorrhage and respiratory obstruction. Seek emergency care if present.

6) Notify the provider if the child develops persistent cough, severe ear pain, or fever.

D. **Bronchitis (Tracheobronchitis)**

1. Inflammation of the trachea and bronchi is usually associated with an upper respiratory section and caused by a virus or *M. pneumoniae* (common in children 6 years and older). It begins with a dry, hacking cough that becomes productive in 2 to 3 days. Symptoms intensify at night. It is treated symptomatically with analgesics, antipyretics, cough suppressants, and humidity. Cough suppressants can interfere with clearing of secretions. It usually resolves in 5 to 10 days. Adolescents who have chronic bronchitis should be screened for marijuana and tobacco use.

2. **Bronchiolitis**

a. Most commonly caused by respiratory syncytial virus, which is the most common lower respiratory infection in children and the most frequent cause of hospitalization of infants. Parainfluenza viruses and adenoviruses are also causes.

b. Contributing Factors

1) Male sex

2) Age younger than 2 years (peaks between 2 and 7 months)

3) Crowded living conditions

4) Chronic disease

5) Daycare

6) Exposure to secondhand smoke

7) Prematurity

c. Expected Findings

1) Rhinorrhea, pharyngitis

2) Fever

3) Coughing, sneezing

4) Possible eye or ear infection

5) Irritability, lethargy

6) Poor feeding or refusal to feed

7) Wheezing, crackles, diminished breath sounds

8) Retractions, nasal flaring

9) Dyspnea

10) Tachypnea, apneic episodes

11) Copious secretions

12) Cyanosis

13) Tests on nasopharyngeal secretions are positive for RSV antigen

d. Laboratory Tests and Diagnostic Procedures

1) Rapid immunofluorescent antibody–direct fluorescent antibody staining

2) Enzyme-linked immunosorbent assay

3) Testing for coexisting infection (urinalysis, lumbar puncture)

4) Arterial blood gases

5) Electrolytes

e. Therapeutic Procedures and Medications

1) Bronchodilators are not recommended.

2) Oxygen, mechanical ventilation

3) Ribavirin (only medication approved for treatment for children hospitalized with RSV; controversial due to high cost)

4) Corticosteroids (controversial but may be used)

5) IV fluids

6) Palivizumab for prevention in at-risk children

f. **Nursing Interventions**

1) Droplet and contact precautions

2) Administer oxygen if oxygen saturation is not consistently maintained at or above 90%, after suctioning and repositioning.

3) Monitor airway and breath sounds.

4) Limit visitors and number of hospital personnel.

5) Assign only to a nurse who has no other at-risk patients.

6) Suction with normal saline before feeding and PRN.

7) Encourage fluids. Offer small amounts (5 to 10 mL) of fluid frequently.

8) Monitor vital signs and oxygenation status.

9) Encourage breastfeeding.

10) Do not administer chest physiotherapy.

g. Client Education

1) Encourage scrupulous handwashing.

2) Discourage smoking in the home.

3) Reinforce teaching about how to instill saline drops and suction with a bulb syringe.

3. **Respiratory Distress Syndrome (RDS)**

   a. A condition of surfactant deficiency and immature thorax, often referred to as hyaline membrane disease, that results in hypoxia. It is most common in premature infants. It is rare in drug-exposed infants or neonates who were exposed to intrauterine stress (preeclampsia, hypertension).

   b. Contributing Factors

      1) Prematurity

      2) Mother who has diabetes, hypoglycemia

      3) Multifetal pregnancy

      4) Cesarean section

      5) Cold stress

      6) Birth asphyxia

      7) Family history of RDS

      8) Sepsis

      9) Cardiac or respiratory abnormality

      10) Premature rupture of membranes

      11) Maternal use of depressants close to delivery

   c. Expected Findings

      1) Tachypnea (respiratory rate greater than 60/min)

      2) Peristernal, pericostal retractions

      3) Nasal flaring

      4) Labored breathing with prolonged expiration

      5) Inspiratory crackles

      6) Expiratory grunt

      7) Mottling

      8) Low oxygen saturation

      9) Respiratory or mixed acidosis, hypercapnia

      10) Atelectasis

      11) As condition worsens: flaccidity unresponsiveness, apnea, decreased breath sounds, central cyanosis

   d. Laboratory Tests and Diagnostic Procedures

      1) Arterial blood gases

      2) Chest x-ray

      3) Cultures of blood, urine, and cerebrospinal fluid

      4) Blood glucose

   e. Therapeutic Procedures and Medications

      1) Mechanical ventilation, CPAP

      2) Oxygen

      3) IV fluids

      4) NPO in acute phase

      5) Total parenteral nutrition

      6) Exogenous surfactant

      7) Prophylactic antibiotics

      8) Caffeine

      9) Inotropes

      10) Electrolytes

      11) Sodium bicarbonate

   f. Nursing Interventions

      1) Monitor response to therapy (respiratory effort, arterial blood gases).

      2) Monitor vital signs, oximetry, color, and pulses.

      3) Place in prone position initially, to increase chest expansion.

      4) Suction only when necessary.

      5) Place clients under radiant warmer or other controlled environment to eliminate heat loss and prevent cold stress.

      6) Encourage parents to hold, touch, and talk to the infant, as status allows.

      7) Encourage parental participation in care (pump and store breast milk; assist with repositioning).

   g. Client Education

      1) Orient to the neonatal intensive care unit.

      2) Explain all procedures.

      3) Encourage kangaroo (skin-to-skin) hold, as condition allows.

      4) Reinforce how to pump and store breast milk.

> **KEY POINT:** Do not give anything by mouth to infants who have a respiratory rate greater than 60/min or to children who have severe respiratory distress.

E. **Neurosensory Disorders**

   1. **Meningitis**

      a. Inflammation of meninges (the covering of the spinal cord and brain) caused by bacterial or viral (also called aseptic) infection. The mortality rate is higher for bacterial meningitis and can result in permanent neurological disability.

      b. Contributing Factors

         1) Premature rupture of fetal membranes

         2) Head trauma

         3) Head, neck, or back surgery

         4) Cochlear implant

         5) More common in late winter, early spring

         6) Crowded living conditions, daycare

         7) Recent viral illness

      c. Expected Findings

         1) Positive cerebral spinal fluid, blood culture (bacterial)

         2) Cerebral spinal fluid

            a) If bacterial: cloudy, elevated white blood cell count, elevated protein, decreased glucose, positive Gram stain

            b) If viral: clear, slightly increased white blood cell count, normal or slightly increased protein, normal glucose, negative Gram stain

         3) Neonates and infants

            a) Poor suck

            b) Poor feeding

            c) Temperature instability

            d) High-pitched cry

            e) Nuchal rigidity (older infants)

            f) Vomiting, diarrhea

g) Bulging fontanels (late)

h) Irritability

i) Seizures

4) Children and adolescents

a) Headache

b) Seizures

c) Nuchal rigidity

d) Photophobia

e) Decreased level of consciousness

f) Vomiting

g) Sensory alterations (seeing spots, halos)

h) Positive Kernig's, Brudzinski's signs (not reliable younger than age 2 years)

i) Irritability, agitation, delirium, stupor, coma

j) Hyperactivity with variable reflex response

k) Fever and chills

KEY POINT: Development of a puerperal or petechial rash in a child who is ill could indicate meningococcemia and requires immediate medical attention.

d. Laboratory Tests and Diagnostic Procedures

1) Lumbar puncture with culture of cerebrospinal fluid

2) Blood culture

3) Nose, throat cultures

4) CT scan

5) MRI

e. Therapeutic Procedures and Medications

1) IV fluids

2) Isolation

3) Oxygen, mechanical ventilation

4) Antibiotics, primarily cephalosporins (if bacterial)

5) Antipyretics

6) Corticosteroids

7) Analgesics

8) Antiepileptics

f. **Nursing Interventions**

1) Droplet precautions as soon as meningitis is suspected.

2) Quiet, low-light, low-stimulus environment.

3) Position with head of bed slightly elevated or side-lying; no pillow.

4) Monitor vital signs, urine output, and neurological status.

5) Maintain NPO until neurological status has improved. Advance to clear-liquid diet as tolerated.

6) Monitor pain level. Provide comfort measures.

7) If fontanels are bulging, measure head circumference.

8) Monitor hydration, fluid volume, and I&O. Restrict fluids if exhibiting signs of increased intracranial pressure.

9) Implement seizure precautions.

10) Provide information and reassurance to the child and parents.

g. Client Education

1) Ensure vaccines are given at the appropriate times. Children should receive the Hib and PCV vaccines at 2, 4, and 6 months of age, then again between 12 and 15 months of age.

2) Explain isolation procedures.

3) Emphasize the importance of adhering to the medication regimen.

2. **Reye Syndrome**

a. Metabolic encephalopathy characterized by significantly decreased level of consciousness, hepatic dysfunction, and fever. The cause is unknown. An association between use of aspirin in children and Reye syndrome has been identified.

b. Contributing Factors

1) Recent viral illness (usually influenza or varicella)

2) Use of aspirin and other salicylates

3) Winter months

c. Expected Findings

1) Cerebral edema

2) Fatty liver, clotting abnormalities

3) Seizures

4) Personality changes, delirium, combativeness

5) Profuse vomiting

6) Lethargy, irritability, coma

7) Elevated liver enzymes

8) Elevated serum ammonia

9) Prolonged clotting times

d. Laboratory Tests and Diagnostic Procedures

1) Liver enzymes (alanine aminotransferase [ALT], aspartate aminotransferase [AST])

2) Electrolytes

3) Serum ammonia

4) Clotting times

5) Liver biopsy

6) Cerebral spinal fluid analysis (to rule out meningitis)

e. Therapeutic Procedures and Medications

1) Oxygen, respiratory support

2) Occupational and physical therapy for resulting neurological deficits

3) Dietary consultation

4) Osmotic diuretic (mannitol)

5) Vitamin K

f. **Nursing Interventions**

1) Position with head of bed elevated 30° and head in neutral position.

2) Monitor seizure precautions.

3) Monitor vital signs, oxygen saturation, and level of consciousness.

4) Monitor bleeding precautions.

5) Monitor strict intake and output.

6) Monitor pain response. Provide comfort measures.

7) Provide information and reassurance to the child and parents.

g. Client Education

   1) Avoid administering aspirin and other salicylates to children.

   2) Assist parents to identify lesser-known sources of salicylates (bismuth subsalicylate, methyl salicylate).

   3) Provide a list of acceptable over-the-counter (OTC) medications for children.

3. **Neonatal Seizure**

a. The most common cause is hypoxic-ischemic encephalopathy secondary to asphyxia. Intracranial hemorrhage is second most common cause. Others include infection, kernicterus, hypoglycemia, birth injury, and electrolyte imbalance.

b. Contributing Factors

   1) Prematurity

   2) Mother who has diabetes, hypoglycemia, or hyperglycemia

   3) Mother who is Rh-negative

   4) Delivery complications (dystocia, prolonged labor, malpresentation, hemorrhage)

   5) Congenital anomaly

   6) Narcotic withdrawal secondary to maternal use

   7) Phenylketonuria (PKU)

   8) Perinatal infection

   9) Intracranial hemorrhage

   10) Uremia, kernicterus

c. Expected Findings

   1) Clonic

      a) Unilateral

      b) Slow, jerking movements

      c) Can migrate from one part of body to another

      d) Last 1 to 3 seconds

      e) Can be focal or multifocal

   2) Tonic

      a) Extension and stiffening of extremities, or stiffened, flexed arms

      b) Sustained posturing of limbs, neck

      c) Can be focal or generalized

   3) Subtle

      a) More common in preterm infants than full-term infants

      b) Repeated blinking

      c) Sucking

      d) Fluttering of eyelids

      e) Pedaling, swimming movements of extremities

      f) Apnea

   4) Myoclonic

      a) Rapid jerking of extremities

      b) Asynchronous twitching

      c) Bilateral jerks of extremities

      d) Can be focal, multifocal, or generalized

d. Laboratory Tests and Diagnostic Procedures

   1) Blood glucose

   2) Serum electrolytes

   3) Cerebrospinal fluid analysis

   4) Electroencephalogram

   5) CT scan

   6) Ultrasound

   7) Electroencephalography

e. Therapeutic Procedures and Medications

   1) Correct underlying problem

   2) Oxygen, respiratory support

   3) Antiepileptics

   4) Benzodiazepines

f. **Nursing Interventions**

   1) Carefully monitor at-risk neonate for seizure activity.

   2) Implement seizure precautions. Implement seizure-response regimen as prescribed.

   3) Monitor vital signs, oxygen status, and level of consciousness.

   4) Keep parents informed of the neonate's condition. Interpret behaviors of the infant.

   5) Encourage parents to participate in care of, hold, talk to, and touch infant.

g. Client Education

   1) Ensure parents understand how to respond if the infant has a seizure.

   2) Discuss medication regimen and expected response.

   3) Stress the importance of maintaining follow-up appointments.

4. Infants Exposed to Substances

a. A substance-exposed neonate will begin to display signs of drug withdrawal 12 to 24 hr after birth, depending on the type of drug, amount, route, and length of exposure. Symptoms can last several weeks.

b. Contributing Factors

   1) Maternal substance use and addiction (prior to knowledge of pregnancy or throughout pregnancy)

c. Expected Findings

   1) Perspiration (highly unusual in the normal neonate)

   2) Hypertonicity, hyperactive reflexes

   3) Tachypnea, tachycardia, apnea, nasal flaring

   4) Cyanosis, mottling

   5) Jitteriness, tremors, frantic movement

   6) Poor feeding, projectile vomiting, diarrhea

   7) Excessive but ineffective sucking

   8) Poor, restless sleep; increased wakefulness

   9) Sneezing, yawning

   10) Intractable, high-pitched cry

   11) Fever

12) Stuffy nose

13) Seizures

14) Excoriated areas on face and knees

15) Positive drug screen

d. Laboratory Tests and Diagnostic Procedures

1) Blood glucose

2) CBC

3) Electrolytes

4) Drug screen of meconium, urine, hair

5) Chest x-ray

e. Therapeutic Procedures and Medications

1) Prenatal drug screening

2) IV fluids, electrolytes

3) Phenobarbital

4) Morphine

5) Tincture of opium

6) Methadone

7) Buprenorphine

8) Clonidine

f. **Nursing Interventions**

1) Provide a quiet, low-light environment.

2) Feed on demand. Monitor amount ingested and response to feedings.

3) Monitor hydration and electrolyte status.

4) Swaddle, but maintain hands close to mouth for sucking.

5) Implement the Neonatal Abstinence Scoring System to evaluate.

6) Monitor reflexes, behavior, and activity in relation to feeding and other stimulation.

7) Involve the mother in care. Remain nonjudgmental.

8) Ensure supervisory care is in place prior to discharge.

g. Client Education

1) Demonstrate bonding behaviors.

2) Discuss options for drug rehabilitation.

3) Identify purpose of referral to Child Protective Services.

F. **Neoplastic Disorders**

1. Cancer in children is rare. Acute lymphoblastic leukemia, lymphoma, and central nervous system tumors are the most common types, all of which occur more frequently in males than females.

2. Contributing Factors

a. Family history of cancer

b. Exposure to cigarette smoke

c. Excessive sun exposure

d. Immunosuppressive medications

e. Radiation exposure

f. Epstein-Barr infection

g. Male sex

h. Caucasian descent

i. Down syndrome

3. Expected Findings

a. Unusual swelling or mass

b. Unexplained fatigue

c. Unexplained pallor

d. Headaches, vomiting with headaches

e. Sudden vision changes

f. Prolonged fever or illness

g. Limp, other change in gait

h. Localized pain

i. Unexplained bruising tendency

j. Sudden unexplained weight loss

k. Anemia

l. Hematuria

m. Thrombocytopenia

n. Neutropenia, leukemic blasts

o. Mass visible on imaging

4. Laboratory Tests and Diagnostic Procedures

a. Complete blood count

b. Urinalysis

c. Blood urea nitrogen, creatinine

d. Bone marrow, organ biopsy

e. CT scan

f. MRI

g. Positron emission tomography (PET) scan

h. Lumbar puncture

i. Serum chemistry

j. Liver function tests

5. Therapeutic Procedures and Medications

a. Chemotherapy

b. Surgery

c. Radiation

d. Bone marrow transplant

e. Analgesics

f. Antiemetics

g. Corticosteroids

h. Cell-stimulating medications (epoetin alfa, filgrastim, oprelvekin)

i. Topical anesthetics (viscous lidocaine, EMLA cream)

j. Antihistamines

k. Antibiotics

6. **Nursing Interventions**

a. Encourage frequent intake of small amounts of fluids.

b. Monitor for anaphylaxis for 20 min after chemotherapy infusion.

c. Maintain strict asepsis.

d. Monitor vital signs.

e. Screen visitors and prohibit those who have signs of infection.

f. Provide favorite foods, but do not pressure the child to eat. Engage the child in menu selection.

g. Institute bleeding and neutropenic precautions.

h. Monitor weight.

i. Premedicate and prepare for painful procedures.

j. Provide pharmacological and nonpharmacological pain relief.

k. Use medical play to demonstrate procedures. Allow the child to safely manipulate equipment.

l. Prepare for hair loss. Let the child decide how to manage.

m. Ensure sun protection when outside.

n. Promote cleanliness and regular hygiene practices.

o. Encourage peer visits and contact.

p. Maintain as normal a routine as possible, including continuation of schooling.

q. Encourage children to dress in their own clothing.

r. Encourage oral hygiene and use of soft toothbrush.

s. Encourage discussion of fears and feelings.

t. Provide uninterrupted time for family.

7. Client Education

a. Carefully explain all procedures to caregiver and child. Adapt to the child's developmental level.

b. Explain what to expect as treatment progresses, including common side effects.

c. Teach ways to handle side effects.

d. Ensure parents understand explanations of medical care and prognostic statistics.

e. Discuss participation in support groups and other support organizations.

COMMON CHILDHOOD CANCERS

	DESCRIPTION	EXPECTED FINDINGS	TREATMENT
Acute lymphocytic leukemia	Most common form of childhood cancer Malignancy of bone marrow and lymphatic system causes over-production of immature WBCs, deficiency in platelets, RBCs Occurs primarily between age 2 to 5 years More common in Caucasian males Greater risk in children who have Down syndrome Relapse most commonly occurs in the testes	Low-grade, unresolving fever Pallor, bruising, petechiae, lethargy, joint pain, headache, nausea, vomiting, weakness, anorexia	IV, intrathecal chemotherapy Corticosteroids Bone marrow transplant Hematopoietic stem cell transplant
Hodgkin disease	Malignancy of the lymph system, primarily lymph nodes Primarily occurs from ages 15 to 19 years	Painless, enlarged subclavicular or cervical nodes Nonproductive cough, abdominal pain, low-grade fever, anorexia, pruritus, night sweats, weight loss	Chemotherapy Radiation
Brain tumor	Most common solid tumor in children (about 25% of childhood cancers) Most occur in brainstem or cerebellum Can originate from any cranial cell; glial tumors are most common, followed by astrocytomas	Depends on location and size Headache upon awakening, vomiting unrelated to food, ataxia, dysmetria, dysarthria, nystagmus, behavioral changes	Radiotherapy prior to surgery Proton radiation Chemotherapy
Neuroblastoma	Most common cancer of infancy Median age is 22 months Solid, extracranial tumor that arises from fetal cells that form the adrenal medulla and sympathetic nervous system Primary site is the abdomen 70% of all cases have metastasized prior to diagnosis	Firm, painless abdominal mass that crosses midline Urinary frequency or retention (due to bladder compression) Manifestations of metastasis: fatigue, hepatomegaly, periorbital edema, supraorbital ecchymosis, respiratory dysfunction, anorexia, weight loss	Surgery followed by radiation Chemotherapy One of few tumors that can spontaneously regress
Osteosarcoma	Most common bone cancer in children Occurs most frequently after age 10 years, after a growth spurt More than half occur in the femur	Localized pain, often relieved with flexion Limping, other gait change	Surgery (limb salvage, amputation) Chemotherapy
Wilms tumor (nephroblastoma)	Most common childhood cancer of the kidney 75% occur under age 5 years 5% are familial	Painless abdominal mass that does not cross the midline Weight loss, enlarged liver, spleen, anemia	Surgery Chemotherapy Note: NEVER palpate the abdomen. Doing so can cause tumor cells to disseminate.

G. **Infectious Disorders**

1. **Otitis Media**

   a. An infection and inflammation of the middle ear. If there is fluid, it is referred to as otitis media with effusion. It is among the most common childhood illnesses.

   b. Contributing Factors

      1) Less than 24 months of age
      2) Cleft lip/palate
      3) Daycare, entering school for the first time
      4) Passive cigarette smoke exposure
      5) Bottle feeding
      6) Propping bottles
      7) Recent upper respiratory infection
      8) Winter and spring months
      9) Allergies
      10) Enlarged adenoids
      11) Nonadherence to vaccine schedule
      12) Down syndrome

   c. Expected Findings

      1) Ear pain, rubbing, tugging at ear, rocking head from side to side
      2) Pain worsens with sucking or chewing
      3) Fever
      4) Enlarged, painful postauricular and cervical lymph glands
      5) Bulging tympanic membrane
      6) Inconsolable crying
      7) Anorexia, nausea, vomiting
      8) Irritability, restlessness, poor sleeping
      9) Purulent drainage from ear
      10) Transient hearing loss, balance problems
      11) Feeling of fullness in the ear
      12) Nonspecific symptoms (rhinitis, cough, diarrhea)
      13) Drainage from ear accompanied by immediate pain relief indicates tympanic rupture
      14) Decreased or no tympanic movement with pneumatic otoscopy

   d. Diagnostic Procedures

      1) Pneumatic otoscopy
      2) Acoustic reflectometry
      3) Tympanometry

   e. Therapeutic Procedures and Medications

      1) Antibiotics
      2) Antipyretics
      3) Analgesics
      4) Topical anesthetics
      5) Myringotomy with tympanostomy tube placement

   f. **Nursing Interventions**

      1) Apply heat over ear and lie on affected side.
      2) Clean drainage from external ear.
      3) Ear wicks should be loose and kept dry.
      4) Monitor for hearing loss.
      5) Provide comfort measures.
      6) Position upright.

   g. Client Education

      1) Stress the importance of adherence to vaccine schedule.
      2) Discourage propping bottles.
      3) Encourage breastfeeding.
      4) Discourage exposure to smoking.
      5) Notify the provider when symptoms initially occur.
      6) If the child has tympanostomy tubes, keep water out of the ears and notify the provider when tubes come out.

2. *Enterobiasis vermicularis* **(pinworms)**

   a. The most common helminthic infection in the U.S. Eggs float through the air and can be ingested or inhaled. They hatch in the upper intestine, mature, migrate out of the intestine, and lay eggs, which are viable for 2 to 3 weeks on indoor surfaces.

   b. Contributing Factors

      1) Close proximity to others (classrooms, daycare)
      2) Hand-to-mouth behavior in children
      3) Temperate climate

   c. Expected Findings

      1) Intense anal itching
      2) Enuresis
      3) Poor sleep, nighttime restlessness
      4) Irritability

   d. Diagnostic Procedure

      1) Tape test: Parents are instructed to wrap a tongue depressor with tape, sticky side out, and firmly press the tape against the perianal area. This is done when the child awakens for three consecutive mornings. The tongue depressors are placed in a jar or plastic bag and brought in for microscopic examination.

   e. Medications

      1) Antihelminths (pyrantel pamoate, pyrvinium pamoate, and albendazole are available OTC)

   f. **Nursing Interventions**

      1) Trim fingernails short.
      2) Dress the child in one-piece pajamas.
      3) Encourage showering rather than bathing.

   g. Client Education

      1) Pyrantel pamoate will turn GI contents red and stain clothing.
      2) Discuss the need for treatment of all family members (initial dose, then repeat 2 weeks later).
      3) Reinforce the importance of good handwashing.

3. *Pediculosis capitis* (head lice)

a. Infestation of the scalp and hair with lice. The louse lays eggs (nits) at night, on the hair shaft, close to scalp, which hatch in 7 to 10 days. The louse sucks blood of the host. With a host, the life span of the louse is around 1 month.

b. Contributing Factors

1) Close proximity to others (classrooms, daycare)

2) School age

3) Common sharing of objects that touch the head (hats, combs)

c. Expected Findings

1) Intense itching of the scalp

2) Small red bumps on the scalp

3) Small white specks attached to hair shaft, usually close to the scalp

d. Medications

1) Permethrin cream rinse (available OTC)

2) Pyrethrin with piperonyl butoxide (available OTC; contraindicated for those who have chrysanthemum or ragweed allergy)

3) Malathion

4) Benzyl alcohol (for children older than 2 years)

5) Spinosad (for children older than 4 years)

6) Ivermectin lotion (for children older than 6 months)

e. **Nursing Interventions**

1) Assure child and caregiver that anyone can get head lice. It is not due to lack of cleanliness.

2) Carefully inspect the head and hair to identify.

3) Use a nit comb on hair after shampooing with pediculicide.

f. Client Education

1) Caution against sharing objects that touch the head (hats, combs, barrettes, scarves, coats).

2) Repeat the treatment in 7 to 10 days.

3) Use a nit comb. Run in sections from scalp to ends.

4) Suggest that the caregiver play "beauty parlor" with the child when treating.

5) Advise covering the child's eyes while treating.

6) Treat all members of the household.

7) Wash linens, towels, and clothing in hot water and dry in a hot dryer. Seal nonwashable objects in a plastic bag for 2 weeks.

8) Thoroughly vacuum carpets, car seats, pillows, and stuffed animals.

9) Soak combs, brushes, and hair accessories in a lice-killing agent for 1 hr.

Nursing Care of the Child Who Has a Chronic Condition

A. **Gastrointestinal Disorders**

1. **Celiac Disease (Gluten–Sensitive Enteropathy)**

a. An immune-mediated disease that causes damage to the small intestine and villi when exposed to foods containing gluten

b. Contributing Factors

1) Type 1 diabetes mellitus or other autoimmune disorder (such as rheumatoid arthritis)

2) Caucasian descent

3) Introduction of solid foods

c. Expected Findings

1) Failure to thrive

2) Chronic diarrhea, steatorrhea

3) Aphthous ulcers (canker sores)

4) Fatigue

5) Abdominal pain and distention

6) Anemia

7) Irritability

8) Muscle wasting

9) Celiac crisis (copious watery diarrhea, vomiting)

10) Positive serologic markers

11) Mucosal inflammation, crypt hyperplasia, and villous atrophy seen with endoscopy

d. Laboratory Tests and Diagnostic Procedures

1) Serologic blood test for tissue transglutaminase and antiendomysial antibodies in children 18 months or older (positive result indicates disease)

2) Gastrointestinal endoscopy and biopsy

e. Medications

1) Nutritional supplements

f. **Nursing Interventions**

1) Restrict gluten from diet.

2) Maintain a high-calorie, high-protein diet.

3) Restrict lactose during periods with acute symptoms.

4) Consult with a dietitian.

5) Encourage the child and parents to express concerns.

g. Client Education

1) Read food labels. Look for hidden sources of gluten.

2) Use the BROWS acronym (barley, rye, oats, wheat, spelt) to recognize major sources of gluten.

3) Assist clients to identify nongluten sources of grains (rice, corn, millet).

4) Discuss support organizations (such as Celiac Support Association).

B. **Respiratory Disorders**

1. **Cystic Fibrosis**

    a. Genetic disorder that affects exocrine (mucous) glands so that secretions are thick and viscous, obstructing organs. It affects multiple systems but manifests primarily in the lungs, GI tract, skin, and pancreas.

    b. Contributing Factors

    1) Caucasian descent

    2) Family history

    c. Expected Findings

    1) Chronic dry cough

    2) Cyanosis, clubbing

    3) Dyspnea, wheezing

    4) Repeated respiratory infections

    5) Meconium ileus in newborn

    6) Abdominal distention, intestinal obstruction

    7) Steatorrhea

    8) Failure to thrive, failure to gain weight

    9) Hypoalbuminemia

    10) Rectal prolapse

    11) Skin tastes salty; tears, sweat, and saliva have excessive sodium and chloride

    12) Hyponatremia, hypochloremia

    13) Atelectasis

    14) Hemoptysis

    15) Voracious appetite

    16) Barrel chest; thin arms and legs

    17) Anemia

    18) Fat-soluble vitamin deficiency

    19) Viscous cervical mucus; decreased or absent sperm

    d. Laboratory Tests and Diagnostic Procedures

    1) Nutritional panel to detect a deficiency of fat-soluble vitamins (A, D, E, K)

    2) Sputum culture

    3) DNA testing

    4) Chest x-ray

    5) Pulmonary function tests

    6) Abdominal x-ray

    7) Stool analysis

    8) Sweat chloride test

    e. Therapeutic Procedures and Medications

    1) Oxygen

    2) IV fluids

    3) Feeding tube (for intractable weight loss)

    4) Chest physiotherapy

    5) High-calorie diet

    6) Vaccines

    7) Palivizumab for RSV prevention

    8) Pancreatic enzymes (must be administered within 30 min of eating)

    9) Multivitamin; vitamins A, D, E, K

    10) Dornase alfa (decreases mucous viscosity)

    11) Antibiotics (including nebulized)

    12) Antifungals

    13) Bronchodilators

    14) Anticholinergics

    15) H_2 blockers, proton pump inhibitors, stool softeners

    16) Surgery for meconium ileus, if indicated

    17) Lung, heart, pancreas, liver transplant for advanced disease

    f. **Nursing Interventions**

    1) Monitor respiratory effort and breath sounds.

    2) Monitor for fatigue.

    3) Monitor for weight loss and muscle wasting.

    4) Involve the child and caregiver in scheduling care activities.

    5) Encourage clients to view care activities as part of a normal daily routine.

    6) Provide airway clearance therapy (ACT) twice daily (more frequently, as indicated).

    7) Perform chest physiotherapy (CPT) (shaker vest, manual cupping) as needed. Avoid doing so right before or after meals.

    8) Encourage a high-protein, high-calorie diet and snacks in between meals.

    9) Monitor blood glucose.

    10) Encourage moderate aerobic exercise.

    11) Refer for dietary consult.

    12) Provide support and reassurance for child and parents.

    g. Client Education

    1) Provide information about access to medical equipment and medications.

    2) Reinforce teaching with the caregiver how to perform airway clearance techniques and chest physiotherapy.

    3) Discuss medication schedule, administration, and therapeutic and side effects.

    4) Monitor for deteriorating respiratory status and notify provider or seek emergency care.

    5) Monitor nutritional status, growth, and weight.

    6) Demonstrate use of a nebulizer.

    7) Reinforce teaching about nasal lavage (used for chronic sinusitis).

    8) Emphasize the importance of adherence to the vaccine schedule.

    9) Reinforce teaching about diet and ways to increase caloric intake.

    10) Provide information about support groups and organizations.

    11) Maintain normalcy in daily routine and the relationship with the child.

C. **Hematologic Disorders**
1. **Sickle Cell Anemia**
   a. A genetic disease in which abnormal sickle hemoglobin (HgS) replaces normal hemoglobin
   b. Contributing Factors
      1) Both parents carry the sickle cell trait.
      2) African, Middle Eastern, Mediterranean, or Indian descent
      3) Family history of the disease
   c. Expected Findings
      1) Organ dysfunction, enlargement (spleen, liver, kidneys), cirrhosis
      2) Osteoporosis
      3) Chronic anemia (hemoglobin less than 10 g/dL)
      4) Hands and feet cool to touch
      5) Increased susceptibility to infection and sepsis
      6) Pallor, pale mucous membranes
      7) Jaundice
      8) Shortness of breath, fatigue
      9) Pain
      10) Retinal detachment
      11) Delayed growth, puberty
      12) Systolic murmur
      13) Enuresis, renal failure
      14) Skeletal deformities; shoulder or hip avascular necrosis
      15) Vaso-occlusive crisis
         a) Extreme pain in joints, hands, and feet
         b) Swelling of joints and extremities
         c) Severe abdominal pain
         d) Priapism
         e) Hematuria
         f) Symptoms of stroke
         g) Dyspnea; acute chest syndrome
         h) Visual disturbances
         i) Shock
         j) Elevated white blood cells, bilirubin, and reticulocytes; decreased hemoglobin
         k) Peripheral blood smear reveals sickled cells
      16) Sequestration
         a) Blood pools excessively in spleen and liver
         b) Reduced blood volume can cause hypovolemia and shock (tachycardia, tachypnea, thready pulse, hypotension)
   d. Laboratory Tests and Diagnostic Procedures
      1) Sickle cell screening of newborn
      2) CBC (for anemia)
      3) Sickle-turbidity: detects presence of HbS; does not differentiate trait from disease
      4) Hemoglobin electrophoresis for definitive diagnosis
      5) DNA sequencing
      6) Transcranial Doppler test detects risk for CVA (performed annually for children 10 to 16 years old who have the disease)

      7) Sickle-cell crisis
         a) CBC
         b) Bilirubin and reticulocyte levels
         c) Peripheral blood smear
   e. Therapeutic Measures and Medications
      1) Hydroxyurea
      2) Penicillin prophylaxis
      3) Exchange transfusion (erythrocytapheresis)
      4) Chelation with deferoxamine, if multiple transfusions required
      5) Splenectomy
      6) Crisis management
         a) IV fluids
         b) Oxygen, if hypoxic (of little value until circulation is improved)
         c) Electrolyte replacement, correction of metabolic acidosis
         d) Opioid analgesia
         e) Blood transfusion
         f) Antibiotics
         g) Bed rest

   > **KEY POINT:** Meperidine is not used for treatment of pain in sickle cell anemia. It produces a metabolite that can cause tremors, anxiety, myoclonus, and generalized seizures as levels rise with repeated doses. Children who have sickle cell disease are particularly at risk for seizures.

   f. **Nursing Interventions**
      1) Use the acronym HOP (hydration, oxygen, pain management) when planning care for vaso-occlusive crisis.
      2) Monitor oxygenation status.
      3) Monitor hydration. Calculate fluid requirements and ensure intake exceeds minimum.
      4) Provide fluids in a specialized cup to encourage fluid intake.
      5) Exclude anyone who has an infection from visiting.
      6) Monitor strict intake and output.
      7) Apply warm compresses to painful joints. Avoid cold compresses.
      8) Monitor for signs of reaction associated with blood transfusion.
      9) Monitor and measure the size of the spleen.
      10) Promote bed rest and conserving energy.
      11) Provide passive range of motion as tolerated.
      12) Weigh the client daily.
      13) Monitor potassium and other electrolyte levels.
      14) Monitor for complications of stroke and chest syndrome (severe thoracic pain, fever, cough, dyspnea, tachycardia, hypoxia).
      15) Refer the client for genetic testing and counseling.
      16) Provide support and information to parents, siblings, and other close family members.

g. Client Education

1) Encourage frequent rest breaks during physical activities.

2) Discourage contact sports if the spleen is enlarged.

3) Avoid low-oxygen environments (nonpressurized airplane, high altitudes).

4) Emphasize the importance of hydration.

5) Reinforce teaching about fluid sources other than water (ice pops, sherbet, soup).

6) Recognize signs of dehydration.

7) Encourage clothing that prevents sweating.

8) Discourage long periods of sun exposure.

9) Discourage limiting fluids if enuresis occurs.

10) Emphasize the importance of scrupulous hand hygiene, adherence to vaccine schedule, and avoiding communicable illnesses.

11) Reinforce teaching about the signs of crisis and infection. Seek medical help immediately.

12) Reinforce teaching with parents how to palpate the spleen to detect sequestration early.

13) Emphasize the importance of good nutrition.

14) Advise wearing a medical alert tag.

15) Discuss support groups and organizations.

2. **Hemophilia**

a. Group of bleeding disorders; the result of a deficiency of a clotting factor, which causes difficulty controlling bleeding, most often as the result of the inheritance of the associated X-linked recessive trait which is passed from a carrier mother to her son

b. Contributing Factors

1) Family history of the disease

2) Affected father; trait-carrying mother

c. Expected Findings

1) Prolonged bleeding (can be first noticed following newborn procedures [injections, heel sticks, circumcision])

2) Epistaxis, bleeding gums, prolonged bleeding after tooth loss

3) Hematuria, tarry stools

4) Bruising, hematoma out of proportion to injury

5) Hemarthrosis, joint pain

6) Anemia

d. Laboratory Tests and Diagnostic Procedures

1) DNA testing

2) aPTT (PT is normal)

3) Factor-specific assay

4) CBC (platelets are within the expected reference range)

e. Therapeutic Procedures and Medications

1) Administer missing factor.

a) Hemophilia A: Factor VIII

b) Hemophilia B: Factor IX

2) Blood transfusion

3) Corticosteroids

4) 1-deamino-8-d-arginine vasopressin (DDAVP)

a) Used for mild cases

b) Can be administered intranasally or parenterally

5) ε-aminocaproic acid (EACA) prevents clot destruction and is used with mouth trauma surgery. The child swishes the medication around in the mouth and then swallows it.

f. **Nursing Interventions**

1) Avoid unnecessary punctures. Venipunctures are preferred to finger or heel sticks. Administer parenteral medications subcutaneously instead of intramuscularly when possible.

2) Monitor urine and stool for blood.

3) Do not administer aspirin or other salicylates. Use of NSAIDs is discouraged. Acetaminophen is acceptable.

4) Provide a soft toothbrush and water irrigation device for oral care.

5) Monitor for signs of bleeding (headache, slurred speech, change in level of consciousness).

6) Respond immediately to an injury.

a) Administer replacement clotting factor immediately.

b) Immobilize, elevate, and apply ice to affected joints.

c) Monitor for adverse response (headache, tachycardia, hypotension, change in level of consciousness).

g. Client Education

1) Encourage regular exercise and physical therapy. (Passive range of motion exercises should not be performed after any acute incident.)

2) Remind parents to create a safe environment that allows for normal development.

3) Encourage participation in noncontact sports (swimming, golf, walking, jogging, fishing, bowling).

4) Reinforce teaching with parents how to administer clotting factor intravenously (beginning when child is 2 to 3 years of age). Reinforce teaching with the child about self-administration at 8 to 12 years of age.

5) Emphasize the need to administer clotting factor without delay if injury occurs.

6) Encourage use of soft toothbrush and electric razor.

7) Work with the school nurse and teach the client to prepare the child for entering school.

8) Emphasize importance of adhering to vaccine schedule.

9) Reinforce teaching about how to identify signs of bleeding.

10) Discuss how to respond to injuries using the RICE acronym (rest, ice, compression, elevation).

11) Inform the family about community resources and support groups.

COMMUNICABLE DISEASES OF CHILDHOOD

	TRANSMISSION, INCUBATION, COMMUNICABILITY	EXPECTED FINDINGS	THERAPEUTIC PROCEDURES	☊ NURSING INTERVENTIONS (STANDARD PRECAUTIONS APPLY TO ALL)
Chickenpox (Varicella zoster)	Contact, airborne Incubation 2 to 3 weeks Communicable 1 day before macule eruption to when all lesions have crusted	Fever, malaise, loss of appetite for first 24 hr; then macule → papules → vesicles → crusts; pruritus, irritability Complications: encephalitis, secondary infection	Medications: Acyclovir, diphenhydramine, or other antihistamine Prevention: Varicella vaccine	Airborne and contact precautions until all lesions are crusted Skin care, tepid oatmeal baths Trim fingernails and keep clean. Lightweight clothing Distract from itching NO aspirin (possible Reye syndrome)
Diphtheria (Corynebacterium diphtheria)	Direct contact, droplet; spread via nasal discharge and lesions Incubation 2 to 5 days Communicable 2 to 4 weeks after disease onset	Malaise, cold-type symptoms, sore throat, epistaxis, thick, white or gray membrane covering throat, fever, hoarseness, lymphadenopathy (bull neck) Complications: Septic shock, myocarditis, neuropathy	Equine antitoxin, penicillin G, strict bed rest, O₂, tracheostomy PRN Prevention: Diphtheria vaccine (series given in infancy and childhood as part of combination vaccine with periodic boosters)	Droplet precautions Contact precautions with skin lesions Provide complete care and conserve client's energy. Monitor vital signs, especially for respiratory obstruction. Suction PRN
Fifth disease (Erythema infectiosum; caused by human parvovirus B19)	Contact with respiratory secretions, blood, and blood products Incubation 4 to 21 days Communicability period not certain	Three stages > Stage I: "Slapped face" erythema on cheeks (days 1 to 4) > Stage II: Appears 1 day after onset of Stage I; maculopapular rash > Stage III: Rash subsides but reappears if skin is irritated Complications: Aplastic crisis (rash usually absent), acute arthritis	Antipyretics, anti-inflammatory medications, analgesics Blood transfusion for aplastic crisis	Usually isolation is unnecessary. Droplet precautions if hospitalized Not likely to be contagious after rash appears May return to school or daycare
Mononucleosis (Epstein-Barr virus)	Direct contact with oral secretions, blood, and blood products Incubation 30 to 50 days Communicability period is unknown Seen primarily in adolescents and young adults	Malaise, sore throat, fever, lymphadenopathy, unusual fatigue, headache, rash (sometimes), epistaxis Complications: Splenic rupture, respiratory failure, neurological events (seizure, meningitis), pancytopenia	IV hydration, rest, analgesics, antipyretics	Monitor airway status. Monitor for hemorrhage secondary to splenic rupture. Encourage saltwater gargles, anesthetic throat spray, or lozenges. Reinforce teaching about the importance of rest.
Mumps (paramyxovirus)	Direct contact with saliva, droplet Incubation 14 to 21 days Communicable immediately before and after swelling of parotid glands	Fever, headache → earache aggravated by chewing Parotitis beginning third day, pain tenderness Complications: Deafness, myocarditis, arthritis, hepatitis, pancreatitis, meningitis, orchitis, oophoritis	Analgesics, antipyretics, IV hydration PRN Prevention: Mumps vaccine (included in MMR)	Droplet and contact precautions Encourage rest and fluids. Provide soft foods. Apply warm or cool compresses to inflamed areas (per client preference).
Pertussis (whooping cough; caused by Bordetella pertussis)	Direct contact with droplets Indirect contact with contaminated objects Incubation 6 to 20 days Communicable during phase with upper respiratory symptoms, before cough	Coryza, sneezing, watery eyes, low-grade fever → paroxysmal "whooping" cough, worse at night, causing bulging eyes, cyanosis, and protruding tongue that can last until mucous plug is dislodged (4 to 6 weeks) Vomiting of mucous Complications: Pneumonia, rib fractures, hemorrhage, seizures, otitis media, atelectasis, hernia, prolapsed rectum	Prophylactic antibiotics, oxygen, IV fluids, mechanical ventilation if needed	Droplet precautions Offer small amounts of fluid frequently. Monitor for airway obstruction.

	TRANSMISSION, INCUBATION, COMMUNICABILITY	EXPECTED FINDINGS	THERAPEUTIC PROCEDURES	NURSING INTERVENTIONS (STANDARD PRECAUTIONS APPLY TO ALL)
Poliomyelitis (three types; caused by enteroviruses)	Direct contact with oropharyngeal secretions or oral–fecal route; less common through sneeze or cough Incubation 7 to 14 days Period of communicability is unknown	Three forms: abortive, nonparalytic, paralytic Fever, headache, vomiting, loss of appetite, nausea, abdominal pain, fatigue Pain in neck, back, legs in more severe form Paralytic: Onset has same symptoms as nonparalytic followed by recovery, then CNS paralysis Complications: Permanent paralysis, respiratory failure, hypertension	Bed rest, mechanical ventilation PRN, physical therapy, sedatives for anxiety, analgesics Prevention: Immunization administered in series in infancy and childhood	Position in alignment. Use footboard and pressure-relieving mattress. Apply moist warm packs. Assist with ROM exercises. Encourage participation in ADLs. Assist with ambulation. Encourage high-protein, high-fiber diet. Encourage fluids.
Roseola (*Exanthem subitum* caused by human herpes virus type 6)	Occurs in children younger than 3 years Transmission is unknown (thought to be from saliva of adults who do not have symptoms) Incubation 5 to 15 days Communicability is unknown	High fever for 3 to 7 days in otherwise healthy child; temperature suddenly drops to normal with appearance of rosy-pink maculopapular rash that begins on trunk and lasts 1 to 2 days; disappears when blanched Bulging fontanels Complications: Febrile seizures, encephalitis	Antipyretics; otherwise supportive Standard precautions	Reinforce teaching to caregiver to monitor temperature and administer antipyretics.
Rubella virus (German measles)	Contact with nasopharyngeal secretions, blood, stool, urine Incubation 14 to 21 days Communicable 7 days before and 5 days after appearance of rash	Prodrome doesn't occur in children; in adolescents consists of low-grade fever, malaise, coryza, and cough lasting 1 to 5 days Rash (maculopapular, begins on face and spreads downward, lasts 3 days) Complications: Rare; greatest risk is teratogenic effect	Supportive Analgesics Antipyretics Prevention: Childhood vaccine (part of MMR)	Droplet precautions Provide comfort measures. Instruct caregiver to keep the child away from people who are pregnant.
Rubeola (measles, virus)	Direct contact More prevalent in winter Incubation 10 to 20 days Communicable 4 days before and 5 days after rash	Fever, malaise, cough, allergy-type nasal irritation, watery eyes, Koplik spots on buccal mucosa Maculopapular rash appears on face third or fourth day and moves down body Anorexia, abdominal pain, lymphadenopathy, photophobia Complications: Otitis media, pneumonia, obstructive laryngitis, encephalitis	Rest, antipyretics Antibiotics in high-risk children Vitamin A Prevention: Rubeola vaccine (included in MMR)	Airborne precautions Encourage rest and quiet activity. Maintain low-light environment. Use a cool-mist vaporizer. Encourage a soft, bland diet and tepid baths.
Scarlet Fever (Group A beta-hemolytic streptococci)	Direct contact with nasopharyngeal secretions Incubation 2 to 5 days, with a range of 1 to 7 Communicable during incubation and throughout illness (about 10 days); can persists for months	Begins with abrupt high fever Generalized rash appears, except on face, about 12 hr after onset Abdominal pain, halitosis Tonsils swollen, very red, and covered in white patches of exudate White strawberry tongue, turns red Face is flushed Circumoral pallor Sandpaper-like rash on torso Sloughing on palms and soles Complications: Peritonsillar abscess, sinusitis, otitis media, acute glomerulonephritis, acute rheumatic fever (arthralgia), rheumatic heart disease (valve damage)	Penicillin (erythromycin if allergic) Analgesics, antipyretics, local anesthetics for throat pain	Droplet precautions until child has been on antibiotic for 24 hr Promote rest and quiet activity. Emphasize importance of full course of antibiotics to the caregiver. Entourage use of gargles and a cool-mist vaporizer. Encourage fluids and soft foods. Reinforce teaching to the family how to prevent spread. (Discard toothbrush.)

D. **Musculoskeletal Disorders**

1. **Idiopathic Scoliosis**

   a. A spinal deformity characterized by lateral curvature and spinal rotation, which causes rib asymmetry. It usually becomes evident at age 10 or older and is the most common spinal deformity.

   b. Contributing Factors

      1) Etiology is unknown, but there appears to be a genetic aspect.

      2) Preadolescent growth spurt

      3) Female

      4) Age 8 to 15 years

   c. Expected Findings

      1) Ill-fitting clothes

      2) Asymmetry in scapula, ribs, flanks, shoulders, and hips

      3) One leg shorter than the other

      4) Head and hips not aligned (uncompensated) or head aligns with gluteal cleft (compensated)

      5) Spinal curvature

   d. Diagnostic Procedures

      1) Screening

         a) Observe from behind.

         b) The child wears clothing that provides a clear view of the spine (shorts, briefs) and bends forward from the waist.

         c) Trunk is parallel to the floor and arms hang freely (Adam's position), making asymmetry apparent.

         d) Screen before and during growth spurts.

      2) Radiography

         a) Cobb technique determines degree of curvature.

         b) Risser scale determines skeletal maturity.

      3) Scoliometry

   e. Therapeutic Procedures and Medications

      1) Bracing and exercise for moderate curvatures of 25° to 45°

      2) Spinal fusion with rod placement if curvature is 45° or more

      3) Postoperative opioid analgesics

   f. **Nursing Interventions**

      1) Bracing and exercise

         a) Assist with fitting brace.

         b) Monitor skin integrity.

         c) Reinforce a positive self-image.

      2) Spinal fusion with rod placement

         a) Preoperative

            (1) Refer for preoperative testing (type and cross-match for blood; pulmonary function testing).

            (2) Orient the adolescent and family to the hospital, including the intensive care unit.

      b) Postoperative

         (1) Monitor neurologic status of extremities. Promptly report any impairment.

         (2) Carefully monitor for pain using an age-appropriate tool.

         (3) Use log-rolling technique to turn frequently.

         (4) Encourage pulmonary hygiene.

         (5) Monitor skin for pressure areas.

         (6) Keep skin clean and dry.

         (7) Monitor surgical sites and drains. Provide wound care as prescribed.

         (8) Monitor bowel function. Monitor for ileus.

         (9) Monitor hematocrit and hemoglobin. Observe for bleeding.

         (10) Monitor for infection.

         (11) Perform range of motion on unaffected extremities. Encourage mobility when tolerated.

         (12) Provide diversionary activities. Encourage visits with family and friends.

   g. Client Education

      1) Bracing and exercise

         a) Explain the process thoroughly and ensure understanding.

         b) Provide guidance when selecting clothing and activities.

         c) Encourage independence and socialization.

      2) Spinal fusion with rod placement

         a) Preoperative

            (1) Discuss options for autologous blood donation.

            (2) Discuss postoperative expectations. Inform clients about monitors, NG tube, chest tubes, urinary catheter, and patient-controlled analgesia.

            (3) Reinforce pulmonary hygiene techniques (turn, cough, deep breathe; incentive spirometry). Discuss respiratory therapy techniques.

            (4) Reinforce teaching about the log-rolling technique.

            (5) Allow time for questions and clarification of medical terms.

         b) Postoperative

            (1) Reinforce the expected course of recovery.

            (2) Encourage the family to arrange the environment to encourage independence.

            (3) Emphasize the importance of follow-up care.

CPR Guidelines for Infants and Children

A. **Cardiac Arrest**

> Refer to the American Heart Association "CPR and ECC Guidelines"

1. C–A–B Sequence
2. Begin compressions and rescue breathing, using a ratio of 15:2 (for one or two rescuers).
3. Compression rate should be approximately 100/min.
4. Chest should be compressed to ⅓ the anteroposterior diameter (1.5 inches in infants; 2 inches in children up to puberty).
5. If available, use AED.
6. Compression–only CPR generally is not effective for children. However, it is preferable to no CPR.

B. **Choking**

1. Infant

    a. Pick up and hold face–down along forearm with infant's head away from the body, angled down.

    b. Administer five back blows.

    c. Turn face up and administer five chest thrusts.

    d. Repeat until obstruction is cleared.

    e. Open the mouth. Remove obstruction if it is visible and can safely be cleared.

    f. Prepare to administer CPR.

2. Child older than 1 year

    a. Observe for signs of choking (hands to throat, inability to talk, dyspnea, ineffective cough, noisy or absent breathing, cyanosis).

    b. Deliver five abdominal thrusts (Heimlich maneuver).

    c. Check for breathing.

    d. Repeat sequence.

    e. If unsuccessful, prepare to perform CPR.

> **KEY POINT:** Never perform a blind finger sweep. The object can be pushed further into the airway.

Activities

Answers for all activities are at the end of the Activities section.

PRIORITIZING NURSING CARE OF THE CHILD

Match each clinical situation to the priority nursing action. Each will be used once.

CLINICAL SITUATION

1. A 3-year-old toddler has diarrhea and has been febrile for 2 days.

2. A 4-week-old infant has hypertrophic pyloric stenosis and is vomiting.

3. A neonate was born with a myelomeningocele in the lumbar region.

4. A 5-year-old child is receiving chemotherapy for acute lymphocytic leukemia.

5. A 10-year-old child has sickle cell anemia and is having a vaso-occlusive crisis.

1. _____
2. _____
3. _____
4. _____
5. _____

PRIORITY NURSING ACTIONS

a. Monitor for hypotension, wheezing, nausea, vomiting, and urticaria.

b. Place on bed rest and minimize activity.

c. Administer oral rehydration fluids.

d. Administer replacement electrolytes intravenously.

e. Monitor respirations and level of consciousness.

INFANT VOCALIZATION

Match the developmental task for vocalization to the age.

CLINICAL SITUATION

1. 2 months
2. 4 months
3. 6 months
4. 8 months
5. 10 months
6. 12 months

1. _____
2. _____
3. _____
4. _____
5. _____
6. _____

PRIORITY ACTIONS

a. Comprehends "bye-bye"

b. Begins to imitate sounds

c. Coos

d. Imitates animal sounds

e. Laughs out loud

f. Combines syllables ("dada") but doesn't understand meaning

NURSING CARE OF THE CHILD WHO HAS A COMMUNICABLE DISEASE

Fill in the blanks with the information that pertains to the identified communicable disease. There are several options for symptoms and interventions.

VARICELLA (CHICKENPOX)

Transmitted via _____ particles

and _____ _____

with open vesicles or lesions.

List three symptoms.

a. _____

b. _____

c. _____

Describe rash: _____ that progresses

to _____

List three nursing interventions.

a. _____

b. _____

c. _____

Report to the Centers for Disease Control: ☐ Yes ☐ No

PERTUSSIS

Transmitted via _____

List three symptoms.

a. _____

b. _____

c. _____

List three nursing interventions.

a. _____

b. _____

c. _____

Report to the Centers for Disease Control: ☐ Yes ☐ No

MEASLES (RUBEOLA)

Transmitted via _____

List three symptoms.

a. _____

b. _____

c. _____

List three nursing interventions.

a. _____

b. _____

c. _____

Report to the Centers for Disease Control: ☐ Yes ☐ No

RESPIRATORY SYNCYTIAL VIRUS (RSV)

Transmitted via _____

List three symptoms.

a. _____

b. _____

c. _____

List three nursing interventions.

a. _____

b. _____

c. _____

Report to the Centers for Disease Control: ☐ Yes ☐ No

ROTAVIRUS

Transmitted via _____

List three symptoms.

a. _____

b. _____

c. _____

List three nursing interventions.

a. _____

b. _____

c. _____

Report to the Centers for Disease Control: ☐ Yes ☐ No

IMMUNIZATIONS

Identify the immunizations to be given based on the developmental stages from the list below. Several will be used more than once.

NEONATE	INFANT	TODDLER	PRESCHOOLER	SCHOOL-AGE	ADOLESCENT

WORD LIST

Diphtheria, tetanus and pertussis (DTaP)

Tetanus, diphtheria and pertussis (Tdap)

Rotavirus (RV)

Influenza

Measles, mumps, rubella (MMR)

Meningococcal (Men)

Human papilloma

virus (vHPV)

Pneumococcal conjugate (PCV13)

Hepatitis B (Hep B)

Hepatitis A (Hep A)

Varicella (VAR)

Inactivated polio virus (IPV)

Haemophilus influenzae type b (Hib)

Answers to Activities

PRIORITIZING NURSING CARE OF THE CHILD ANSWERS

CLINICAL SITUATION	PRIORITY NURSING ACTIONS	RATIONALE
1. A 3-year-old toddler has diarrhea and has been febrile for 2 days.	c. Administer oral rehydration fluids.	Fluid volume deficit, which could lead to hypovolemic shock, is the primary concern. Oral rehydration replaces fluid loss from diarrhea and is preferred to intravenous therapy.
2. A 4-week-old infant has hypertrophic pyloric stenosis and is vomiting.	d. Administer replacement electrolytes intravenously.	Children who have this condition are especially prone to depletion of potassium, sodium, and chloride. All of these electrolytes are contained within gastric secretions. A serious imbalance could be life-threatening.
3. A neonate was born with a myelomeningocele in the lumbar region.	e. Monitor respirations and level of consciousness.	Of children who are born with a myelomeningocele, 80% to 85% develop hydrocephalus, which can affect respiration and neurological function. Feeding difficulties, irritability, lethargy, seizures, and episodes of apnea should be reported immediately.
4. A 5 year-old child is receiving chemotherapy for acute lymphocytic leukemia.	a. Monitor for hypotension, wheezing, nausea, vomiting, and urticaria.	Many chemotherapeutic agents have anaphylactic potential. Children should be monitored carefully while the medication is infusing and for 1 hr afterward for signs of anaphylaxis. Emergency equipment and medications must be immediately available.
5. A 10-year-old child has sickle cell anemia and is having a vaso-occlusive crisis.	b. Place on bed rest and minimize activity.	The primary objective in treatment of a vaso-occlusive crisis is to minimize oxygen expenditure and improve oxygen use, which occurs by limiting physical activity.

INFANT VOCALIZATION ANSWERS

CLINICAL SITUATION	VOCALIZATION
1. 2 months	c. Coos
2. 4 months	e. Laughs out loud
3. 6 months	b. Begins to imitate sounds
4. 8 months	f. Combines syllables ("dada") but doesn't understand meaning
5. 10 months	a. Comprehends "bye-bye"
6. 12 months	d. Imitates animal sounds

VARICELLA (CHICKENPOX)

Transmitted via airborne particles and direct contact with open vesicles or lesions.

List three symptoms.

> Fever

> Lymphadenopathy

> Intense pruritus

Describe rash: Maculopapular rash that progresses to vesicles

List three nursing interventions.

> Place client on airborne and contact precautions until all vesicles are dried and crusted over.

> Bathe and change sheets and clothes daily.

> Apply calamine lotion.

> Keep fingernails short. Apply mittens.

> Maintain a cool environment.

> Provide diversionary activities to distract from scratching.

> Teach the child to apply pressure instead of scratching.

> Remove loose crusts.

> Avoid use of aspirin.

Report to the Center for Disease Control: Yes

PERTUSSIS

Transmitted via droplet

List three symptoms.

> Coryza

> Sneezing

> Watery eyes

> Low-grade fever

> Dry hacking cough that becomes paroxysmal

> Cough followed by a sudden inspiration that produces a whooping sound

> Flushed cheeks or cyanosis during cough

> Mucous plug dislodged by cough

> Vomiting after coughing

List three nursing interventions.

> Place the child on droplet precautions.

> Offer small amounts of fluids frequently.

> Position the child on side.

> Provide humidified oxygen.

> Monitor for airway obstruction and hypoxia.

> Emphasize the need for the child to finish the entire course of antibiotics.

Report to the Center for Disease Control: Yes

MEASLES (RUBEOLA)

Transmitted via airborne particles

List three symptoms.

> Fever and malaise

> Coryza, cough, conjunctivitis

> Koplik spots on buccal mucosa before rash

> Maculopapular rash that starts on the face and spreads down

> Anorexia, abdominal pain

> Lymphadenopathy

> Photophobia

List three nursing interventions.

> Place on airborne precautions.

> Encourage rest.

> Provide antipyretics.

> Maintain low-light environment.

> Clean eyes with warm saline.

> Provide a cool-mist vaporizer.

> Encourage fluids and soft foods.

> Bathe in tepid water.

Report to the Center for Disease Control: Yes

RESPIRATORY SYNCYTIAL VIRUS (RSV)

Transmitted via droplet, direct, or indirect contact

List three symptoms.

> Rhinorrhea

> Low-grade fever

> Cough

> Respiratory symptoms: wheezing, retractions, crackles, dyspnea, tachypnea, crackles, diminished breath sounds

> Lethargy

> Poor feeding

> Apneic episodes

List three nursing interventions.

> Place on droplet and contact precautions.

> Screen visitors for illness.

> Encourage breastfeeding clients to pump and store milk.

> Provide small amounts of fluid frequently.

> Monitor oxygenation.

> Suction PRN.

> Reinforce teaching to parents to suction nares using saline drops and a bulb syringe.

> Administer antipyretics.

Report to the Center for Disease Control: No

ROTAVIRUS

Transmitted via fecal-oral, contact

List three symptoms.

> Watery diarrhea

> Vomiting

> Fever

> Abdominal pain

> Anorexia, poor feeding

> Irritability

> Signs of dehydration (absence of tears; dry mucous membranes; decreased output; weight loss; warm, dry skin; sunken fontanel)

List three nursing interventions.

> Place the client on contact precautions.

> Administer oral rehydration in small amounts (1 to 2 tsp) frequently (every 5 to 10 min while awake).

> Administer and monitor IV fluids if unable to tolerate oral fluids.

> Weigh the client daily.

> Monitor intake and output.

> Monitor for signs of hypovolemic shock (lethargy, pallor, tachycardia, tachypnea).

> Monitor specific gravity.

> For infants, reinforce teaching to parents to alternate oral rehydration solution with breast milk or formula.

> Progress diet as tolerated.

Report to the Center for Disease Control: No

IMMUNIZATIONS ANSWERS

NEWBORN	INFANT	TODDLER	PRESCHOOLER	SCHOOL-AGE	ADOLESCENT
Hepatitis B (Hep B)	Hepatitis B (Hep B)	Hepatitis B (Hep B)	Diphtheria, tetanus, and pertussis (DTaP)	Influenza	Influenza
	Rotavirus (RV)	Diphtheria, tetanus, and pertussis (DTaP)	Inactivated polio virus (IPV)	Meningococcal	Meningococcal
	Diphtheria, tetanus, and pertussis (DTaP)	*Haemophilus influenzae* type b (Hib)	Influenza	Tetanus, diphtheria, and pertussis (Tdap)	
	Haemophilus influenzae type b (Hib)	Pneumococcal conjugate (PCV13)	MMR	Human papilloma virus (vHPV)	
	Pneumococcal conjugate (PCV13)	Inactivated polio virus (IPV)			
	Inactivated polio virus (IPV)	Influenza			
	Influenza	Measles, mumps, rubella (MMR)			
		Varicella (VAR)			
		Hepatitis A (Hep A)			

Source: https://www.cdc.gov/vaccines/schedules/hcp/imz/child-adolescent.html

Practice Questions

Coordinated Care

1. A nurse reinforces teaching to a client about end-of-life decisions. Which information about advance directives is correct?

   A. Informed consent should be verified.

   B. A health care proxy can be designated.

   C. Specific dietary restrictions are identified.

   D. Legal counsel is needed to make changes.

2. A client who has a terminal illness decides to discontinue treatment. What is the appropriate response from the nurse?

   A. "Why are you giving up?"

   B. "Tell me about your decision."

   C. "What does your family want?"

   D. "You have other available options."

3. A nurse recognizes an increase in client falls in a long-term care facility. Which step should the nurse use to begin the quality improvement process?

   A. Collect data.

   B. Identify causes.

   C. Initiate corrective action.

   D. Analyze possible solutions.

4. A student nurse provides care to an 18-year-old client. Which action maintains confidentiality?

   A. Takes a picture of client's wound to use for classroom discussion

   B. Prints a copy of the client's medical record for educational purposes.

   C. Encourages a parent to be present during physical examination of client.

   D. Discloses client status over the phone when caller provides correct code

5. A licensed practical nurse (LPN) provides care to a group of clients. Which client should be reassigned to the RN? Client who has

   A. a nasogastric tube and pH of the gastric aspirate is 3

   B. asthma and prescribed oxygen via nonrebreather mask

   C. diabetes mellitus and a blood glucose level of 160 mg/dL

   D. a stage III pressure ulcer and requires a sterile dressing change

6. A charge nurse conducts an in-service on documentation. Which abbreviation is acceptable for use in client medication prescriptions?

   A. cc

   B. SQ

   C. D/C

   D. mcg

7. A nurse plans to provide change-of-shift report for a client. Which action is appropriate?

   A. Describe current status.

   B. Ask family to participate.

   C. Give report in the hallway.

   D. Include past admission data.

8. When given a scheduled medication, the client states, "This blue pill looks different than the one I take at home." Which response by the nurse is appropriate?

   A. "You can refuse to take it."

   B. "Let me verify the prescription."

   C. "This is what the pharmacy sent."

   D. "It is important for you to take this."

9. A nurse plans care for an assigned group of clients. Which intervention is the priority?

   A. Administer insulin to a client who has hyperglycemia.

   B. Suction a tracheostomy for a client who has pneumonia.

   C. Provide emotional support to a client who has breast cancer.

   D. Reinforce dietary teaching for a client who has a peptic ulcer.

10. A newly hired nurse prepares to insert an indwelling urinary catheter for the first time. Which action is appropriate?

    A. Review policy and procedure manual.

    B. Read and follow instructions provided.

    C. Ask preceptor to observe the procedure.

    D. Request another nurse to complete the skill.

11. A nurse participates in the process of informed consent with a client who is considering a surgical procedure. Which ethical principle is being demonstrated?

    A. Justice

    B. Autonomy

    C. Beneficence

    D. Nonmaleficence

12. A nurse provides care to a client who requires informed consent for an elective surgery. What is the appropriate action?

    A. Explain the procedure.

    B. Identify risks involved.

    C. Answer client questions.

    D. Witness client signature.

13. A preceptor is discussing computer documentation with a new nurse. Which statement should be included?

    A. "Sharing your password during an emergency situation may be required."

    B. "Access to all client records will be granted when orientation is completed."

    C. "Move the computer to prevent your client's family from viewing the screen."

    D. "Logging off the computer terminal is not necessary when in a private room."

14. A nurse observes a staff member who falsifies client documentation. What is the appropriate action?

    A. Discuss findings with the staff member.

    B. Continue to monitor the staff member's actions.

    C. Report the staff member's action to the charge nurse.

    D. Request the staff member to complete an incident report.

15. A nurse provides care for a client who has type 2 diabetes mellitus. Which members of the interdisciplinary team should be involved in promoting self-management for a foot ulcer? (Select all that apply.)

    A. Case manager

    B. Wound specialist

    C. Exercise therapist

    D. Registered dietitian

    E. Speech-language pathologist

Pharmacology in Nursing

1. A nurse reinforces discharge instructions to a client prescribed carbidopa/levodopa. Which instruction should be included?

   A. Urine may turn a dark color.

   B. The risk of falls is decreased.

   C. A high protein diet is encouraged.

   D. Medication should be taken at bedtime.

2. A nurse provides care for a client who has type 1 diabetes mellitus and is prescribed propranolol HCL. Which finding should be recognized as a sign of hypoglycemia?

   A. Fluid loss

   B. Diaphoresis

   C. Tachycardia

   D. Increased thirst

3. A client who has rheumatoid arthritis reports taking several herbal supplements. Which supplement would be of concern to the nurse?

   A. Flaxseed

   B. Green tea

   C. Echinacea

   D. Saw palmetto

4. A nurse provides care to a client who has chronic kidney disease. Which prescription should be questioned?

   A. Furosemide 20 mg PO, twice daily

   B. Insulin detemir 8 units subcutaneous at bedtime

   C. Lactated Ringer's 50 mL/hr by continuous IV infusion

   D. Acetaminophen 650 mg rectal suppository every 6 hr PRN pain

5. A client has a new prescription for bethanechol. The nurse is aware of potential risk if which medication is also administered?

   A. Digoxin

   B. Cephalexin

   C. Neostigmine

   D. Acetaminophen

6. A nurse reinforces teaching related to valproic acid. Which client statement indicates understanding?

   A. "I will continue to take an aspirin daily."

   B. "My kidney function will need to be monitored."

   C. "Taking oral contraceptives is not recommended."

   D. "It is important to report stools changing to a lighter color."

7. A nurse prepares to administer a beta blocker to a client. Which finding indicates the medication should be withheld?

   A. Confusion

   B. Pedal edema

   C. Pulse rate 52/min

   D. Blood pressure 102/70 mm Hg

8. A client receives an IV infusion of cefazolin. The nurse should be most concerned about the sudden onset of which finding?

   A. Urticaria

   B. Diarrhea

   C. Hoarse voice

   D. Dull headache

9. A nurse prepares to dispose of unused client medications. A witness is required for discarding which medications? (Select all that apply.)

   A. Diazepam

   B. Methadone

   C. Benzocaine

   D. Phenobarbital

   E. Methylphenidate

10. A nurse provides care for a client prescribed nitrofurantoin. Which finding is of concern?

    A. Fatigue

    B. Dry cough

    C. Bladder spasms

    D. Brown discoloration of urine

11. A nurse provides care for a 5-year-old child who is prescribed 2 drops of ofloxacin 0.3% solution to the left ear twice daily. Which action is appropriate?

    A. Wash hands and apply sterile gloves.

    B. Position left lateral following instillation.

    C. Pull auricle upward and outward during administration.

    D. Instill medication by positioning a dropper inside the auditory canal.

12. A nurse reinforces teaching for a client who has a continuous subcutaneous insulin infusion (CSII) via pump. Which information should be included?

    A. Remove pump when sleeping.

    B. Change the needle every 2 to 3 days.

    C. Prime pump and tubing with long-acting insulin.

    D. Test urine ketones if blood glucose level is greater than 150 mg/dL.

13. A nurse prepares to administer memantine to a client and is unsure of the desired effect. Which action should be taken?

    A. Call the pharmacist.

    B. Ask the charge nurse.

    C. Use a website.

    D. Review a drug reference.

14. A nurse reinforces teaching for a client who is prescribed patient-controlled analgesia. Which statement should be included?

    A. "You will be able to adjust the dose limits if in pain."

    B. "Family members can administer the medicine for you."

    C. "An overdose can occur if the button is pushed too often."

    D. "This method can decrease the amount of medication needed."

15. A nurse provides care for a client who has multiple sclerosis and is prescribed diazepam. Which finding indicates a therapeutic response to the medication?

    A. Decreased appetite

    B. Increased hair growth

    C. Increased mental acuity

    D. Decreased muscle spasms

16. A nurse prepares to administer medications for a client. Which action does not follow safe practice guidelines?

    A. Verify any client allergies.

    B. Open medication package at the bedside.

    C. Give within 2 hr of scheduled time.

    D. Provide information about purpose of the medication.

17. A nurse reinforces teaching to a client who is prescribed polyethylene glycol-electrolyte solution in preparation for a scheduled colonoscopy. Which statement indicates teaching was effective?

    A. "I must drink 240 mL of the liquid each hour."

    B. "I may experience mild abdominal discomfort."

    C. "I will increase my salt intake prior to ingesting."

    D. "I should expect a bowel movement within 4 hours."

18. A nurse prepares to administer latanoprost ophthalmic drops to a client. Which action is appropriate?

    A. Rest dropper on the lower conjunctiva.

    B. Apply pressure to the nasolacrimal duct.

    C. Pull the eyelid upward to expose cornea.

    D. Do not repeat instillation if drops fall on the outer lid.

19. A nurse provides care to a client prescribed cephalexin. A history of an allergic reaction to which medication should be of concern?

    A. Amoxicillin

    B. Doxycycline

    C. Sulfadiazine

    D. Erythromycin

20. A client who is 24 hours post appendectomy reports a pain level of 6 on a 0-to-10 scale. Which PRN medication should the nurse plan to administer?

    A. Fentanyl

    B. Ibuprofen

    C. Hydrocodone

    D. Acetaminophen

21. A nurse monitors effectiveness of pain medication for a client who is receiving mechanical ventilation. Which response indicates a therapeutic effect?

    A. Relaxed facial expression

    B. Spontaneous eye opening

    C. Heart rate within normal limits

    D. Ability to respond to command

22. A nurse prepares to administer ampicillin 250 mg intermittent IV bolus to a client who has a continuous infusion of 0.9% sodium chloride. Which action should be taken?

    A. Apply a cool compress to infusion site.

    B. Apply a warm compress to infusion site.

    C. Position piggyback above primary infusion bag.

    D. Position piggyback below primary infusion bag.

23. A nurse provides care to a client who is prescribed warfarin. When reviewing the home medication list, which supplement is of concern?

    A. Flaxseed

    B. Echinacea

    C. Valerian root

    D. Glucosamine

24. A nurse reinforces teaching for a client who is prescribed lithium carbonate. Which instruction should be included?

    A. Take prior to meals.

    B. Choose foods low in sodium.

    C. Hold if abdominal pain occurs.

    D. Maintain adequate fluid intake.

25. A client is prescribed a continuous infusion of dextrose 5% in water (D_5W) at 75 mL/hr. The IV tubing drop factor is 15 gtt/mL. The nurse should set the manual IV infusion to deliver how many gtt/min? (Round the answer to the nearest whole number.) _____gtt/min

Fundamentals for Nursing

1. A nurse provides care for a client who has expressive aphasia. Which intervention should be used to gather data?

    A. Use communication board.

    B. Ask open-ended questions.

    C. Provide only verbal information.

    D. Request a trained medical interpreter.

2. A nurse prepares to administer an intramuscular injection. Which client identifiers can be used? (Select all that apply.)

    A. Full name

    B. Date of birth

    C. Room number

    D. Telephone number

    E. Photo identification

3. A nurse provides care to a client who has *Clostridium difficile* infection. Which technique is appropriate for hand hygiene?

    A. Apply an alcohol-based sanitizer.

    B. Use a chlorine bleach solution.

    C. Wash with an antibacterial soap.

    D. Cleanse with hydrogen peroxide.

4. A nurse provides care to a client who has a new prescription for the application of restraints. Which information should be included in documentation? (Select all that apply.)

    A. Time of application

    B. Nurse-to-client ratio

    C. Location and type of restraint

    D. Behavior of client making restraints necessary

    E. Client's response when restraints are removed

5. What sequence should a nurse use to perform wound irrigation for a client who has a pressure ulcer? (Place the following steps for the procedure in the correct order. All steps must be used.)

    A. Obtain culture.

    B. Apply appropriate dressing.

    C. Dry wound edges with gauze.

    D. Flush wound using continuous pressure.

    E. Fill 30 mL syringe with irrigation solution.

    F. Attach 19-gauge angiocatheter to the syringe.

6. A nurse reinforces teaching to a client about isometric exercises. Which activity should the nurse recommend?

    A. Walking

    B. Swimming

    C. Aerobic dance

    D. Gluteal contractions

7. A nurse provides care to a client who is in balanced-suspension traction. Which action should be implemented?

    A. Remove weights if the client reports severe pain.

    B. Adjust screws twice a day to maintain alignment.

    C. Insert an indwelling catheter to prevent incontinence.

    D. Encourage incentive spirometer use every hour while awake.

8. A nurse provides care for a client who has *Haemophilus influenzae* type B. Which type of personal protective equipment (PPE) is required?

    A. Mask

    B. Gown

    C. Gloves

    D. Goggles

9. A nurse participates in a staff education session at a skilled nursing facility. Which items found in a client's room are a potential fire hazard? (Select all that apply.)

    A. New hair dryer

    B. Portable oxygen tank

    C. Multiple infusion pumps

    D. Cracked electrical cords

    E. Chest tube to wall suction

10. A nurse reinforces home safety with an older adult client. Which finding in the home environment poses a safety risk?

    A. Grab bars near the toilet

    B. Fire extinguisher in the garage

    C. Commode close to the bedside

    D. Extension cord under the carpet

11. A nurse inserts a nasogastric tube for a client who requires continuous enteral feeding. The initial gastric pH is 3.3. Which action should the nurse perform next?

    A. Connect the tube to the suction device.

    B. Advance the tube until drainage appears.

    C. Confirm placement of the tube with an x-ray.

    D. Inject air into the tube while listening for a bubbling sound.

12. A nurse transfers a client who is partially weight-bearing from the bed to a chair using a transfer belt. Which action is appropriate?

    A. Place chair near foot of the bed.

    B. Use side rails for support.

    C. Position the chair on the client's weaker side.

    D. Grasp under the belt along the client's sides.

13. Evacuation is required because of a fire in a long-term care facility. Which client should the nurse evacuate first?

    A. A client who is receiving mechanical ventilation.

    B. A client who has decreased strength and uses a walker.

    C. A client who has mild Alzheimer's disease and is ambulatory.

    D. A client who is receiving continuous gastrostomy tube feeding.

14. A nurse transports a newborn to the wrong mother. Upon identifying the error, which nursing action is the priority?

    A. Notify the provider.

    B. Inform risk management.

    C. Return the newborn to the nursery.

    D. Document the error in an incident report.

15. A nurse reinforces teaching for a client who has diverticulitis. Which foods are for a low-residue diet? (Select all that apply.)

    A. White rice

    B. Wheat toast

    C. Canned fruit

    D. Vegetable juice

    E. Hard-boiled egg

16. A nurse reinforces teaching to a client about the use of a walker. Which information should be included?

    A. Pull on the walker when rising from chair.

    B. Advance the walker, then the affected leg.

    C. Line the top of the walker up to waist height.

    D. Advance the walker, then the unaffected leg.

17. A nurse reinforces home safety about bathing for an older adult client. Which statement demonstrates understanding?

    A. "Grab bars will be installed in the shower."

    B. "The bathroom door should remain locked."

    C. "A towel will be placed in the bottom of the shower."

    D. "Water should be turned on after entering the tub."

18. A client who is receiving intermittent tube feedings reports that the alarm on the pump is continually sounding. Which action should the nurse take?

    A. Silence the alarm and continue the feeding.

    B. Stop the feeding and obtain a new pump.

    C. Notify the charge nurse and primary care provider.

    D. Identify the cause and verify pump is operating properly.

19. A nurse implements triage for a mass casualty. Which client should be recommended for discharge first? A client who

    A. has a long bone fracture

    B. has a small bowel obstruction

    C. reports new onset of chest pain

    D. is scheduled for elective surgery

20. What sequence should the nurse use in providing postmortem care to a client? (Place the steps in selected order of performance. All steps must be used.)

    A. Remove all equipment.

    B. Apply identifying tags.

    C. Inquire about cultural preferences.

    D. Identify client using two identifiers.

    E. Cleanse the body.

Adult Medical Surgical Nursing

1. A nurse discovers a client who is leaving against medical advice. Which action is appropriate?

    A. Notify the provider.

    B. Contact hospital security.

    C. Reinforce discharge instructions.

    D. Administer prescribed medications.

2. A client who has a cervical collar in place following a fall asks "Can I take this off when sleeping?" The nurse should respond with which statement?

    A. "You may remove the brace during naps and just prior to bedtime."

    B. "The brace is protecting your airway and may be removed in a few days."

    C. "I will remove the brace as soon as I see normal movement in your extremities."

    D. "The brace must remain in place until it can be determined there is no spinal injury."

3. A client reports leg pain when walking short distances. After noting hair loss on the lower left leg, which action should the nurse take?

    A. Check for edema in both legs.

    B. Compare bilateral posterior tibial pulses.

    C. Look for brown discoloration along the ankles.

    D. Monitor warmth and redness on lower extremities.

4. A nurse provides care for a client who has a NG tube to intermittent suction. Which action should be included in the plan of care?

    A. Clamp the air vent.

    B. Elevate head of bed 15°.

    C. Check residual every 4 hr.

    D. Monitor for abdominal distension.

5. A nurse provides care to a client who has a chest tube and observes fluctuations in the water seal chamber. What is the appropriate action?

    A. Locate air leak.

    B. Reinforce dressing.

    C. Continue to monitor.

    D. Increase wall suction.

6. A nurse performs wound care for a client who has a stage II pressure ulcer. Which action is appropriate?

    A. Apply vacuum-assisted closure.

    B. Cover with hydrocolloid dressing.

    C. Debride with proteolytic enzymes.

    D. Clean using povidone-iodine solution.

7. A nurse reinforces teaching for a client about a fecal occult blood test to be performed in the home setting. Which instruction should be included?

    A. Three different stool samples will be required.

    B. Restrict all dietary meat for 7 days prior to the test.

    C. Refrain from eating at least 24 hours before the test.

    D. A rectal exam will be necessary to obtain a stool sample.

8. A nurse prepares to remove an indwelling urinary catheter for a client. Which action is the priority when performing this task?

    A. Position supine

    B. Document urine output

    C. Drain fluid from balloon

    D. Wrap tube in waterproof pad

9. A nurse prepares to perform a venipuncture on an older adult client. Which action is appropriate to enhance venous access?

    A. Use a BP cuff to dilate veins.

    B. Use the largest catheter possible.

    C. Apply tourniquet tightly above site.

    D. Vigorously clean site in a circular motion.

10. A nurse prepares to insert an NG tube for a client. Which action is appropriate?

    A. Have client blow nose.

    B. Place in supine position.

    C. Measure distance from tip of nose to chin.

    D. Remove if client reports nasal burning sensation.

11. A nurse prepares to assist the provider with a bronchoscopy. What is required for the procedure?

    A. Benzocaine spray

    B. Supplemental oxygen

    C. Vacuum collection bottle

    D. Emergency tracheostomy tray

12. A nurse reinforces teaching for a client who has an ileal conduit. Which information should be included? (Select all that apply.)

    A. Self-catheterization is necessary.

    B. Bowel movements will contain urine.

    C. Stoma should appear pink and moist.

    D. Low-residue foods are recommended.

    E. Urine is collected in an external pouch.

13. A nurse provides care for a client who had abdominal surgery. Which actions are appropriate when applying compression stockings? (Select all that apply.)

    A. Smooth wrinkles from stocking.

    B. Monitor pulses and skin integrity.

    C. Remove and reapply stockings daily.

    D. Measure legs to determine correct size.

    E. Fold stockings to avoid covering the toes.

14. A nurse provides care for a client who has an NG tube for gastric decompression. Which findings indicate a need for intervention?

    A. pH value of gastric aspirate of 4

    B. Tube secured to nose with tape

    C. Absence of drainage for 8 hr

    D. Green fluid observed in suction container

15. A nurse provides care for a client who has a Penrose drain. Which action is appropriate?

   A. Keep safety pin secure in the drain.

   B. Place drain above level of the wound.

   C. Use sterile technique when emptying the drain.

   D. Notify RN if drainage is observed on the dressing.

16. A nurse provides care for a client who has COPD and is experiencing dyspnea during hygiene activities. Which action is appropriate?

   A. Increase supplemental oxygen.

   B. Encourage pursed-lip breathing.

   C. Obtain an oxygen saturation level.

   D. Auscultate bilateral breath sounds.

17. A nurse reinforces teaching for a client who has a prescription for bumetanide. Increased intake of which food should be recommended?

   A. Celery

   B. Lettuce

   C. Cabbage

   D. Avocados

18. A nurse assists with the removal of a Jackson-Pratt abdominal drain. Which action should be implemented following the procedure?

   A. Obtain and document the client's weight.

   B. Record the amount and color of drainage.

   C. Measure and report the client's abdominal girth.

   D. Apply an occlusive dressing over the drainage site.

19. A nurse provides care for a client who has an open fracture of the femur. The client suddenly develops shortness of breath and tachypnea. Which action is most appropriate?

   A. Suction the client.

   B. Obtain blood culture.

   C. Prepare for chest tube insertion.

   D. Place client in high-Fowler's position.

20. A nurse reinforces teaching to a client about glucose monitoring. Which action is appropriate?

   A. Clean site with alcohol.

   B. Use first drop of blood for testing.

   C. Puncture site immediately after cleaning.

   D. Hold finger in dependent position prior to puncturing.

21. A client returns to the room following a CT scan with contrast. What should the nurse monitor to identify potential complications?

   A. Pain level

   B. Urine output

   C. Daily weight

   D. Bowel sounds

22. A nurse prepares to remove a peripheral IV catheter. Which finding is most important to report to the RN?

   A. Purulent drainage

   B. Non-intact catheter

   C. Bruising after removal

   D. Redness around the site

23. A nurse reinforces teaching for a client who has a new colostomy. Which instruction should be included?

   A. Report any bleeding from the surgical site.

   B. Clean the skin around the stoma with mild soap and water.

   C. Keep unused ostomy pouches and wafers in the refrigerator.

   D. Use an alcohol-based skin sealant when attaching the appliance.

24. A nurse reinforces teaching to a client about a creatinine clearance test. Which of the following information should be included?

   A. Urine will be saved for 24 hr.

   B. Each sample is obtained midstream.

   C. Expected reference range is 60 to 80 mL/min.

   D. Timing begins with collection of the first void.

25. A nurse provides care for a client following abdominal surgery. Which action is appropriate regarding staple removal?

   A. Use a hemostat to gently remove each staple.

   B. Use sterile scissors to lift each side of the staple.

   C. Pull staple through one side of the skin after clipping.

   D. Insert tip of staple remover under the middle of the staple.

Mental Health Nursing

1. A nurse provides care for a client who has depression and anorexia. Which actions should the nurse take? (Select all that apply.)

   A. Weigh client daily.

   B. Monitor eating patterns.

   C. Encourage the client to sit with family while eating.

   D. Offer small portions of high-calorie foods frequently.

   E. Include client preferences when developing eating plan.

2. A client who practices Judaism reports a disruption in sleep patterns following the death of a loved one. The nurse should recommend which intervention to promote spiritual health?

   A. Delay discussion of recent loss.

   B. Limit family visitation to brief times.

   C. Encourage the client to spend time alone.

   D. Offer to contact the client's personal rabbi.

3. A nurse reinforces teaching regarding the benefits of a bereavement support group for a client who has experienced the death of a spouse. Which benefits should the nurse include? (Select all that apply.)

   A. Provides mutual support

   B. Offers networking resources

   C. Decreases feelings of isolation

   D. Integrates role-playing to act out emotions

   E. Allows an opportunity to meet a new companion

4. A nurse provides care for a client who is experiencing symptoms of alcohol withdrawal 12 hr after admission. Which intervention is the priority?

   A. Offer food and fluids.

   B. Document observations.

   C. Dim lights and reduce noise.

   D. Implement seizure precautions.

5. A nurse provides care for a client who has alopecia after 4 weeks of chemotherapy. Which statement reflects acceptance of body image?

   A. "I miss brushing my hair."

   B. "My family loved my long hair."

   C. "Imagine losing all of your hair."

   D. "The new wig looks like my own hair."

6. A nurse provides care for a client who is in a residential treatment program following cocaine withdrawal. Which findings indicate symptoms of relapse? (Select all that apply.)

   A. Euphoria

   B. Insomnia

   C. Tachycardia

   D. Hypotension

   E. Constricted pupils

7. A nurse provides care for a client who has a dependent personality disorder. Which behavior should the nurse expect?

   A. Maintains a rigid schedule

   B. Engages in splitting behaviors

   C. Views self as inferior to others

   D. Struggles with initiating projects

8. A licensed practical nurse (LPN) provides care to a client who recently received methadone. Which finding must the nurse report to the RN immediately?

   A. Pulse oximetry 90%

   B. Urine output 25 mL/hr

   C. Temperature 37.3° C (99.1° F)

   D. Blood pressure 100/62 mm Hg

9. A client who has schizophrenia screams, "Don't strangle me with that thing in your hand!" Which response by the nurse indicates a focus on reality orientation?

   A. "Don't worry. I won't hurt you."

   B. "This is a stethoscope. I use it to listen to your lungs."

   C. "You are being paranoid. That is a symptom of your illness."

   D. "You sound frightened. You will feel better after taking your medication."

10. A nurse provides care for a client receiving treatment for chronic back pain who states, "I cannot go on living like this anymore." Which response is therapeutic?

    A. "You should feel relief soon."

    B. "I know how overwhelming this can be."

    C. "Is there a minister or priest I can contact?"

    D. "Have you been thinking about ending your life?"

Maternal and Newborn Nursing

1. A nurse assists with the care of an intrapartum client. Which action should be implemented for the following fetal monitoring strip?

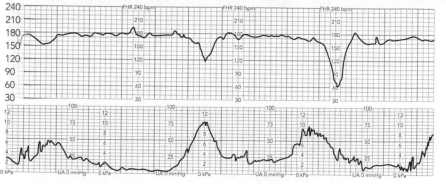

    A.   Notify the provider.

    B.   Reposition the client.

    C.   Elevate the client's legs.

    D.   Prepare for cesarean birth.

2. A nurse provides care to a client who has eclampsia. After observing brief seizure activity and calling for help, which priority action should the nurse implement?

    A. Raise and pad side rails.

    B. Suction airway secretions.

    C. Monitor blood pressure and heart rate.

    D. Apply oxygen via nonrebreather face mask.

3. A nurse collects data from a client who is receiving terbutaline. Which finding should be reported immediately?

    A. Heart rate 125/min

    B. Dyspnea and crackles

    C. Tremors and headache

    D. Blood pressure 100/60 mm Hg

4. A client who is at 32 weeks of gestation is prescribed terbutaline. Which condition should cause the nurse to question this medication?

    A. Pre-eclampsia

    B. Preterm labor

    C. History of asthma

    D. Allergy to macrolides

5. A nurse provides care for a client who is at 20 weeks of gestation. Which finding supports emotional preparedness and adaptation to pregnancy?

    A. Shows emotional lability

    B. Displays effective communication

    C. Identifies multiple support systems

    D. Verbalizes feelings of ambivalence

6. A nurse repositions a client who is in labor and observes the umbilical cord protruding from the vagina. Which action is the priority?

    A. Call for immediate assistance.

    B. Place in Trendelenburg position.

    C. Apply oxygen via nonrebreather mask.

    D. Wrap cord in a saline-soaked sterile towel.

7. A nurse performs cord care for a newborn. Which action should be included?

    A. Keep cord clean and dry.

    B. Cover cord with diaper and clothing.

    C. Remove cord clamp within 1 hr of birth.

    D. Administer acetaminophen prior to cord care.

8. A nurse prepares a client for a non-stress test. Which action should be included?

    A. Verify NPO status.

    B. Ensure bladder is empty.

    C. Confirm consent is signed.

    D. Place in semi-Fowler's position.

9. A nurse monitors the recovery of a client who is stable 48 hr after delivery. Which finding is expected?

    A. Firm fundus and small clots

    B. Elevated pulse and respirations

    C. Decreased desire to eat and drink

    D. Moderate amount of lochia serosa and no odor

10. A nurse provides care for a client who is 2 days postpartum. Which finding of positive maternal adaptation is expected?

    A. Demonstrates apathy when the infant cries

    B. Maintains close physical contact with the infant.

    C. Asks other members of the family to feed the infant

    D. Expresses concern when infant needs a diaper change

Nursing Care of Children

1. A nurse provides care to a 6-month-old infant. Which finding should be reported to the health care provider?

    A. Absent grasp reflex

    B. Inability to hold a bottle

    C. Does not pull up to stand

    D. Closed posterior fontanel

2. A nurse provides care to a 14-year-old client admitted with pelvic inflammatory disease. Which guideline is appropriate for communication?

    A. Begin with personal questions.

    B. Listen attentively without judgment.

    C. Explain that all information is confidential.

    D. Include parents in every conversation.

3. A nurse provides care to a 6-month-old infant. Which observation should be reported?

    A. Demonstrates head lag.

    B. Birth weight has doubled.

    C. Grasps objects voluntarily.

    D. Posterior fontanel is closed.

4. A nurse plans to administer an injection to a 4-year-old child. Which nursing action demonstrates age-appropriate communication?

    A. Describe the shot as feeling like a bee sting.

    B. Explain that some medicine will be put under the skin.

    C. Direct the explanation of the procedure to the caregiver.

    D. Share that all kids who go to school must have this medication.

5. A nurse provides care to a preschooler who is hospitalized. Which activity is age-appropriate?

    A. Shaking a colorful rattle

    B. Putting a puzzle together

    C. Arranging a coin collection

    D. Building a model spaceship

6. A nurse provides care to a 6-month-old infant hospitalized with dehydration. Which action should be included?

    A. Provide frequent cuddling.

    B. Suggest time in the playroom.

    C. Encourage multiple caregivers.

    D. Promote separation from parents.

7. A nurse assists with an annual physical examination for an 11-year-old child. Which immunization should be administered?

    A. Herpes zoster

    B. Pneumococcal (PPSV)

    C. Inactivated poliovirus (IPV)

    D. Human papilloma virus (HPV)

8. A nurse provides care to an 8-year-old child who has bacterial pneumonia. Which action is appropriate?

    A. Suggest the child go to the playroom.

    B. Assist the child in completing homework.

    C. Encourage the child to participate in care.

    D. Provide the child with detailed information.

9. A nurse reinforces discharge teaching for a school-aged child following a tonsillectomy. Which instruction should be included?

    A. Remove packing in 3 days.

    B. Gargle with salt water at bedtime.

    C. Avoid placing objects in the mouth.

    D. Notify provider if bad breath develops.

10. A nurse reinforces teaching about fiberglass cast care to an adolescent who has a fractured tibia. Which information should be included? (Select all that apply.)

    A. Expect complete drying in 24 hr.

    B. Pad the edges of the cast if irritation occurs.

    C. Use an ice pack on the cast to relieve itching.

    D. Stand with crutches 30 to 45 minutes each day.

    E. Report any changes in skin color below the cast.

Comprehensive Assessment

1. A nurse reviews laboratory results for a client who is receiving heparin therapy. Which laboratory values should be reported to the RN? (Select all that apply.)

   A. Hct 29%

   B. Hgb 15 g/dL

   C. aPTT 70 seconds

   D. WBC 8,600/mm³

   E. Platelet 115,000/mm³

2. A client who has fibromyalgia has a new prescription for imipramine. Which statement is of concern to the nurse?

   A. "I take naproxen at bedtime."

   B. "I drink several cups of coffee daily."

   C. "I usually eat smoked sausage for breakfast."

   D. "I use an antihistamine during allergy season."

3. A nurse notes redness, cracks, and blisters on the skin around a client's intravenous site. Which action should the nurse take first?

   A. Administer diphenhydramine.

   B. Document findings in medical record.

   C. Remove transparent adhesive dressing.

   D. Ask about previous reactions after eating kiwi.

4. A home health nurse reinforces availability of community resources for the caretaker of a client who is in hospice care. Which resources should the nurse include? (Select all that apply.)

   A. Respite care

   B. Meals on Wheels

   C. Adult day care services

   D. Anticipatory grief counseling

   E. Alzheimer's Association

5. A nurse prepares to perform a central venous catheter dressing change for a client. Which item should be used?

   A. Sterile gloves

   B. Antibiotic ointment

   C. Normal saline flush

   D. Hydrogen peroxide

6. A nurse prepares to administer medication though a gastrostomy tube to a client. Which interventions are appropriate? (Select all that apply.)

   A. Administer each medication separately.

   B. Use cranberry juice to prevent tube clogging.

   C. Verify placement using air bolus auscultation.

   D. Flush the tube before and after each medication.

   E. Crush extended-release and enteric-coated tablets.

7. A nurse provides care to a 10-year-old child who has a terminal illness. Which statement can the nurse expect from the child?

   A. "I am afraid of dying."

   B. "Will I be dead forever?"

   C. "What did I do to cause this disease?"

   D. "I do not want my appearance to change."

8. A client declines to take a prepared dose of oxycodone. Which action should the nurse take to discard the unused medication?

   A. Encourage the client to take the medication.

   B. Place the medication in the sharps container.

   C. Request another nurse to witness medication disposal.

   D. Return medication to the automated dispensing system.

9. A nurse provides care for a client who has a tracheostomy. Which action is appropriate?

   A. Reposition every 4 hr.

   B. Keep padded hemostat at bedside.

   C. Provide methods for communication.

   D. Clean the stoma site every 24 hr.

10. A client asks the nurse, "Who will have access to my medical information?" Which response by the nurse is appropriate?

    A. "Authorized persons."

    B. "All hospital employees."

    C. "Direct family members."

    D. "Your immediate supervisor."

11. A nurse reinforces teaching to a client who is postpartum and reports perineal discomfort. Which instruction should be included?

    A. Use a sitz bath.

    B. Massage fundus.

    C. Ambulate with assistance.

    D. Cleanse perineum with a squeeze bottle.

12. A licensed practical nurse (LPN) has been asked to provide initial teaching to a client who has a prescription for lisinopril. Which action should be taken?

    A. Refer this task to the RN.

    B. Request a change in assignment.

    C. Use an approved medication reference.

    D. Provide information about adverse effects.

13. A nurse reinforces teaching for a client who had a permanent pacemaker inserted. Which information should be included?

    A. Maintain a clear liquid diet.

    B. Resume showers after 2 weeks.

    C. Take pulse for 1 full minute each day.

    D. Apply pressure to site if dizziness occurs.

14. A nurse reviews effective use of client care materials with a group of assistive personnel (AP). Which statement is accurate?

    A. "Dirty linen should be held close to your body."

    B. "Enteral feeding bags should be replaced weekly."

    C. "Clean gloves should be used for medical asepsis."

    D. "Isolation stethoscopes should be recycled if needed."

15. A nurse provides care for a client who is receiving IV therapy. Which finding indicates fluid volume excess?

    A. Presence of tactile fremitus

    B. Crackles noted upon auscultation

    C. Capillary refill less than 2 seconds

    D. Urine output of 250 mL over 8 hours

16. A nurse recognizes a need for a speech-language pathology referral if the client develops which manifestation?

    A. Ataxia

    B. Aphonia

    C. Alopecia

    D. Akinesia

17. A nurse provides care for a client who reports difficulty sleeping while in the hospital. Which interventions should the nurse implement? (Select all that apply.)

    A. Dim overhead lights.

    B. Keep room door open.

    C. Cluster nursing activities.

    D. Silence monitor alarms.

    E. Provide fluids just prior to bedtime.

18. The nurse should place the client in which position prior to insertion of a nontunneled percutaneous central venous catheter?

    A. Fowler's

    B. Left lateral

    C. Semi-prone

    D. Trendelenburg

19. A nurse monitors a client's response to heat therapy. Which outcome is expected?

    A. Increased flexibility

    B. Increased strength

    C. Decreased edema

    D. Decreased sensation

20. A nurse cares for a client who reports using a stress management technique to visualize a peaceful scene near a stream of running water. Which method is the client using?

    A. Biofeedback

    B. Mindfulness

    C. Guided imagery

    D. Muscle relaxation

21. An assistive personnel (AP) obtains vital signs for a group of clients. Which findings should be reported to the nurse? (Select all that apply.)

    A. Heart rate 120/min

    B. Pulse oximetry 90%

    C. Temperature 37.3° C (99.1° F)

    D. Respiratory rate 10/min

    E. Blood pressure 115/75 mm Hg

22. A nurse reinforces client teaching regarding stress injuries at work. Which instruction is appropriate?

    A. Use a narrow stance to lift.

    B. Alternate tasks and postures.

    C. Pull rather than push objects.

    D. Bend and twist to reach items.

23. Identify the sequence a nurse should follow when setting up a sterile field for a client who requires an indwelling urinary catheter. (Place the steps in selected order of performance. All steps must be used.)

    A. Open the inner flap.

    B. Open the outer flap.

    C. Open the side flaps.

    D. Apply sterile gloves.

    E. Place the package on clean surface.

24. A nurse plans care for a group of clients. Which task should be delegated to the licensed practical nurse (LPN)?

    A. Admit a client who has *Clostridium difficile*.

    B. Titrate IV heparin for a client who has aPTT of 30 seconds.

    C. Suction a client who had a tracheostomy placed 4 hr ago.

    D. Change the sterile dressing for a client who has a foot ulcer.

25. A nurse monitors the neurological status of a client. Which finding should be reported to the RN?

    A. States name and date of birth

    B. Asymmetry observed when smiling

    C. Pupils are equal and reactive to light

    D. Shrugs shoulders against resistance

26. A caregiver of a client who has moderate Alzheimer's disease expresses feelings of increased stress and helplessness. Which coping strategy should the nurse recommend?

    A. Establish a routine schedule.

    B. Plan daily time away from the client.

    C. Place the client in a skilled nursing facility.

    D. Participate in supportive behavioral therapy.

27. A nurse observes increased bloody drainage on the dressing of a client who is 48 hr postoperative following abdominal surgery. Which action is priority?

    A. Obtain vital signs.

    B. Notify the provider.

    C. Document findings.

    D. Monitor urine output.

28. A client who follows Catholicism is scheduled for chemotherapy treatment. Which nursing action is appropriate?

    A. Avoid eye contact during conversation.

    B. Allow at least 3 feet of personal space.

    C. Support use of traditional prayer beads.

    D. Provide privacy during prayer five times daily.

29. Which laboratory data should be collected prior to administration?

    A. Calcium

    B. Sodium

    C. Potassium

    D. Magnesium

30. A client who has schizophrenia is experiencing auditory hallucinations. Which intervention should the nurse implement?

    A. Report the findings to the provider.

    B. Tell the client the voices will go away soon.

    C. Explain that hearing voices is part of the illness.

    D. Ask the client if a medication dose has been skipped.

31. A nurse provides care to a 10-year-old child who has a broken leg. Which of the following activities is age-appropriate?

    A. Board game

    B. Puppet show

    C. Pretend play

    D. Coloring book

32. A 13-year-old adolescent who has type 1 diabetes mellitus is reluctant to self-administer insulin during school. Which of the following responses by the school nurse demonstrates understanding of age-appropriate concerns?

    A. "Do not be afraid of needles."

    B. "This will upset your parents."

    C. "You will be given extra time at lunch."

    D. "There is a private area available to use."

33. A nurse reviews the postpartum medical records for a group of clients. Who is in need of an immunization?

    A. A client who has immunity to varicella

    B. A client who has no immunity to rubella

    C. A client who is Rh-negative with a Rh-negative newborn

    D. A client who is positive group B beta-hemolytic streptococcus

34. A client who has benign prostatic hypertrophy (BPH) has a new prescription for doxazosin mesylate. Which of the following instructions should the nurse reinforce?

    A. Take the initial dose at bedtime.

    B. Carry an albuterol inhaler at all times.

    C. Measure oral temperature every morning.

    D. Stop the medication if headaches develop.

35. A nurse observes flapping of the hands and a decreased level of consciousness in a client who has cirrhosis. Which medication should be administered?

    A. Ribavirin

    B. Lactulose

    C. Octreotide

    D. Furosemide

36. A client who has lower-back pain is prescribed ketorolac tromethamine. The nurse should monitor for which adverse reaction?

    A. Diarrhea

    B. Bronchospasm

    C. Respiratory depression

    D. Gastrointestinal bleeding

37. A nurse reinforces teaching to a client who is 1 day postpartum and breastfeeding. Which instruction should the nurse include?

    A. Start each feeding with the same breast.

    B. Breastfeed at least 8 to 12 times per day.

    C. Allow 10 minutes to fully empty each breast.

    D. Expect moderate breast pain with a proper latch.

38. A client who is experiencing adverse effects of neostigmine methylsulfate is prescribed atropine sulfate. The nurse should expect a decrease in which finding after medication administration?

    A. Muscle spasms and pain

    B. Salivation and diaphoresis

    C. Respiratory and heart rate

    D. Potassium and calcium level

39. A nurse reinforces teaching to the parents of an infant scheduled for a cleft palate repair. Which statement should be included regarding postoperative care?

    A. "Avoid holding your child until fully awake."

    B. "Pacifiers can be used to soothe your child."

    C. "Restraints will be applied to your child's arms."

    D. "Your child must remain positioned on the abdomen."

40. A nurse reinforces teaching regarding the use of mindfulness as a stress management technique. Which action demonstrates client understanding?

    A. Progressively tenses muscles then relaxes

    B. Writes extensively in a journal at the bedside

    C. Concentrates on an object and deep breathes

    D. Uses senses to focus on environmental surroundings

41. A nurse provides care for a client who has placenta previa. Which finding is expected?

    A. Decreased estrogen level

    B. Painful, dark-red vaginal bleeding

    C. Elevated serum progesterone level

    D. Painless, bright-red vaginal bleeding

42. A nurse provides care for a client and auscultates bowel sounds occurring 50 times per minute. Which description should the nurse use for these findings?

    A. Absent

    B. Infrequent

    C. Hypoactive

    D. Hyperactive

43. A nurse is assisting with scoliosis screening of a school-age child. Which instruction should be given?

    A. "Bend at the waist with your arms folded."

    B. "Stand with your arms positioned on your hips."

    C. "Stand with your arms extended horizontally."

    D. "Bend at the waist with your arms hanging down."

44. A nurse reinforces discharge teaching for a client who is 2 days postpartum. Which instruction would be appropriate regarding newborn positioning?

    A. Position on left side after feeding.

    B. Support back and buttocks when lifting.

    C. Hold and position under running water to bathe.

    D. Place supine on a firm crib mattress when sleeping.

45. A client who has an indwelling urinary catheter is diagnosed with a urinary tract infection. Which actions should the nurse include in the client's care? (Select all that apply.)

    A. Monitor urinary output.

    B. Increase oral fluid intake.

    C. Discontinue urinary catheter.

    D. Administer antipyretics as needed.

    E. Irrigate catheter with pressure syringe.

Practice Answers

COORDINATED CARE

1. **Correct: B**

   Advance directives are written instructions concerning desired care at end of life. The health care surrogate/proxy is the individual authorized to make decisions regarding health care should the client be unable to do so. This individual is named as a durable power of attorney for healthcare.

2. **Correct: B**

   The nurse must advocate for the client and his decisions. The client has verbalized a choice and it should be supported. The option provides an opportunity for the nurse to explore further discussion.

3. **Correct: A**

   Quality issues are identified by staff. Data is collected and analyzed, causes are identified, and a root-cause analysis may be done. Solutions or corrective actions are analyzed, and a solution is chosen for implementation. Educational or corrective actions are implemented and then the issue is re-evaluated.

4. **Correct: D**

   Many hospitals use a code system in which information is only disclosed to individuals who can provide the code. Nurses should ask any individual inquiring about a client's status for the code and disclose information only when an individual can give the code.

5. **Correct: B**

   The client who has asthma and requires a nonrebreather mask is unstable and will require further assessment, evaluation, and interventions. The client should be reassigned to the RN.

6. **Correct: D**

   Acceptable use includes mcg rather than μg. To help reduce medication errors, some abbreviations (cc, SQ, D/C) should not be used.

7. **Correct: A**

   Change-of-shift report includes the current health status of the client, informs the oncoming nurse of pertinent client information, and provides an opportunity to clarify and ask questions. It should be given in a private area, such as a conference room or at the client's bedside (as long as the client does not have a roommate and no unsolicited visitors are present).

8. **Correct: B**

   Clients have the right to question medications and treatments. The nurse should compare the medication available with the provider's prescription.

9. **Correct: B**

   Suctioning the tracheostomy will clear the client's airway. Using the priority-setting frameworks of Maslow's hierarchy of needs and airway, breathing, circulation (ABC), airway is the priority.

10. **Correct: A**

    The nurse is legally required to complete skills in accordance to the agency policy and procedure manual. This ensures the safety of the client and is the appropriate action.

11. **Correct: B**

    Autonomy is the ability of the client to make decisions. Autonomy refers to the commitment to include clients in the decision-making process. Informed consent demonstrates the principle of autonomy and the client's independence to make decisions.

12. **Correct: D**

    The nurse's role is to witness the client's signature and ensure the consent has been properly obtained.

13. **Correct: C**

    Once logged into the computer, the nurse should not leave the screen unattended. The nurse should log out when leaving the computer, and be sure the computer screen is not visible for public viewing. A computer password should not be shared with anyone under any circumstances.

14. **Correct: C**

    Staff members who witness an inappropriate action by a coworker should follow the chain of command in reporting. The unit manager should also be notified.

15. **Correct: A, B, C, D**

    Type 2 diabetes mellitus is a complex disease affecting glucose regulation and requires a collaborative approach to manage behavioral and lifestyle changes. The case manager coordinates the plan of care. An exercise therapist helps develop an exercise plan to maintain weight control and minimize cardiovascular complications. The wound specialist assesses and promotes skin integrity and develops a plan to promote healing and prevent complications. The registered dietitian assists with meal planning to maintain glycemic control.

PHARMACOLOGY IN NURSING

1. **Correct: A**

   Carbidopa/levodopa can cause dark discoloration of urine and sweat. The client should be informed this effect is harmless.

2. **Correct: B**

   Propranolol HCL is classified as a nonselective beta blocker of both cardiac and bronchial receptors used in the management of hypertension, angina, and myocardial infarction. Side effects include bradycardia and mild hypotension. Propranolol HCL can mask tachycardia as an early sign of hypoglycemia. Clients should be instructed to monitor other signs such as sweating, hunger, fatigue, and poor concentration. Clients should also closely monitor blood glucose.

3. **Correct: C**

   Echinacea is taken to stimulate the immune system for protection from infection and is contraindicated for clients who have autoimmune disorders. The herb can cause leukopenia and hepatomegaly, as well as interfere with immunosuppressant medications used to manage rheumatoid arthritis.

4. **Correct: C**

   Lactated Ringer's (LR) is an isotonic solution with electrolytes (sodium chloride, calcium, and potassium) added. LR should not be administered to clients who have chronic kidney disease due to the risk of hyperkalemia.

5. **Correct: C**

   Bethanechol is a direct-acting cholinergic. Giving neostigmine (a cholinergic muscle stimulant/cholinesterase inhibitor) concurrently with bethanechol can increase cholinergic effects and toxicity, resulting in increased salivation, bowel movements, and urination. It can also cause blurred vision.

6. **Correct: D**

   Valproic acid is an antiepileptic medication. It is important to monitor for signs of liver impairment, such as dark urine, pale stools (gray or white), jaundice, or altered liver function tests.

7. **Correct: C**

   Beta-adrenergic blocking agents (metoprolol, carvedilol) are commonly used to treat hypertension and heart disease. Medications in this class should be withheld and the provider notified if the client has a heart rate less than 60/min or a systolic BP less than 100 mm Hg.

8. **Correct: C**

   Cefazolin is a first-generation cephalosporin antibiotic. Signs of anaphylaxis include urticaria and hoarse voice. The client's voice being hoarse is the highest priority, as it can indicate impending respiratory distress.

9. **Correct: A, B, D, E**

   Diazepam (Schedule IV), methadone (Schedule II), phenobarbital (Schedule IV), and methylphenidate (Schedule II) are controlled substances, which have a potential for abuse and dependence and have a "Schedule" classification. These medications should be kept in a secure area and another nurse should witness the discarding.

10. **Correct: B**

    Nitrofurantoin is a broad-spectrum antibiotic used to treat urinary tract infections. Nitrofurantoin can cause pulmonary hypersensitivity reactions resulting in dyspnea, cough, chest pain, fever, chills, and alveolar infiltration. The client should stop the medication and notify the provider. Symptoms resolve 2 to 4 days after discontinuing the medication.

11. **Correct: C**

    Straighten the ear canal by pulling the auricle down and back for children younger than 3 years old. Pull upward and outward for children 4 years of age and older.

12. **Correct: B**

    The needle should be changed every 2 to 3 days to prevent infection.

13. **Correct: D**

    Drug references are compiled for nurses and contain information about medication administration, nursing implications, and client education.

14. **Correct: D**

    Patient-controlled analgesia (PCA) is a delivery system that allows clients to self-administer safe doses of opioids. Clients experience less time between identified need and delivery of medication, which increases a sense of control. This can decrease the amount of medication needed.

15. **Correct: D**

    Diazepam is a benzodiazepine and anticonvulsant used in the management of muscle spasms in clients who have multiple sclerosis.

16. **Correct: C**

    To prevent medication errors, the nurse follows the rights of safe medication administration. The nurse verifies client allergies by asking the client, looking at the allergy bracelet, and reviewing the medication administration record. The medication should be administered within 1 hr of the scheduled time (30 minutes before or 30 minutes after). Unit-dose medication is left in the package until administration. Accurate information is provided to the client about the medication purpose and adverse effects.

17. **Correct: B**

    Polyethylene glycol-electrolyte solutions (CoLyte, GoLYTELY) are prescribed prior to colonoscopy to evacuate the bowel and permit good visualization. The most common adverse effects are mild abdominal cramping, nausea, bloating, and flatulence. The client is instructed to drink 8 oz every 10 minutes until the prescribed amount is ingested. The first bowel movement is expected within 1 hr after the start of the solution.

18. **Correct: B**

    Latanoprost is an ophthalmic medication used to lower intraocular pressure in open angle glaucoma or intraocular hypertension. Gentle pressure should be applied to the nasolacrimal duct for 30 to 60 seconds to prevent systemic absorption of the medication.

19. **Correct: A**

    Cephalexin is a cephalosporin, and there is a possible cross-sensitivity to penicillin. Amoxicillin is a broad-spectrum penicillin. An alternate classification of antibiotic should be prescribed.

20. **Correct: C**

    Hydrocodone is a narcotic opiate used in the management of moderate to moderately severe pain. Onset of medication is 10 to 20 minutes with duration of 3 to 6 hr. Because of the high potential for abuse and addiction, it is intended for short-term use in clients experiencing acute pain postoperatively.

21. **Correct: A**

    According the Hierarchy of Pain Measures, if a client cannot self-report pain, the nurse should observe for changes in pain behaviors (facial expression, restlessness, crying) as indications of pain.

22. **Correct: C**

    The intermittent (piggyback) IV bolus should be placed above the primary bag to facilitate infusion of the fluid.

23. **Correct: D**

    Glucosamine, garlic, ginger, and ginkgo biloba can increase the risk of bleeding and should be used with caution in clients who take warfarin.

24. **Correct: D**

    Clients should maintain adequate fluid intake by consuming at least 1.5 to 3 L/day of fluid from beverages and food sources. Dehydration can alter therapeutic lithium levels.

25. **Correct: 19**

    If an electronic infusion pump is not available, regulate the IV flow rate using the roller clamp on the IV tubing. When setting the flow rate, count the number of drops that fall into the drip chamber over the period of 1 min.

    Formula:

    $$\frac{\text{Volume (mL)}}{\text{Time (min)}} \times \frac{\text{Drop Factor}}{\text{(gtt/mL)}} = \frac{Y \text{ (Flow Rate}}{\text{in gtt/min)}}$$

    Calculation:

    $$\frac{75 \text{ mL}}{60 \text{ min}} \times 15 \text{ gtt/mL} = 18.75 = 19 \text{ gtt/min}$$

FUNDAMENTALS FOR NURSING

1. **Correct: A**

   Expressive aphasia is the inability to produce language. Utilization of a communication board would aid in efforts for communication.

2. **Correct: A, B, D, E**

   The nurse should verify the client's identification prior to each medication administration. Acceptable identifiers include the client's name, telephone number, birth date, photo identification card, and assigned hospital identification number.

3. **Correct: C**

   Only hand hygiene with soap and water is effective to physically remove *Clostridium difficile* spores from the skin.

4. **Correct: A, C, D, E**

   Nursing documentation should include behaviors that make the restraint necessary, attempts to use alternatives to restraints and the client's response to those attempts, the client's level of consciousness, type and location of restraint used, education and explanations given to the client and family, exact time of application and removal, client behavior while restrained, type and frequency of care, and client's response when the restraint is removed.

5. **Correct: E, F, D, A, C, B**

   Fill a 30 to 60 mL syringe with irrigation solution, attach a soft 19-gauge angiocatheter, hold syringe tip above the upper end of the wound and over the area to be cleaned, and use continuous pressure to flush the wound. Repeat steps as needed to clean the wound. Obtain the culture as prescribed. Assess the wound bed, dry the wound edges with gauze, and apply the appropriate dressing.

6. Correct: D

Gluteal contractions are isometric exercises that involve tightening or tensing of muscles without movement of body parts. The goal is to improve muscle mass, tone, and strength.

7. Correct: D

The client is at risk of pulmonary secretions collecting in the lungs' lower lobes because of the immobility. An incentive spirometer should be used every hour while awake to facilitate lung expansion and coughing, thereby decreasing the risk of a buildup of pulmonary secretions.

8. Correct: A

Haemophilus influenza requires droplet precautions. Droplet precautions protect against droplets larger than 5 mcg and that travel 3 to 6 feet from the client. Providers and visitors should wear a mask to prevent transmission of the disease.

9. Correct: A, B, C, D

Any electrical appliances or devices are a fire risk hazard and must be evaluated by the safety inspection department before use in a health care facility.

10. Correct: D

An extension cord under the carpet is an electrical hazard and poses a risk for fire. The client should be made aware of this environmental factor, and a suggestion for modification should be made.

11. Correct: C

Confirming initial placement with an x-ray is the accepted practice of ensuring proper placement of the tubing. Subsequent placement is verified using the pH method. A pH of 4 or less is expected.

12. Correct: D

The nurse should grasp the belt from underneath and along the client's sides to promote movement of the client at his or her center of gravity. This provides stability for the client during transfer and reduces the risk for falling.

13. Correct: C

This is a safety issue. The most ambulatory resident will be evacuated first, followed by those who need assistance with mobility (wheelchairs) or equipment (tubes, catheters), and finally those who need to be moved by stretcher or in their beds. The prevailing concept is to move as many clients as quickly (and safely) as possible from the area.

14. Correct: C

Returning the newborn to the nursery and verifying the identification bracelets are priority. Acknowledgment and corrective action must be taken first when a practice error occurs.

15. Correct: A, C, D, E

Low-residue foods include ground and well-cooked meats, chicken, fish, eggs (not fried), mild cheeses, fruit and vegetable juice without pulp, pureed or strained vegetables, canned fruit and firm bananas, white rice, plain pasta and potatoes, and refined white bread.

16. Correct: B

Advance the walker, then the affected leg, using the walker for support on the weaker side. For the correct size, the top should line up with the crease on the inside of the wrist. Do not pull on the walker to rise, as the bottom of the walker could slip and allow the client to fall.

17. Correct: A

Grab bars should be placed near the toilet and in the tub or shower to reduce the risk of injury.

18. Correct: D

Potential causes should be identified, which could include the client and equipment. It is the nurse's responsibility to ensure that all client care equipment is functioning properly.

19. Correct: D

In the event of a mass casualty, ambulatory and self-care clients who need little or no assistance are the first clients to be safely discharged, transferred, or relocated. Clients who are considered stable (such as those scheduled for elective surgery) can be discharged.

20. Correct: D, C, A, E, B

Identify the client using two identifiers and confirm the information using the client's medical record. Verify the family's wishes regarding cultural, religious, and spiritual preferences. Remove all equipment and tubes. An autopsy or organ donation can be an exception to this step. Cleanse the body using proper personal protective precautions, and cover the body with a clean sheet. Prepare the environment. Offer family time to view the body and say goodbye. Apply identifying name tags. Complete the documentation. Transport the body.

ADULT MEDICAL SURGICAL NURSING

1. Correct: A

The client who is legally competent has the right to leave the facility at any time. The nurse should immediately notify the provider.

2. Correct: D

The cervical spine must be stabilized following any trauma that can result in injury to the spine. Radiological testing is required to determine the presence and extent of spinal injuries. Cervical collars should not be removed without a specific prescription to do so.

3. Correct: B

Leg pain while walking short distances is a symptom of peripheral arterial disease. The client can also experience hair loss on the lower calf, ankle, and foot. Other symptoms include dry, scaly skin; thickened toenails; cold and cyanotic extremities; and dependent rubor. The nurse should compare the strength of the posterior tibial pulses bilaterally as an indication of arterial function.

4. Correct: D

Placing the NG tube to intermittent suction removes gastric secretions and provides gastric decompression. The client's abdomen should be monitored for distention to determine adequate functioning of the tube.

5. Correct: C

This finding is expected and indicates appropriate function of the chest tube.

6. Correct: B

A stage II pressure ulcer is a partial-thickness loss of dermis, such as a shallow open ulcer with a red-pink wound bed without slough. A hydrocolloid dressing is an occlusive dressing that forms a seal at the wound's surface to prevent evaporation of moisture from the skin and supports healing in clean, granulating wounds.

7. Correct: A

An occult blood test of stool is performed to detect if GI bleeding is present. The test can be performed by a nurse or guaiac cards sent home with the client. If these cards are used, three stool samples are usually required to confirm GI bleeding.

8. Correct: C

The balloon should be drained prior to removal to prevent urethral trauma. This is the priority action.

9. Correct: A

Using a BP cuff is recommended for older adults and clients who have fragile veins.

10. Correct: A

Blowing the nose removes nasal secretions to clear nasal passages for ease of insertion and optimizes airflow through the other naris.

11. Correct: B

A bronchoscopy involves the insertion of a tube into the airways for visualization and to obtain specimens for analysis. The client's BP, pulse, respirations, and oxygen saturation should be continuously monitored during the procedure and supplemental oxygen administered.

12. Correct: C, E

An ileal conduit is a surgically placed permanent urinary diversion. The ureters are placed in a portion of the small intestine, which is opened onto the skin as a stoma. An external pouch covers the stoma and collects urine. A healthy stoma should appear pink and moist.

13. Correct: A, B, D

Smoothing wrinkles from the stocking will help prevent alterations of skin integrity and circulation. Pulses and skin integrity should be monitored to ensure circulation and skin integrity are not impaired. A tape measure is used to measure leg size to identify the correct stocking size.

14. Correct: C

The absence of drainage can indicate the NG tube is no longer in the stomach or obstructed. The amount and color of gastric secretions should be monitored while the tube is in place.

15. Correct: A

A pin is placed through the Penrose drain to prevent it from slipping into the wound.

16. Correct: B

It is common for clients who have COPD to experience exertional dyspnea. Pursed-lip breathing can be useful in managing a dyspneic episode as it facilitates expansion of the alveoli. It should be encouraged not only during the episode but also during any physical activity that can cause dyspnea to occur.

17. Correct: D

Bumetanide is a loop diuretic that has a potassium-depleting effect. The client should consume potassium-rich foods such as avocados, spinach, apricots, prunes, broccoli, dried beans, mushrooms, potatoes, oranges, bananas, kiwis, and cantaloupe.

18. Correct: B

Surgical drains are commonly placed to provide an exit of air, blood, and fluid following surgery. They can help prevent infections and abscess formation. The amount and color of drainage should be observed and documented as output and also at the time of drain removal.

19. Correct: D

The client is experiencing signs of fat embolism. Initial treatment is aimed at maximizing oxygenation to the client. The client should be repositioned to high-Fowler's position and oxygen administered. Additional treatment includes bed rest, hydration, and possible steroid therapy.

20. Correct: D

Holding the finger in a dependent position will improve blood flow.

21. Correct: B

The IV contrast used in many radiologic procedures increases the risk of renal damage, placing the client at high risk of kidney failure.

22. Correct: B

The IV catheter should be inspected to assure the tip has not broken off. The tip can move into the circulatory system resulting in an embolism.

23. Correct: B

The client should be instructed to clean around the stoma with mild soap and water prior to the application of the appliance. Soap with alcohol or lotion is to be avoided.

24. Correct: A

Creatinine clearance test requires urine collected over a specific time period (8, 12, or 24 hr) to measure glomerular filtration rate and kidney function. All urine voided during the prescribed time period is collected.

25. Correct: D

Insert the tip of the staple remover under the center of each wire staple. Slowly close ends of staple remover to free the staple from the skin.

MENTAL HEALTH NURSING

1. Correct: B, C, D, E

Clients who have depression can experience decreased appetite. Careful observation of eating patterns will provide needed information in establishing interventions. Providing preferred foods can encourage an increase of intake. Small, high-calorie portions are more easily tolerated than larger plates of food. Eating with others present can reinforce caring, increase self-esteem, and serve as an incentive to eat.

2. Correct: D

The role of spirituality or religion affects the restoration of health in a client, especially during spiritual distress. Spiritual leaders, such as a rabbi, have skills that offer reassurance and a sense of hope during time of pain and loss. Beliefs and practices encourage resilience and create new meaning of one's journey and all of its challenges.

3. Correct: A, B, C

A bereavement support group is a community service for those who have experienced the loss of a loved one. Health education and networking for resources are shared. Mutual support for members who share grief decreases feelings of isolation and offers coping strategies during the various stages of grief.

4. Correct: D

Clients experiencing alcohol withdrawal are at high risk of developing seizures. Manifestations usually start within 4 to 12 hr of the last intake of alcohol. Seizure precautions should be implemented immediately to reduce injury to the client.

5. Correct: D

Clients often experience a disturbance in body image due to losses related to chemotherapy. Willingness to use strategies to enhance one's appearance is significant and indicates progress toward acceptance.

6. Correct: A, B, C

Cocaine is a central nervous stimulant that produces feeling of euphoria. Indications of intoxication reflect a stimulated CNS such as tachycardia, insomnia, dilated pupils, hypertension, nausea, vomiting, and anxiety.

7. Correct: D

Dependent personality disorder is characterized by extreme dependency in close relationships. This can lead to clinging behavior, fear of separation, and difficulty initiating projects or doing things due to lack of confidence in decision-making, judgment, and abilities.

8. Correct: A

Methadone can cause respiratory depression. The pulse oximetry of 90% must be reported immediately to the RN as it indicates a low oxygenation level. Decreased oxygenation is the priority finding.

9. Correct: B

Delusions of persecution are alterations in thought causing the client to feel singled out for harm by others. The thoughts are false, fixed beliefs that cannot be corrected by reasoning. The nurse should not argue or agree with a client's delusions, but offer reality orientation.

10. Correct: D

Using direct communication that addresses suicide ideation shows support, empathy, and understanding. Acknowledging the client's feelings provides relief to talk openly about thoughts of defeat, despair, and hopelessness. This direct, closed-ended question is necessary to assess the immediate risk of self-injury and to convey a willingness to talk about feelings of despair to ensure client safety.

MATERNAL AND NEWBORN NURSING

1. **Correct: B**

   The pattern identifies variable decelerations indicating cord compression. The nurse should reposition the client to side-lying or knee-to-chest position to improve cardiac output and apply oxygen to improve oxygenation.

2. **Correct: B**

   Suctioning airway secretion will ensure a patent airway. After calling for help and remaining at the bedside, the priority action is to ensure a patent airway.

3. **Correct: B**

   Dyspnea and crackles should be reported immediately. Terbutaline stimulates cardiopulmonary effects including bronchodilation. Any signs of pulmonary edema (dyspnea, crackles, decreased SaO_2) require immediate action.

4. **Correct: A**

   Terbutaline is a tocolytic and should not be used for clients who have pre-eclampsia. Terbutaline can cause pulmonary edema, palpitations, chest pain, and myocardial ischemia.

5. **Correct: C**

   Support systems and perception of pregnancy are critical elements for emotional preparedness and adaptation to pregnancy. Ambivalence is common during the first trimester. During the second trimester, the focus is on the pregnancy and relationships with the client's mother and other pregnant clients.

6. **Correct: A**

   A prolapsed cord is a medical emergency. Calling for assistance is priority. The nurse would then place in Trendelenburg or modified Sim's position, wrap the cord loosely in a sterile towel saturated with warm saline, apply oxygen, administer IV fluids, and monitor FHR. The RN will perform a sterile vaginal exam and push the presenting part off the cord.

7. **Correct: A**

   The umbilical stump should be kept clean and dry to promote drying and minimize infection.

8. **Correct: D**

   A non-stress test is a noninvasive procedure. The test requires placing the client in a reclining chair, or bed in a semi-Fowler's or left-lateral position. Other preparation measures include applying the tocotransducer and fetal heart monitor to the client's abdomen and assessing for accelerations with fetal movement.

9. **Correct: A**

   The fundus should be firm, midline, and at the level of the umbilicus during the recovery stage. Small clots with lochia rubra are also expected.

10. **Correct: B**

   Touching the infant and maintaining close physical contact is a sign of effective maternal-infant bonding. It is essential for the nurse to observe emotional readiness and mother's ability to provide infant care before discharge.

NURSING CARE OF CHILDREN

1. **Correct: B**

   A 6-month-old infant should have motor development that includes rolling from back to front, holding a bottle, and picking up objects if dropped. Inability to do so can indicate a developmental delay and should be more thoroughly investigated.

2. **Correct: B**

   Appropriate guidelines for communicating with adolescents include listening attentively without judging. The nurse should begin with nonthreatening questions and provide for privacy from parents. Explain that there are limits to confidentiality, such as duty to report abuse.

3. **Correct: A**

   Head lag in a 6-month-old is unexpected. It would be expected in a 1-month-old infant. By 3 months of age, infants can hold their head well beyond the plane of the body.

4. **Correct: B**

   According to Erik Erikson, the expected psychosocial development of the preschooler is initiative versus guilt. Children at this age experience variations in thinking and focus on one aspect instead of the whole concept. The nurse should use neutral words to provide clear and simple explanations, appropriate to the child's developmental stage.

5. **Correct: B**

   Examples of age-appropriate activities for a preschooler include playing ball, doing puzzles, riding a tricycle, pretend play and dress-up, painting, role-playing, and musical toys.

6. **Correct: A**

   Based on Erikson's stages of growth and development, the infant is in the stage of trust vs. mistrust. Tactile stimulation is important in the process of acquiring trust.

7. **Correct: D**

   The routine vaccination schedule for an 11- to 12-year-old child includes yearly influenza; meningococcal; human papilloma virus; and tetanus, diphtheria, and acellular pertussis.

8. **Correct: C**

   Based on Erikson's stages of growth and development, the school-age child is in the stage of industry vs. inferiority. The nurse should encourage the child to assist with care to help achieve industry.

9. **Correct: C**

   Caregivers should be instructed to ensure the child does not put objects in the mouth to prevent injury to the surgical site.

10. **Correct: B, C, E**

   Padding the edge of the cast protects the skin from irritation and breakdown. An ice pack placed on the cast can decrease itching. Changes in skin color below the cast can indicate ischemia and should be reported immediately. To reduce risk of infection, remind the client to avoid placing objects down the cast.

COMPREHENSIVE ASSESSMENT

1. **Correct: A, E**

   Decreased Hct can indicate bleeding. Low platelet count (thrombocytopenia) can increase the risk of bleeding.

2. **Correct: D**

   Imipramine is a tricyclic antidepressant used in the management of depression and is prescribed for off-label use for enuresis, generalized anxiety disorder, neuropathic pain, fibromyalgia, and neuralgia. Tricyclic antidepressants exert an anticholinergic effect. As a result, all medications that potentiate this effect, including antihistamines, should be avoided.

3. **Correct: C**

   Transparent dressings, tape, tourniquet, and tubing products can contain latex. The assessment data indicates a potential latex sensitivity. The priority is client safety. Remove all latex products from the client's skin. The food allergies most likely to cause a latex sensitivity include apple, avocado, banana, carrot, celery, chestnut, kiwi, melons, papaya, raw potato, and tomato.

4. Correct: A, D

Providing care for a loved one who is terminally ill can be overwhelming emotionally, spiritually, and physically. Respite care allows the caregiver time to restore energy, manage stress, and perform self-care. Once hospice care is determined, family members begin a type of grief that anticipates the effect of the future loss of their loved one. Anticipatory grief counseling services provide information and support to assist with staying connected with the loved one during the dying process and to explore ways of coping with emotions.

5. Correct: A

The dressing of a central venous catheter should be changed using sterile technique. Therefore, sterile gloves should be obtained for the application of the dressing. The nurse should follow the agency policy and procedure, which often includes a prepackaged kit for central venous catheter care.

6. Correct: A, D

Each medication should be administered separately. To prevent clogging, the gastrostomy tube should be flushed with 15 to 30 mL of water (sterile water for clients who have weakened immune system) before and after each medication.

7. Correct: A

School-age children experience fear of the disease and death process, loss of control, and the unknown. They begin to have an adult concept of death.

8. Correct: C

Discarding of a controlled substance should be witnessed by a second nurse. Agency protocol should be followed for appropriate waste of narcotics.

9. Correct: C

A tracheostomy is an artificial airway. The client will need a method to communicate with staff. The nurse can use methods such as a communication board, paper and pen, or dry-erase board.

10. Correct: A

Only health care members who are directly responsible for the client's care should have access to the client's records. Client information should not be given to unauthorized persons, including family members who request it. The client can designate to whom information can be released.

11. Correct: A

Perineal discomfort results from perineal lacerations or episiotomies. A sitz bath is a nonpharmacological intervention to promote perineal comfort.

12. Correct: A

The RN should provide initial teaching, and the LPN reinforces teaching for the client.

13. Correct: C

The client should be instructed to take a daily pulse for 1 full minute to ensure proper functioning of the pacemaker. The client should know the rate at which the pacemaker is set and notify the provider if symptoms of pacemaker failure occur.

14. Correct: C

Medical asepsis refers to clean technique. It applies to common nursing tasks, such as administering oral medication, managing nasogastric tubes, and providing personal hygiene.

15. Correct: B

Crackles in the dependent portions of the lungs is a sign of circulatory overload.

16. Correct: B

Aphonia is the inability to produce normal speech sounds. Etiology includes overuse of vocal cords, laryngeal trauma, or organic disease. A client demonstrating aphonia is a candidate for referral to speech therapy.

17. Correct: A, C

Sleep is often disrupted by noise, lighting, and client care activities. The nurse should implement actions to promote rest and sleep, such as dimming lights, closing client doors when possible, clustering nursing activities to decrease interruptions, limiting fluids 2 to 4 hr prior to bedtime, and reducing noise.

18. Correct: D

The client should be placed in Trendelenburg or supine position to decrease the risk of air embolus. This position also produces dilation of neck and shoulder vessels, making insertion easier.

19. Correct: A

Heat application is most effective with chronic pain. Heat works by increasing blood flow and helping the muscles relax, alleviating both pain and stiffness.

20. Correct: C

Guided imagery is based on mentally envisioning images that are calming and health-enhancing.

21. Correct: A, B, D

Findings outside of the expected reference range should be reported to the nurse. The heart rate is increased, and the pulse oximetry and respiratory rates are decreased.

22. Correct: B

Alternating tasks and postures that use different motions and muscles groups, such as sitting and standing, helps to avoid stress injuries. If motions are repeated frequently (such as every few seconds) and for prolonged periods, fatigue and injury can result.

23. Correct: E, B, C, A, D

Place the package on a clean surface. Open the outer flap away from your body while keeping your arm outstretched and away from the field. Open the side flaps using the right hand for the right flap and the left hand for the left flap. Stand away from the field and open the inner flap toward your body, never crossing the sterile field with your arm. Apply sterile gloves and begin the procedure.

24. Correct: D

It is within the scope of practice of the LPN to provide wound care that requires a sterile dressing change.

25. Correct: B

Asymmetry of facial features can indicate impairment of cranial nerve VII.

26. Correct: B

The caregiver is expressing symptoms of role strain. Exploring ways of coping, such as taking time off from the client and arranging for assistance in caring for the client, can provide relief for both the client and caregiver.

27. Correct: A

Obtaining vital signs is the priority action. The client should be checked first and the findings then communicated to the provider.

28. Correct: C

Followers of Catholicism use rosary (prayer beads) as a traditional practice that provides comfort and peace. Practice of religious traditions promote resilience and create meaning from experiences and life challenges.

29. Correct: C

Digoxin is a cardiac glycoside. Potassium and digoxin compete for the same receptor sites. Hypokalemia places a client at risk for digoxin toxicity.

30. Correct: C

Therapeutic communication aims to decrease the client's anxiety, provide a safe environment, and focus on reality-based conversations such as, "The voice you hear is part of your illness. You are safe." Hallucinations are an alteration in perception involving a sensory experience without the presence of an external stimulus (hearing voices when no one speaks).

31. Correct: A

Age-appropriate activities for children from 9 to 12 years old include making crafts, building models, collecting things, solving jigsaw puzzles, playing board and card games, and playing organized competitive sports.

32. Correct: D

Adolescents are preoccupied with body changes, causing them to imagine that everyone notices them and their actions. By giving the injection in private, the adolescent can feel a sense of autonomy and maintain a positive self-image.

33. Correct: B

A client who has a titer of less than 1:8 or is nonimmune should receive a subcutaneous injection of rubella vaccine or a measles, mumps, and rubella vaccine during the postpartum period. The client should be instructed to avoid pregnancy for 1 month following the immunization.

34. Correct: A

Doxazosin is an alpha adrenergic blocker used to treat BPH and hypertension. The initial dose can cause profound hypotension, and the client is discouraged from driving or engaging in hazardous activities 12 to 24 hr after the initial dose. These effects are minimized by taking the initial medication dose at bedtime.

35. Correct: B

Flapping of the hands and decreased level of consciousness are manifestations of hepatic encephalopathy, which results from an elevated ammonia level. Lactulose promotes a reduction in ammonia levels via intestinal excretion.

36. Correct: D

Ketorolac tromethamine is a nonnarcotic analgesic, NSAID, and antipyretic. As with other NSAIDs, ketorolac tromethamine can cause peptic ulcers, perforation of stomach/intestines, and GI bleeding. This medication is contraindicated in clients who have peptic ulcer disease or a history of GI bleeding.

37. Correct: B

Breastfeeding should be done at least 8 to 12 times per day to ensure adequate intake in a newborn.

38. Correct: B

Neostigmine is a cholinesterase inhibitor used to manage myasthenia gravis with the therapeutic effect of muscle nerve stimulant. Adverse effects of neostigmine include excessive salivation, increased gastric secretions, increased tone and motility of the GI tract, urinary urgency, bradycardia, diaphoresis, and miosis. Atropine is given to counter these effects.

39. Correct: C

The parents should be informed that the infant will have elbow restraints in place to prevent the infant from reaching the mouth area. The infant can require elbow restraints for 4 to 6 weeks following surgery.

40. Correct: D

Mindfulness is a stress management technique where the client is encouraged to stop and become mindful of the surroundings (such as the warmth of sunlight or the sound of a breeze), using seeing, hearing, and feeling. The client learns to restructure negative thoughts into positive ones.

41. Correct: D

Painless, bright -ed vaginal bleeding during the second or third trimester is a common finding with placenta previa. The uterus is typically soft, relaxed, and nontender to touch.

42. Correct: D

Hyperactive bowel sounds occur greater than 35 sounds per minute. These are considered abnormal findings and should be reported to the RN.

43. Correct: D

Scoliosis is characterized by spinal curvature and spinal rotation resulting in rib asymmetry. The child is asked to bend over with arms hanging down and is observed for asymmetry of ribs and flank. Findings of scoliosis include ill-fitting clothes; one leg shorter than the other; spinal curvature; and head and hips misaligned. Therapeutic management depends on the degrees of spine curvature.

44. Correct: D

A newborn/infant should be placed in the supine position when sleeping, on a firm crib mattress, with a fitted sheet, during the first year of life to prevent sudden infant death syndrome.

45. Correct: A, B, C, D

Urinary catheters should be removed at the earliest possible opportunity. Catheters significantly increase the risk for urinary tract infections in hospitals and long-term care facilities.

References

American Cancer Society. (n.d.). www.cancer.org.

American Diabetes Association. (n.d.). www.diabetes.org.

American Heart Association. (n.d.). www.heart.org.

Berman, A. J., Frandsen, G., & Snyder S. (2015). *Kozier & Erb's fundamentals of nursing: Concepts, process, and practice* (10th ed.). Upper Saddle River, NJ: Prentice-Hall.

Burchum, J. R., & Rosenthal, L. D. (2016). *Lehne's pharmacology for nursing care* (9th ed.). St. Louis, MO: Elsevier.

Centers for Disease Control and Prevention. (n.d.). www.cdc.gov.

Halter, M. J. (2014). *Varcarolis' foundations of psychiatric mental health nursing: A clinical approach* (7th ed.). St. Louis, MO: Saunders.

Hinkle, J. L., & Cheever, K. H. (2014). *Brunner and Suddarth's textbook of medical-surgical nursing* (13th ed.). Philadelphia: Lippincott Williams & Wilkins.

Hockenberry, M.J., & Wilson, D. (2015). *Wong's nursing care of infants and children* (10th ed). St. Louis, MO: Mosby.

Ignatavicius, D. D., & Workman, M. L. (2015). *Medical-surgical nursing: Patient-centered collaborative care* (8th ed.). St. Louis, MO: Saunders.

Lowdermilk, D. L., Perry, S. E., Cashion, M.C., & Alden, K.R. (2015). *Maternity & women's health care* (11th ed.). St. Louis, MO: Mosby.

Marquis, B.L., & Huston, C. J. (2017). *Leadership roles and management functions in nursing: Theory and application* (9th ed.). Philadelphia: Lippincott Williams & Wilkins.

National Institutes of Health. (n.d.). www.nih.gov.

Pagana, K. D., & Pagana, T. J. (2014). *Mosby's manual of diagnostic and laboratory tests* (5th ed.) St. Louis, MO: Mosby.

Potter, P. A., Perry, A. G., Stockert, P., & Hall, A. (2017). *Fundamentals of nursing* (9th ed.). St. Louis, MO: Mosby.

Stanhope, M., & Lancaster, J. (2014). *Foundations of nursing in the community: Community-oriented practice* (4th ed.). St. Louis, MO: Mosby.

Wilson, B. A., Shannon, M. T., & Shields, K. M. (2017). *Pearson nurse's drug guide 2017*. Upper Saddle River, NJ: Prentice-Hall.

Index

Breast cancer, 219
Breastfeeding, 29, 208, 213
Breath tests, 98
Breech presentation, 199
Broad-spectrum antibiotics, 29
Bronchitis, 88-89, 253
Bronchodilators, 88
Bronchoscopy, 87
B12 deficiency anemias, 127-128
Buck's traction, 115
Buddhism, 25
Budget process, 12
Buerger's disease (thromboangiitis obliterans), 135
Bulb syringes, 213
Bulimia nervosa, 184
Burns, 163-165, 226, 228, 229, 231, 232
Butterfly rash (erythematosus), 163
BV (bacterial vaginosis), 218

C

CABG (coronary artery bypass graft), 136
CAD (coronary artery disease), 131
Calcium-channel blockers, 33, 134
Calcium gluconate, 196, 202
Calcium imbalances, 84
Calcium-modified diets, 169
Calculations and conversions, 28
Cancer
    breast, 219
    cervical, 218
    in children, 257-258
    classification of, 159
    disease-related consequences of, 159
    endometrial, 218
    laryngeal, 90-91
    leukemia, 159, 258
    lung, 91
    management of, 159-161
    manifestations of, 159
    ovarian, 219
    overview, 159
    pancreatic, 110-111
    prostate, 148
    risk factors for, 159
    testicular, 148
Canes, 69
CAPD (continuous ambulatory peritoneal dialysis), 146-147
Carbamazepine, 57
Carbohydrate recommendations, 167
Carbon dioxide toxicity, 89
Carcinomas, 159

Cardiac arrest, 267
Cardiac catheterization, 130
Cardiac enzyme testing, 129
Cardiac glycosides, 35
Cardiogenic shock, 136
Cardiopulmonary resuscitation (CPR), 137, 267
Cardiovascular system disorders, 129-141
    adjunctive management of, 137-138
    angina, 131
    aortic aneurysm, 133
    Buerger's disease (thromboangiitis obliterans), 135
    congenital heart disease, 237-239
    CPR for, 137, 267
    diagnostic procedures for, 129-130
    heart failure, 132-133, 239
    hypertension, 133-134, 195-196
    medications for, 32-36
    myocardial infarction, 132
    overview, 129
    peripheral vascular disease, 134
    pregnancy and, 194-196
    Raynaud's syndrome, 135-136
    shock, 96, 136
    surgical procedures for, 136
    valvular disorders, 133
    varicose veins, 135
    venous thromboembolism, 135
Cardioversion, 137
Car seats. See Motor vehicle safety
Case management, 12
Casts, 114
CAT (computerized adaptive testing), 2
Cataracts, 157
Categories of bioterrorism agents, 23
Catheterization, 130, 143, 199
Catholicism, 25
CBC (complete blood count), 170
Celiac disease, 260
Centers for Disease Control and Prevention (CDC)
    communicable disease list from, 17
    in disaster relief, 21
    on health care associated infections, 70
    HIV/AIDS information from, 161
    on immunizations, 225, 227, 229-231
Centrally acting alpha2 agonists, 33-34, 134
Central venous catheters, 30
Cephalic presentation, 199
Cephalopelvic disproportion, 199
Cephalosporins, 50

Cerebral arteriography, 150
Cerebral palsy, 243
Cerebrovascular accidents (CVAs), 152-153
Cervical cancer, 218
Cervical diaphragms, 59
Cervical dilation, 199
Cervical insufficiency, 198
Cervical traction, 115
Cesarean births, 199, 206, 213
Chain of infection, 70
Chart questions, 3
Chemical agent guidelines, 67
Chemotherapy, 159-160, 219
Chest tubes, 92
Chickenpox. See Varicella
Child and adolescent nursing, 223-273. See also Newborn nursing
    abuse and neglect concerns in, 17, 232-233
    for acute conditions, 246-260
    adapting care for children, 233-237
    ADHD and, 55, 178
    for adolescents, 231-232
    age-related nursing interventions, 233
    autism spectrum disorders and, 179
    for chronic conditions, 260-263, 266
    communicable diseases in, 264-265
    for congenital anomalies, 237-246
    CPR guidelines for, 267
    death and dying in, 236-237
    family involvement in, 224
    growth and development in, 224-233
    hospitalization effects on children, 233, 234
    immunizations in, 49, 225, 227, 229-231
    for infants, 224-226
    intellectual development disorder and, 178
    medication administration in, 29, 235-236
    mental health disorders and, 178-179
    motor disorders and, 178
    pain management in, 234-235
    for preschoolers, 228-229
    safety concerns in, 226, 228, 229, 231, 232
    for school-age children, 230-231
    substance abuse and, 231, 232
    therapeutic play in, 234
    for toddlers, 227-228
    vital sign expectations, 211-212, 233
    worksheets on, 268-273

CST (contraction stress test), 191

CT (computed tomography), 87, 149

Culturally and linguistically appropriate services standards (CLAS), 24

Culturally competent care, 23-26

Cultures of specimens, 29

Cushing's disease and syndrome, 120

CVAs (cerebrovascular accidents), 152-153

Cycle of violence, 185

Cystic fibrosis, 261

Cystitis, 143-144

Cystoscopy, 143

D

Data security, 18

Date rape, 185

Day of exam procedures, 7

DDH (developmental dysplasia of the hip), 241

Death and dying, 25-26, 166, 236-237

Debriefing process, 23

Decerebrate posturing, 149

Decision-making process, 16

Decongestants, 39

Decorticate posturing, 149

Deep-vein thrombosis (DVT), 135

De-escalation strategies, 185

Defense mechanisms, 176

Defibrillation, 137

Definitive therapy, 29

Defusing process, 23

Dehydration, 81

Delayed wound healing, 97

Delegation and prioritization, 13-15

Delirium, 182, 183

Delivery date calculation, 189. See also Labor and delivery

Delusions, 177, 178

Dementia, 182, 183

Democratic leadership, 10

Denial, 176

Dental care for children and adolescents, 228-230, 232

Dental caries, 100

Department of _____. See specific name of department

Dependent personality disorder, 180, 181

Depressants, 182

Depression, 53-54, 179-180, 210

Detached retina, 157

Developmental dysplasia of the hip (DDH), 241

DEXA (dual-energy x-ray absorptiometry) scans, 111

Diabetes insipidus (DI), 118

Diabetes mellitus, 123-125, 196-197

Diabetic ketoacidosis, 125

Diagnosis
of cardiovascular system disorders, 129-130
of gastrointestinal system disorders, 97-99
of genitourinary system disorders, 142-143
of mental health issues, 174
of musculoskeletal system disorders, 111
of neurosensory disorders, 149-150
of respiratory system disorders, 87

Dialysis, 146-147

Diarrhea, 247

Diet and nutrition
for children and adolescents, 225-226, 228-230, 232
cultural considerations in, 24
for diarrhea and vomiting, 247
guidelines for healthy eating, 167
overview, 166-167
religious/spiritual influences on, 25-26
therapeutic diets, 167-169

Dietary Supplement Health and Education Act of 1994, 61

Dietary supplements, 61-63

Digestive system disorders. See Gastrointestinal system disorders

Digoxin and digoxin toxicity, 35, 239

Dilation of cervix, 199

Dilemmas, ethical, 16

Dinoprostone, 203

Diphtheria, 264

Disasters and disaster planning, 20-23

Discectomy, 156

Disclosure of information. See Confidentiality

Disease-modifying antirheumatic drugs (DMARDs), 52

Disease prevention strategies, 74. See also specific types and names of diseases

Distractors, 3, 4

Distributive shock, 136

Disulfiram, 55-56

Diuretics, 47-48, 134

Diverticular disease, 105

Docusate sodium, 47

Donation of organs and tissue, 16

Dosage calculations, 28

Down syndrome, 239-240

Drag-and-drop questions, 3

Drills in disaster planning, 21

Droplet precautions, 71, 73

Drowning, 226, 228, 229, 231

Drug abuse. See Substance abuse and dependence

Drug class suffixes, 31. See also Medications; Pharmacology

Dual-energy x-ray absorptiometry (DEXA) scans, 111

Due date calculation, 189. See also Labor and delivery

Durable power of attorney for health care, 16

DVT (deep-vein thrombosis), 135

Dwarfism, 118

Dysentery, 73

Dystocia, 208

E

Ear infections, 259

Ear medications, 236

Eating disorders, 160, 184

Eating habits. See Diet and nutrition

ECG (electrocardiogram), 130, 139-141

Echinacea (Echinacea purpurea), 61

Echocardiogram, 130

Echolalia, 177

Eclampsia, 195

Ecological disasters, 20

Economic abuse, 185

ECT (electroconvulsive therapy), 179, 186

Ectopic pregnancy, 198

Edrophonium chloride, 155

EEG (electroencephalogram), 150

Effacement, 199

EGD (esophagogastroduodenoscopy), 98

Ego, 172, 173

Elderly populations. See Gerontologic considerations

Electrical equipment guidelines, 67

Electrocardiogram (ECG), 130, 139-141

Electroconvulsive therapy (ECT), 179, 186

Electroencephalogram (EEG), 150

Electrolytes and fluids, 81-87, 167, 170

Electromyography (EMG), 111

Emergency childbirth, 207

Emergency contraception, 58

Emergency management systems, 21

Emergency Medical Treatment and Active Labor Act of 1986 (EMTALA), 199

Potassium imbalances, 83

Potassium-modified diets, 169

Potassium-sparing diuretics, 47, 134

Potty training, 227

PPE (personal protective equipment), 70, 71

PPIs (proton pump inhibitors), 46

PPN (peripheral parenteral nutrition), 100

Preeclampsia, 195, 196

Pregestational diabetes mellitus, 196

Pregnancy, 188-198. See also Labor and delivery
    abortion, 25-26, 198
    anticipatory care during, 194
    complications of, 194-198
    delivery date calculation, 189
    fertilization process in, 188
    fetal development and assessment during, 188, 190-192
    medications and, 29, 193
    prenatal period and care, 188-193
    psychological and physiological adaptations of, 188-189, 194
    signs and symptoms of, 189
    terminology related to, 193
    verification of, 189

Preinfarction angina, 131

Prenatal period and care, 188-193

Preoperative phase, 95

Presbyopia, 156

Preschoolers, 228-229. See also Child and adolescent nursing

Present-oriented perspective, 24

Preterm births, 193, 206, 216

Preventive care, 74

Primary hypertension, 133

Primary prevention strategies, 74

Prinzmetal's angina, 131

Prioritization and delegation, 13-15

Priority-setting guidelines, 5

Privacy. See Confidentiality

Progesterone, 188

Projection, 176

Promethazine, 46

Prostate cancer, 148

Prostatic hyperplasia, 147

Protein-modified diets, 168

Protein recommendations, 167

Proton pump inhibitors (PPIs), 46

Psychoanalytic models of development, 172, 173

Psychosocial development, 225, 227, 229-231

Psyllium, 47

PTSD (posttraumatic stress disorder), 22, 185, 186

PUBS (percutaneous umbilical blood sampling), 192

PUD (peptic ulcer disease), 102-103

Pudendal blocks, 204

Puerperal infections, 211

Puerperal rash, 255

Pulmonary embolism (PE), 91-92, 135

Pulmonary emphysema, 88

Pupil checks, 149

Pureed diets, 167

Purging, 184

Q

Quality control, 11

QuantiFERON-TB Gold test (QFT-GT), 87

Quasi-intentional torts, 17

Questions. See Test questions

R

Radiation therapy, 67, 160-161, 219

Radiographic studies, 99

Radiologic tests, 142

Rape and rape trauma syndrome, 185

Rashes, 163, 255

Raynaud's syndrome, 135-136

RDS (respiratory distress syndrome), 216, 254

Reactions to medications, 29, 32

Reactivity periods of newborns, 213

Rectal route of administration, 236

Red Cross, 21

Red tag injuries, 22

Referrals, 12, 20

Reflection technique, 175

Reflexes, 149, 212-213

Regional blocks, 204

Registered nurses (RNs), 6, 13, 14, 29, 192, 194

Registration process, 2

Regression, 176

Religion and spirituality, 24-26

Renal angiography, 143

Renal biopsy, 143

Renal failure, 145

Renal function tests, 142, 170

Reporting requirements, 12, 17

Reproductive system, 58-60, 188. See also Maternal nursing; Women's health

Resource management, 12

Respirators, 71

Respiratory acidosis, 86

Respiratory alkalosis, 86

Respiratory depression, 96

Respiratory distress syndrome (RDS), 216, 254

Respiratory syncytial virus (RSV), 73, 253

Respiratory system disorders, 87-94
    airway management for, 93-94
    asthma, 87-88
    bronchitis, 88-89, 253
    carbon dioxide toxicity, 89
    in children, 252-254, 261
    COPD, 88-89
    cystic fibrosis, 261
    diagnostic tests for, 87
    hemothorax, 92
    laryngeal cancer, 90-91
    lung cancer, 91
    medications for, 37-39
    pneumonia, 73, 89-90, 94, 96
    pneumothorax, 30, 92, 94
    pulmonary embolism, 91-92, 135
    pulmonary emphysema, 88
    respiratory distress syndrome, 216, 254
    respiratory syncytial virus, 73, 253
    status asthmaticus, 88
    tension pneumothorax, 92
    tonsillitis, 252-253
    tuberculosis, 73, 87, 90
    worksheet on, 94

Restatement technique, 175

Restraints, 66, 185, 186, 196

Retina detachment, 157

Reversal agents, 31

Reye syndrome, 255-256

Rheumatoid arthritis, 112-113

Rho(D) immune globulin, 60, 192, 193, 198, 210

Rhythm method of contraception, 58

Ritodrine hydrochloride, 203

RNs. See Registered nurses

Rolling walkers, 69

Room assignments, 70, 71

Root cause analysis, 11

Roseola, 265

Rotavirus, 73, 247